Malaria

Maria M. Mota • Ana Rodriguez
Editors

Malaria

Immune Response to Infection and Vaccination

Springer

Editors
Maria M. Mota
Instituto de Medicina Molecular
Faculdade de Medicina Universidade de Lisboa
Lisbon, Portugal

Ana Rodriguez
Division of Parasitology
Department of Microbiology
New York University School of Medicine
New York, NY, USA

ISBN 978-3-319-45208-1 ISBN 978-3-319-45210-4 (eBook)
DOI 10.1007/978-3-319-45210-4

Library of Congress Control Number: 2016957986

Printed on acid-free paper

This Springer imprint is published by Springer Nature
The registered company is Springer International Publishing AG
The registered company address is: Gewerbestrasse 11, 6330 Cham, Switzerland

Contents

Part I Immune Response to Infection

Innate Immunity to Malaria 3
Anton Götz, Maureen Ty, Angelo Ferreira Chora, Vanessa Zuzarte-Luís, Maria M. Mota, and Ana Rodriguez

Mechanisms of Adaptive Immunity to *Plasmodium* Liver-Stage Infection: The Known and Unknown 27
Stina L. Urban, Katherine L. Doll, and John T. Harty

Adaptive Immunity to *Plasmodium* Blood Stages 47
Michelle N. Wykes, Robin Stephens, and Ian A. Cockburn

Pathogenetic Immune Responses in Cerebral Malaria 67
Georges Emile Raymond Grau and Samuel Crocodile Wassmer

A Role for Autoimmunity in the Immune Response Against Malaria 81
Juan Rivera-Correa and Ana Rodriguez

Part II Immune Response to Malaria Vaccines: Liver Stage Vaccines

Whole-Sporozoite Malaria Vaccines 99
António M. Mendes, Anja Scholzen, Ann-Kristin Mueller, Shahid M. Khan, Robert W. Sauerwein, and Miguel Prudêncio

Immune Responses to the RTS,S/AS01 Malaria Vaccine Candidate: Lessons from Human Immunology, Parasitologic and Clinical Evaluations 139
Johan Vekemans

Viral Vector Vaccines for Liver-Stage Malaria 157
Cristina Fernández-Arias and Moriya Tsuji

Epitopic Malaria Vaccines Comprised of Minimal T- and B-Cell Epitopes of the *P. falciparum* CS Protein 171
Elizabeth H. Nardin

Part III Immune Response to Malaria Vaccines: Blood Stage Vaccines

Immune Responses to Whole-Organism Blood-Stage Malaria Vaccines 197
Amber I. Raja, Danielle I. Stanisic, and Michael F. Good

Subunit Blood-Stage Malaria Vaccines 211
Alexander D. Douglas

Part IV Immune Response to Malaria Vaccines: Transmission Blocking Vaccines

Antimalarial Transmission-Blocking Vaccines 241
R.E. Sinden, Sumi Biswas, and A.M. Blagborough

Index 273

Part I
Immune Response to Infection

Innate Immunity to Malaria

Anton Götz, Maureen Ty, Angelo Ferreira Chora, Vanessa Zuzarte-Luís, Maria M. Mota, and Ana Rodriguez

Contents

1 *Plasmodium* Infection and Disease 4
2 Parasite- and Host-Derived Inflammatory Molecules 4
3 Cellular Responses During Malaria 9
3.1 Hepatocytes 9
3.2 Granulocytes 9
3.3 Monocytes and Macrophages 10
3.4 Dendritic Cells 10
3.5 NK Cells 11
3.6 γδ T Cells 11
4 Cytokine Responses in Malaria 12
References 13

Abbreviations

DCs	Dendritic cells
GPI	Glycosylphosphatidylinositol
IFN	Interferon
Ifnar	Interferon alpha receptor
ISG	Interferon-stimulated gene

A. Götz • M. Ty • A. Rodriguez (✉)
Division of Parasitology, Department of Microbiology, New York University School of Medicine, New York, NY, USA
e-mail: Anton.Goetz@nyumc.org; MaureenMichelle.Ty@nyumc.org; Ana.Rodriguez@nyumc.org

A.F. Chora • V. Zuzarte-Luís • M.M. Mota
Instituto de Medicina Molecular, Faculdade de Medicina Universidade de Lisboa, Lisbon, Portugal
e-mail: angelochora@medicina.ulisboa.pt; vluis@medicina.ulisboa.pt

M.M. Mota, A. Rodriguez (eds.), *Malaria*, DOI 10.1007/978-3-319-45210-4_1

MAVS	Mitochondrial antiviral-signaling protein
MDA5	Melanoma differentiation-associated protein 5
NK	Natural killer cells
NKT	Natural killer T cells
PBMC	Peripheral blood mononuclear cells
ROS	Reactive oxygen species
TLR	Toll-like receptors

1 *Plasmodium* Infection and Disease

Malaria infection starts when an infected *Anopheles* mosquito injects *Plasmodium* sporozoites into the skin of the vertebrate host. After traversing the dermis, the parasites enter the circulation and home to the liver, initiating the hepatic stage of infection. Within the liver, hepatocyte traversal precedes parasite invasion and replication in the host cell, ultimately maturing into erythrocyte-infectious merozoites [1]. These are later released into the lumen of liver sinusoids [2] invading, developing, and multiplying inside erythrocytes, the blood stage of infection, associated with the establishment of disease and all its complications.

The blood stage of malaria is characterized by high cyclical fevers and elevated levels of inflammatory mediators in the circulation. Excessive and persistent inflammation during *P. falciparum* infections contributes to severe pathology and to the development of associated complications such as cerebral malaria and severe malarial anemia [3].

Acute malaria is always characterized by high fevers, but it is known that different species of *Plasmodium* need to reach higher parasitemias to induce inflammatory responses in the host. Although the mechanisms underlying this effect are not clear, it seems apparent that *P. vivax* is more effective at inducing inflammation and therefore needs lower parasitemias to induce a high fever response compared to *P. falciparum* [4]. This difference has also been observed in the levels of TNF compared to parasitemia in patients, where *P. vivax* or *P. ovale* induce much higher levels of inflammation per infected erythrocyte compared to *P. falciparum* [5, 6], although this observation has been recently challenged [7, 8].

2 Parasite- and Host-Derived Inflammatory Molecules

The asymptomatic nature of the liver stage, the first step of *Plasmodium* infection in the mammalian host, has led to the long-lasting view that the parasite can establish and replicate within the host hepatocyte without being detected [1]. However, such notion has been challenged by the presence of inflammatory cell foci in the liver during exoerythrocytic parasite development [9–12], as well as by the mounting of a strong inflammatory reaction aiming at controlling *Plasmodium* hepatic burden, as is the case of the rate-limiting enzyme of heme catabolism heme oxygenase 1 [9]. Taken together, these findings suggest that the host is able to sense *Plasmodium* hepatocyte infection and respond to it.

In contrast, the inflammatory nature of the blood stage of infection has long been recognized. As described by Golgi [13], the synchronized rupture of infected erythrocytes in the peripheral circulation is followed by a peak of fever in malaria patients. This observation led to the hypothesis that the high levels of inflammation in malaria during the blood stage of infection were caused by molecules released from infected erythrocytes during parasite egress, including merozoites and erythrocyte cellular contents. The search for these molecules for the past century has led to the identification of several pro-inflammatory molecules that are either derived directly from *Plasmodium* or generated as a result of infection from erythrocyte components.

Among the molecules generated by the parasite, glycosylphosphatidylinositol (*GPI*) anchors were identified early as inflammatory mediators [14]. These glycolipid structures anchor parasite proteins to the plasma membrane in the merozoite [15] and activate toll-like receptors (TLR), preferentially TLR-2/TLR-6 and TLR-2/TLR-1 heterodimers, but also TLR-4 homodimers [16]. Although purified GPI anchors induce an inflammatory response in mice [14], in vitro this response is downregulated in the presence of other *P. falciparum* lipids [17], which may explain why in vitro inflammatory responses do not require TLR-2 or TLR-4 [18]. The association of TLR-4 [19], TLR-2, TLR-1, and TLR-6 [20, 21] polymorphisms with malaria severity may be compatible with a role for GPI anchors in malaria inflammation, but this association may also be caused by other *Plasmodium*-derived inflammatory mediators. The role of GPI in malaria-induced inflammation in patients remains unclear.

Another parasite-derived molecule with inflammatory effects is *hemozoin*, a crystal polymer of heme that *Plasmodium* generates after degradation of hemoglobin within infected erythrocytes. Hemozoin is generated in the parasite's food vacuole and is released after erythrocyte rupture and merozoites egress. It is important to consider than the inflammatory properties of crystals, such as hemozoin, depend on the size, charge, and association with protein, lipids, or other elements of the crystal [22]. Different groups have found conflicting results regarding the inflammatory effects of hemozoin, which are probably due to the variations in the protocols used to obtain hemozoin that would result in crystals with different inflammatory characteristics. When synthetic hemozoin, or also hemozoin purified from infected erythrocytes and stripped of any binding molecules, was used as starting material, activation and binding to TLR-9 [23, 24] was observed. Inflammatory pathways dependent on nitric oxide and NF-kB [25], as well as activation of the NLRP3 inflammasome [26, 27], were also identified.

It is likely that hemozoin obtained from cultured parasites that naturally rupture and release their contents would more accurately resemble the characteristics of the hemozoin generated during disease. This kind of hemozoin was used in studies that found parasite and host components bound to it, including *Plasmodium DNA* [28] and host fibrinogen [29]. The bound materials DNA and fibrinogen, not the hemozoin per se, were found to mediate the inflammatory response observed in vitro through the activation of TLR-9 and TLR-4 or the integrin CD11b/CD18, respectively [28, 30]. Indeed, the inflammatory activity of hemozoin was lost after treatment to remove associated proteins or DNA, probably because the proteins provide a link to bind DNA to the hemozoin crystal [31]. These results indicate that hemozoin could act as a "carrier" for other molecules, increasing their inflammatory potential. Another effect of hemozoin, also caused by other crystals, is the destabilization of the phagosome [32], which results in the release of hemozoin and DNA to the cytosol of the phagocytic cell and in the activation of the AIM2 and NLRP3 inflammasomes, respectively [31]. Accordingly, synthetic hemozoin is being developed as a vaccine adjuvant for other diseases [33, 34].

The "carrier" effect was also proposed for *Plasmodium* histones, which are bound to parasite DNA and mediate inflammation in vitro [35]. Additionally, immune complexes formed by DNA and anti-DNA antibodies, which are found in high concentrations in the sera of malaria patients, were found to induce cytokine secretion from immune cells in vitro [36], suggesting that another *Plasmodium* DNA-carrier complex is also contributing to the inflammatory pathway. *Plasmodium* DNA can activate not only TLR-9, which recognizes CpG motifs, but also an alternative inflammatory pathway that recognizes AT-rich hairpin motifs, involves STING/TBK1/IRF3 signaling, and results in the production of type I interferon [37].

Interestingly, whole lysates of *P. falciparum*-infected erythrocytes injected into mice are more immunogenic in *wt* compared to TLR-9-deficient mice, independently of *Plasmodium* DNA [24]; however, infection of TLR-9-deficient mice with *P. berghei* did not show a reduction in inflammatory cytokine response [38, 39]. Studies in malaria patients have found an association of TLR-9 polymorphisms with malaria susceptibility and development of anemia [40, 41], but not with malaria severity [19, 40, 42]. The role of hemozoin and *Plasmodium* DNA in the inflammatory response in malaria patients is still not well defined.

Plasmodium RNA is probably also an inflammatory activator during the blood stage of infection, since TLR-7, which recognizes ssRNA, was found to be essential for cytokine production in mice [39]. Since TLR-7 and 9, which recognize ssRNA and dsDNA, respectively, are not found in the plasma membrane of immune cells, the "carrier" effect is thought to facilitate phagocytosis of the nucleic acids, allowing the contact with the endosomes in the phagolysosome. In the liver stage, however, it is established that *Plasmodium* dsRNA is sensed by the host hepatocyte by a mechanism involving the intracellular RIG-I-like receptor melanoma differentiation-associated protein 5 (MDA5 also known as IFIH1), its adaptor protein mitochondrial antiviral-signaling protein (MAVS), and the transcription factors IRF3 and IRF7. Notwithstanding, the ensuing immune response is partially MDA5 independent, supporting the idea that several parallel mechanisms could contribute to *Plasmodium* recognition by the host during the liver stage of infection [43]. The question remains, however, on how *Plasmodium spp.* dsRNA becomes accessible to the host cytosolic receptors. Several hypotheses can be put forward including: (1) the active transport of this ligand across the parasitophorous vacuole, (2) passive release of dsRNA through vacuolar membrane pores, (3) leakage of dsRNA into the cytosol from nonviable parasites, and/or (4) vesicular transfer of parasite dsRNA from infected cells to liver-resident immune cells, such as Kupffer cells. Overall, we cannot exclude that several of these mechanisms operate simultaneously to trigger the immune response against *Plasmodium* during the liver stage of infection.

Another pro-inflammatory mediator that could contribute to the inflammatory response to *Plasmodium* infection is precipitated *uric acid. Plasmodium*-infected erythrocytes import hypoxanthine, which is the precursor of uric acid, for the synthesis of nucleic acids required during parasite replication. After requirements for hypoxanthine decrease at the end of the replication cycle, hypoxanthine accumulates in the infected erythrocyte [44, 45]. Precipitates of uric acid are also observed in the cytoplasm of the *Plasmodium* parasitophorous vacuole [46]. Upon rupture of infected erythrocytes, precipitates of uric acid and soluble hypoxanthine, which would be degraded into uric acid in the tissues, are released and can become inflammatory [44–46]. Indeed, activation of the NLRP3 inflammasome by uric acid precipitates is well characterized [47], and activation of both NLRP3 and NLRP12 inflammasomes has been observed in infected mice and malaria patients [48], possibly caused by hemozoin and/or uric acid crystals. Uric acid was also found to mediate the activation of mast cells in a mouse model of malaria, leading to the regulation of a subset of dendritic cells, which then activate pathogenic $CD8^+$ T cell responses directed against the parasite [49]. Interestingly, treatment of malaria patients with an inhibitor of xanthine oxidase, an enzyme that produces uric acid, results in a more rapid decrease of the inflammatory response [50], suggesting that uric acid may be involved in the inflammatory response in patients.

Microvesicles are shed by almost all cell types in response to different stimuli, such as activation or response to environmental stress [51]. Microvesicles derived from *Plasmodium*-infected erythrocytes, induced probably in response to oxidative stress during infection [52], can activate macrophages and trigger the secretion of inflammatory cytokines in vitro through the activation of TLR-4 [53, 54]. Endothelial microvesicles can also induce the proliferation of T cells [55]. In malaria patients, increased levels of circulating microvesicles are derived preferentially from uninfected erythrocytes, but also infected erythrocytes, lymphocytes, platelets, and endothelial cells [52, 56, 57]. Correlations of microvesicle levels with inflammatory markers or disease severity has been observed in malaria patients. Microvesicle levels correlate with TNF in cerebral malaria patients [58], erythrocyte [52] and endothelial [57] microvesicles correlate with the severity of *P. falciparum* malaria, and platelet microvesicles also correlate with fever in *P. vivax* infections [56]. It is still not clear whether microvesicles are causing inflammation and malaria severe pathology in patients or their formation is induced as a consequence of the high inflammation [59], which is characteristic of severe malaria.

Although *Plasmodium* converts *heme* derived from hemoglobin degradation into nontoxic hemozoin, which in itself can be inflammatory (see below), up to 40 % of the hemoglobin of an infected red blood cell can be released and oxidized. This leads to the formation of toxic heme in the circulation of infected individuals [60]. In vitro and in vivo experiments suggest that heme induces apoptosis of brain vascular endothelial cells, which affects the stability of the blood-brain barrier in experimental cerebral malaria [61, 62]. Heme-induced apoptosis of brain vascular endothelial cells or endothelial progenitor cells was shown to be mediated by the transcription factor STAT3 [61, 62], the tumor protein p73 [63], or TLR-4-induced CXCL10 [64].

Another source of inflammation in malaria appears to be *oxidative stress* that is generated during infection. Malaria patients exhibit high levels of oxidative stress, as measured by lipid peroxidation, and at the same time lower anti-oxidative factors compared to healthy controls [65–68]. The source of increased reactive oxygen species (ROS) leading to oxidative stress has been subject of speculation. While some reports suggest that ROS might be produced by the parasite [69–71], others indicate that the human host can be a potent source of ROS to combat *Plasmodium*, most notably through the oxidative burst of phagocytes [72, 73] and ROS-producing enzymes like xanthine oxidase [74]. This implicates that ROS production by the host might be an important inflammatory response to control parasitemia; however, elevated levels of oxidative stress also correlate with increased disease severity during the infection [75, 76], suggesting a role in pathology. It is not clear whether oxidative stress is a cause or consequence of inflammation during malaria. Given the severe nature of complications often leaving traces of oxidative damage like impaired memory after cerebral malaria, the use of antioxidants as adjunctive therapy has been discussed. Although of great potential benefit, antioxidants could increase parasite survival by interfering with the host inflammatory response or the action of antimalarial drugs (reviewed in [77]).

All the parasite and host components described above are able to induce inflammatory reactions in vitro and/or when injected in mice, but their relative importance in the inflammation observed in malaria patients remains unclear. Assessing their real contribution during disease has not been possible because of the difficulties in specifically inhibiting each of them in vivo; therefore, most of the available evidence comes from correlations of inflammatory parameters in the blood of malaria patients that cannot establish a causative relation. In vitro inhibition of DNA and/or uric acid is possible using *P. falciparum* lysates or merozoites treated with DNAse and/or uricase, which suggest an important role for these molecules in the activation of human dendritic cells [18, 46]. The role of hemozoin in the inflammatory response in vivo may now be tested in mice using *P. berghei* parasites that produce very low levels of hemozoin [78]. Inhibition of uric acid formation in vivo is possible by treatment of malaria patients with allopurinol, an inhibitor of the enzyme that produces uric acid. In this case, a more rapid decrease of the inflammatory response was observed in treated patients [50].

There is an unsolved paradox in the study of the innate immune response to malaria blood stage, where patients present all signs of an intense inflammatory response, including high fevers and circulating inflammatory cytokines, but innate immune cells in vitro respond weakly to the parasite when incubated together. When naïve peripheral blood mononuclear cells (PBMCs), isolated dendritic cells, or macrophages are incubated with *P. falciparum*-infected red blood cells in vitro, the levels of inflammatory cytokines released, such as TNF, are undetectable or substantially lower than responses triggered by well-characterized activators (LPS, CpG, or β-hematin [79, 80]) or inflammasome activators (uric acid). Conversely, cells from infected individuals were much more responsive to parasite stimuli in the secretion of cytokines [81, 82] when compared to cells from healthy individuals or recovered patients. These results suggest that there still may be components of the innate immune response to blood-stage *Plasmodium* infection that have not been identified yet and play an important role during infection.

3 Cellular Responses During Malaria

3.1 Hepatocytes

Within hepatocytes, *Plasmodium* parasites settle inside a parasitophorous vacuole where it undergoes a remarkable transformation differentiating into highly metabolically active merozoites. By the end of the liver stage, as the vacuole expands, a single parasite generates thousands of merozoites. During this process plasmodial dsRNA gains access to the host cell cytosol and activates the MDA5/MAVS/IRF3/7 cytosolic signaling pathway leading to the release of type I interferon (IFN) into the extracellular environment. The initial signal is consequently propagated in an autocrine and paracrine manner through the activation of the interferon alpha receptor (Ifnar) in neighboring hepatocytes via the production of interferon-stimulated genes (ISGs). This type I IFN-mediated response enables the host to control hepatic parasite burden. However such control does not seem to be mediated directly by hepatocytes but rather relies on the recruitment of accessory immune cells [43, 83]. In fact, liver-stage infection results in the recruitment of natural killer T (NKT) cells in an IFNAR-dependent manner, that through an IFNγ-mediated mechanism are responsible for the control of *Plasmodium* liver infection [83]. Although IFNγ has been shown to directly kill liver-stage parasites [84, 85], it is possible that an IFNγ-independent killing mechanism within the hepatocyte could also take place.

3.2 Granulocytes

The levels of circulating *neutrophils* during malaria are significantly increased [86] and correlate with inflammation and severe disease [87, 88]. Adoptive transfer of neutrophils from infected rats provided partial protection against infection, suggesting that they play a role in protection against malaria [89]. However, the chemokine CXCL10 that is secreted by neutrophils during *P. berghei* infection in mice inhibits the control of blood-stage parasitemia and is required for the development of experimental cerebral malaria [90], although depletion of neutrophils did not prevent the development of this pathology [91]. Interestingly, activated neutrophils correlate with cerebral malaria vasculopathy, which presents with higher cytoadhesion levels of infected erythrocytes to endothelial cells in the brain [92], suggesting a role for neutrophils in *P. falciparum* malaria-induced pathology. In *P. vivax* infections expression of type I interferon in neutrophils was correlated with liver damage [93]; however, neutrophils present an atypical activation profile since phagocytic activity and superoxide production were increased but molecular markers of activation and secretion of cytokines are very low in response to stimulation [94].

Mast cells contribute to parasite clearance and TNF production in rodent malaria [95] and appear to have a role in promoting innate immune activation since they produce Flt3 ligand during malaria in mice, which, in turn, induces proliferation of a subpopulation of dendritic cells. Both Flt3 ligand and this subpopulation of dendritic cells are also elevated in malaria patients [49].

3.3 Monocytes and Macrophages

Macrophages are essential for clearance of infected erythrocytes as observed in mouse models of infection [96, 97]. Macrophages efficiently phagocytose infected erythrocytes, as early as ring stage [98], which are subsequently degraded in acidic phagosomes [99]. Non-opsonic phagocytosis is mediated by binding of infected erythrocytes to CD36 [100], while opsonic phagocytosis is mediated by complement receptor-1 [101, 102] and Fc-γ receptors [103].

3.4 Dendritic Cells

Dendritic cells (DCs) are crucial for the initiation of the adaptive immune responses and regulate both innate and adaptive immunity to infections. DCs activate, or mature, in response to different pathogen signals, enabling their capacity as antigen-presenting cells that efficiently activate naïve T cells [104]. In vitro studies incubating DCs with Plasmodium showed efficient phagocytosis and phagosomal maturation of infected erythrocytes [99], but demonstrate that there is a dose-dependent inhibition of DC maturation [105] that takes place only at high concentrations of infected erythrocytes, where DCs do not upregulate co-stimulatory molecules [106]. Studies using isolated human DCs and *Plasmodium* lysates have found upregulation of classical co-stimulatory molecules in DCs [46, 79]. Also, plasmacytoid DCs are activated through TLR-9 by infected erythrocytes [79]. During early infection [107] and in asymptomatic patients [108], the level of expression of surface HLA-DR in circulating DCs maintains normal levels, but during the acute phase of disease, these levels are reduced [49, 109, 110]. The decreased levels of HLA-DR could affect antigen presentation and T cell activation during disease, although their role in malaria immune response remains unclear.

The dendritic cell cytokine response to *Plasmodium* in vitro was found to be low for common cytokines such as IL-12, IL-8, IL-6, IL-1β, IL-10, and TNF [80, 105], with the exception of IFN-α that is secreted by plasmacytoid DCs [79]. However, other authors found upregulation of inflammatory cytokines upon incubation with infected erythrocytes [111, 112].

When DCs were extracted from malaria patients, they show an impaired capacity to mature, capture, and present antigens to T cells. They also undergo high levels of apoptosis probably as a result of increased IL-10 during infection [113, 114]. It appears that malaria, despite the high levels of inflammation, does not induce classical activation of DCs. However, studies in patients are limited to circulating DCs, and it is possible that effective, mature DCs are migrating into tissues and lymphatic organs and are not being detected in the studies.

During severe malaria, the numbers of BDCA3 DCs, which are a minor subset of myeloid DCs, are increased in peripheral blood [115] and correlate with high levels of Flt3L, a factor that induces expansion of DCs. Other DC populations, BDCA1 and plasmacytoid DCs (BDCA2), were not increased in malaria patients [49]. Conversely, in early uncomplicated human malaria infections, the frequency of BDCA3 DCs was not increased, but plasmacytoid DCs were [116], suggesting that the DC response may vary at different stages of infection.

3.5 NK Cells

In vitro studies show that incubation of PBMC with *P. falciparum*-infected erythrocytes results in the rapid activation of natural killer (NK) cells to secrete IFN-γ [117]. This activation requires the help of cytokines such as IL-2, IL-12, and IL-18 [117–119] from T cells but also contact-dependent signals from monocytes and dendritic cells [120]. In mice, NK cells are important for the control of parasitemia during early infection probably through the production of IFN-γ [121, 122]. Also in human malaria infections, restimulation of PBMCs show that NK cells contribute moderately to the production of IFN-γ [107].

3.6 γδ T Cells

γδ T cells are a minor population of T cells in the peripheral circulation that recognize self and non-self antigens without the restriction of MHC antigen presentation. γδ T cells expand during malaria to constitute a high percentage of circulating T cells in humans infected with *P. falciparum* [123, 124]. They get activated by parasite phosphoantigens produced by *Plasmodium* apicoplast [125] and release cytotoxic granules containing granulysin that are effective against merozoites [126]. γδ T cells proliferate and produce IFNγ and TNF after in vitro stimulation with *P. falciparum*-infected red blood cells which is dependent on IL-2 or autologous irradiated PBMC [127–131]. γδ T cells are the main producers of IFNγ in response to *P. falciparum* in vitro [127] and upon in vitro restimulation of PBMCs from humans infected with *P. falciparum* [107]. In mice, γδ T cells contribute to parasite clearance [132–134], probably due to the high production of IFNγ and their role in activation of dendritic cells [132].

In human malaria patients, γδ T cells are important contributors to inflammatory cytokines and have been associated with severe malaria [129]. When single experimental *P. falciparum* infections were analyzed, both γδ T cells and NK cells showed an enhanced IFNγ response upon restimulation with *P. falciparum*-infected red blood cells, even several weeks after the parasite clearance, indicating a memory-like activation [107, 135]. However, when patients with repeated exposure to malaria in endemic areas were analyzed, loss and dysfunction of γδ T cells was observed in the most exposed patients, which is associated with reduced symptoms and clinical tolerance upon reinfection [136]. This suggests that γδ T cells have roles in both clearance of the parasite as well as pathology.

4 Cytokine Responses in Malaria

The inflammatory response during acute malaria is often described as a "cytokine storm" to convey that there are high levels of a broad range of cytokines in the circulation. Earlier studies already correlated the levels of IFN-α and IFN-γ with levels of parasite [137, 138] that were followed up by the confirmation that plasma levels of inflammatory cytokines—IFN-γ, TNF, IL1β, and IL-6—are elevated in patients with malaria and directly correlate with disease severity in *P. falciparum* and *P. vivax* infections [139–150]. Gene expression profiles also confirm high levels of inflammatory cytokines in peripheral blood mononuclear cells [148] and in tissues such as the brain of cerebral malaria patients [151, 152]. The use of mice models of malaria has allowed the continued evaluation of cytokine production during a self-resolving infection, where it was observed that there is an early production of pro-inflammatory cytokines that start decreasing before the parasitemia [153].

TNF is a pro-inflammatory cytokine produced early in mouse *Plasmodium* infection that is important in the clearance of parasites both in the liver and blood stages [154–157]. This protection is induced through the generation of nitric oxide [158]. Studies on malaria patients showed that TNF not only correlates with disease severity but was ten times as high in fatal cases of cerebral malaria [144]. Further studies confirmed the importance of TNF in malaria pathology showing that different alleles of the promoter region of TNF confer either decreased or increased susceptibility to cerebral malaria and severe anemia in populations of children in endemic areas [159–163]. High levels of TNF are also correlated with a rapid parasitological cure in patients supporting the hypothesis that inflammatory cytokines were effective and necessary for clearance of the parasite, but could also lead to severe forms of the disease [143]. Based on the evidences for the strong association of TNF with malaria severity, a clinical trial for the use of anti-TNF antibodies as adjunctive treatment for cerebral malaria patients was performed. However, no improvement in survival was found in the patients [164], a finding that revealed the complexity of the antimalarial immune response and our limited knowledge in the mechanisms underlying immune-mediated pathology.

Another inflammatory cytokine that has been implicated in parasite clearance and is highly increased during acute malaria is *IFN-γ*, with the particularity that increased levels of this cytokine during liver-stage infection were correlated with lack of blood-stage development in humans [165] and monkeys [166], suggesting that this cytokine may be important to inhibit progression of the disease, a finding that is specially relevant for vaccines targeting the liver stage. Studies in mice have shown that IFN-γ is key in the elimination of *Plasmodium*, since infected mice given exogenous IFN-γ showed lower parasitemias and delayed mortality, while mice deficient in the IFN-γ gene or treated with anti-IFN-γ monoclonal antibodies had higher parasitemia and increased mortality [153, 155, 156, 167–175].

Mouse studies on *IL-12* and *IL-18* have established that these cytokines contribute to parasite clearance [176]. The increased protection granted by these cytokines is probably mediated by the positive effect on IFN-γ production [175, 177, 178]. However, high IFN-γ levels can be dangerous, since experimental *Plasmodium* infections also induce liver injury mediated by IL-12-dependent IFN-γ production [179, 180].

Regulatory, or anti-inflammatory, cytokines such as *IL-10* are also highly increased during malaria and correlate with severe disease [149, 181, 182]; although in fatal severe cases, low IL-10 was observed in late stages as death approached [183]. Since regulatory cytokines are probably elevated as a response to the high levels of pro-inflammatory cytokines, it is considered more informative to study the ratio between both types of cytokine responses rather than the absolute levels of each specific cytokine. Different studies have confirmed that, in general, high pro-inflammatory versus regulatory cytokine ratios are indicative of severe disease, with specific examples such as high ratios of IL-6/IL-10 or IFN-γ/IL-10 being associated with severe *P. falciparum* malaria [139, 183]. However, the ratios of TGF-β1/IL-12 and IL-10/IL-12 were significantly higher in the severe malaria patients, suggesting that the generally considered pro-inflammatory cytokine IL-12 could have protective effects [184]. Further studies have shown that high IL-10/TNF ratios were found in children with uncomplicated malaria, while a low IL-10/TNF ratio is associated with malarial anemia in falciparum patients [184–187]. The role of IL-10 in malaria anemia is also supported by the finding that different IL-10 promoter haplotypes that result in low levels of IL-10 increase susceptibility to severe anemia in falciparum patients [188]. As observed before for inflammatory cytokines that contribute to parasite clearance but can promote malaria-associated pathologies, high levels of regulatory cytokines appear to be protective against severe malaria complications but induce a less effective clearance of *P. falciparum* parasites [189, 190].

References

1. Prudencio M, Rodriguez A, Mota MM (2006) The silent path to thousands of merozoites: the *Plasmodium* liver stage. Nat Rev Microbiol 4(11):849–856. doi:10.1038/nrmicro1529
2. Sturm A, Amino R, van de Sand C, Regen T, Retzlaff S, Rennenberg A, Krueger A, Pollok JM, Menard R, Heussler VT (2006) Manipulation of host hepatocytes by the malaria parasite for delivery into liver sinusoids. Science 313(5791):1287–1290. doi:10.1126/science.1129720
3. Mackintosh CL, Beeson JG, Marsh K (2004) Clinical features and pathogenesis of severe malaria. Trends Parasitol 20(12):597–603

4. Kwiatkowski D (1995) Malarial toxins and the regulation of parasite density. Parasitol Today 11(6):206–212
5. Hemmer CJ, Holst FG, Kern P, Chiwakata CB, Dietrich M, Reisinger EC (2006) Stronger host response per parasitized erythrocyte in *Plasmodium vivax* or ovale than in *Plasmodium falciparum* malaria. Trop Med Int Health 11(6):817–823. doi:10.1111/j.1365-3156.2006.01635.x
6. Yeo TW, Lampah DA, Tjitra E, Piera K, Gitawati R, Kenangalem E, Price RN, Anstey NM (2010) Greater endothelial activation, Weibel-Palade body release and host inflammatory response to *Plasmodium vivax*, compared with *Plasmodium falciparum*: a prospective study in Papua, Indonesia. J Infect Dis 202(1):109–112. doi:10.1086/653211
7. Goncalves RM, Scopel KK, Bastos MS, Ferreira MU (2012) Cytokine balance in human malaria: does *Plasmodium vivax* elicit more inflammatory responses than *Plasmodium falciparum*? PLoS One 7(9), e44394. doi:10.1371/journal.pone.0044394
8. Branch O, Casapia WM, Gamboa DV, Hernandez JN, Alava FF, Roncal N, Alvarez E, Perez EJ, Gotuzzo E (2005) Clustered local transmission and asymptomatic *Plasmodium falciparum* and *Plasmodium vivax* malaria infections in a recently emerged, hypoendemic Peruvian Amazon community. Malar J 4:27
9. Epiphanio S, Mikolajczak SA, Goncalves LA, Pamplona A, Portugal S, Albuquerque S, Goldberg M, Rebelo S, Anderson DG, Akinc A, Vornlocher HP, Kappe SH, Soares MP, Mota MM (2008) Heme oxygenase-1 is an anti-inflammatory host factor that promotes murine *Plasmodium* liver infection. Cell Host Microbe 3(5):331–338. doi:10.1016/j.chom.2008.04.003
10. Khan ZM, Ng C, Vanderberg JP (1992) Early hepatic stages of *Plasmodium berghei*: release of circumsporozoite protein and host cellular inflammatory response. Infect Immun 60(1):264–270
11. Leiriao P, Mota MM, Rodriguez A (2005) Apoptotic *Plasmodium*-infected hepatocytes provide antigens to liver dendritic cells. J Infect Dis 191(10):1576–1581. doi:10.1086/429635
12. van de Sand C, Horstmann S, Schmidt A, Sturm A, Bolte S, Krueger A, Lutgehetmann M, Pollok JM, Libert C, Heussler VT (2005) The liver stage of *Plasmodium berghei* inhibits host cell apoptosis. Mol Microbiol 58(3):731–742. doi:10.1111/j.1365-2958.2005.04888.x
13. Golgi C (1893) Sulle febbri malariche estivo-autunnali di Roma. Gazzetta Medica di Pavia 2:2:481–493; 505–520; 553–559
14. Schofield L, Hackett F (1993) Signal transduction in host cells by a glycosylphosphatidylinositol toxin of malaria parasites. J Exp Med 177(1):145–153
15. Bautista JM, Marin-Garcia P, Diez A, Azcarate IG, Puyet A (2014) Malaria proteomics: insights into the parasite-host interactions in the pathogenic space. J Proteome 97:107–125. doi:10.1016/j.jprot.2013.10.011
16. Krishnegowda G, Hajjar AM, Zhu J, Douglass EJ, Uematsu S, Akira S, Woods AS, Gowda DC (2005) Induction of proinflammatory responses in macrophages by the glycosylphosphatidylinositols of *Plasmodium falciparum*: cell signaling receptors, glycosylphosphatidylinositol (GPI) structural requirement, and regulation of GPI activity. J Biol Chem 280(9):8606–8616. doi:10.1074/jbc.M413541200
17. Debierre-Grockiego F, Schofield L, Azzouz N, Schmidt J, Santos de Macedo C, Ferguson MA, Schwarz RT (2006) Fatty acids from *Plasmodium falciparum* down-regulate the toxic activity of malaria glycosylphosphatidylinositols. Infect Immun 74(10):5487–5496. doi:10.1128/IAI.01934-05
18. Wu X, Gowda NM, Kumar S, Gowda DC (2010) Protein-DNA complex is the exclusive malaria parasite component that activates dendritic cells and triggers innate immune responses. J Immunol 184(8):4338–4348. doi:10.4049/jimmunol.0903824
19. Mockenhaupt FP, Cramer JP, Hamann L, Stegemann MS, Eckert J, Oh NR, Otchwemah RN, Dietz E, Ehrhardt S, Schroder NW, Bienzle U, Schumann RR (2006) Toll-like receptor (TLR) polymorphisms in African children: common TLR-4 variants predispose to severe malaria. Proc Natl Acad Sci U S A 103(1):177–182. doi:10.1073/pnas.0506803102
20. Panigrahi S, Kar A, Tripathy S, Mohapatra MK, Dhangadamajhi G (2016) Genetic predisposition of variants in TLR2 and its co-receptors to severe malaria in Odisha, India. Immunol Res 64(1):291–302. doi:10.1007/s12026-015-8749-7

21. Manning L, Cutts J, Stanisic DI, Laman M, Carmagnac A, Allen S, O'Donnell A, Karunajeewa H, Rosanas-Urgell A, Siba P, Davis TM, Michon P, Schofield L, Rockett K, Kwiatkowski D, Mueller I (2016) A Toll-like receptor-1 variant and its characteristic cellular phenotype is associated with severe malaria in Papua New Guinean children. Genes Immun 17(1):52–59. doi:10.1038/gene.2015.50
22. Franklin BS, Mangan MS, Latz E (2016) Crystal formation in inflammation. Annu Rev Immunol 34:173–202. doi:10.1146/annurev-immunol-041015-055539
23. Coban C, Ishii KJ, Kawai T, Hemmi H, Sato S, Uematsu S, Yamamoto M, Takeuchi O, Itagaki S, Kumar N, Horii T, Akira S (2005) Toll-like receptor 9 mediates innate immune activation by the malaria pigment hemozoin. J Exp Med 201(1):19–25
24. Coban C, Igari Y, Yagi M, Reimer T, Koyama S, Aoshi T, Ohata K, Tsukui T, Takeshita F, Sakurai K, Ikegami T, Nakagawa A, Horii T, Nunez G, Ishii KJ, Akira S (2010) Immunogenicity of whole-parasite vaccines against *Plasmodium falciparum* involves malarial hemozoin and host TLR9. Cell Host Microbe 7(1):50–61
25. Jaramillo M, Gowda DC, Radzioch D, Olivier M (2003) Hemozoin increases IFN-gamma-inducible macrophage nitric oxide generation through extracellular signal-regulated kinase- and NF-kappa B-dependent pathways. J Immunol 171(8):4243–4253
26. Shio MT, Eisenbarth SC, Savaria M, Vinet AF, Bellemare MJ, Harder KW, Sutterwala FS, Bohle DS, Descoteaux A, Flavell RA, Olivier M (2009) Malarial hemozoin activates the NLRP3 inflammasome through Lyn and Syk kinases. PLoS Pathog 5(8), e1000559. doi:10.1371/journal.ppat.1000559
27. Dostert C, Guarda G, Romero JF, Menu P, Gross O, Tardivel A, Suva ML, Stehle JC, Kopf M, Stamenkovic I, Corradin G, Tschopp J (2009) Malarial hemozoin is a Nalp3 inflammasome activating danger signal. PLoS One 4(8), e6510. doi:10.1371/journal.pone.0006510
28. Parroche P, Lauw FN, Goutagny N, Latz E, Monks BG, Visintin A, Halmen KA, Lamphier M, Olivier M, Bartholomeu DC, Gazzinelli RT, Golenbock DT (2007) Malaria hemozoin is immunologically inert but radically enhances innate responses by presenting malaria DNA to Toll-like receptor 9. Proc Natl Acad Sci U S A 104(6):1919–1924
29. Barrera V, Skorokhod OA, Baci D, Gremo G, Arese P, Schwarzer E (2011) Host fibrinogen stably bound to hemozoin rapidly activates monocytes via TLR-4 and CD11b/CD18-integrin: a new paradigm of hemozoin action. Blood 117(21):5674–5682. doi:10.1182/blood-2010-10-312413
30. Pichyangkul S, Saengkrai P, Webster HK (1994) *Plasmodium falciparum* pigment induces monocytes to release high levels of tumor necrosis factor-alpha and interleukin-1 beta. Am J Trop Med Hyg 51(4):430–435
31. Kalantari P, DeOliveira RB, Chan J, Corbett Y, Rathinam V, Stutz A, Latz E, Gazzinelli RT, Golenbock DT, Fitzgerald KA (2014) Dual engagement of the NLRP3 and AIM2 inflammasomes by *Plasmodium*-derived hemozoin and DNA during malaria. Cell Rep 6(1):196–210. doi:10.1016/j.celrep.2013.12.014
32. Tyberghein A, Deroost K, Schwarzer E, Arese P, Van den Steen PE (2014) Immunopathological effects of malaria pigment or hemozoin and other crystals. Biofactors 40(1):59–78. doi:10.1002/biof.1119
33. Onishi M, Kitano M, Taniguchi K, Homma T, Kobayashi M, Sato A, Coban C, Ishii KJ (2014) Hemozoin is a potent adjuvant for hemagglutinin split vaccine without pyrogenicity in ferrets. Vaccine 32(25):3004–3009. doi:10.1016/j.vaccine.2014.03.072
34. Uraki R, Das SC, Hatta M, Kiso M, Iwatsuki-Horimoto K, Ozawa M, Coban C, Ishii KJ, Kawaoka Y (2014) Hemozoin as a novel adjuvant for inactivated whole virion influenza vaccine. Vaccine 32(41):5295–5300. doi:10.1016/j.vaccine.2014.07.079
35. Gowda NM, Wu X, Gowda DC (2011) The nucleosome (histone-DNA complex) is the TLR9-specific immunostimulatory component of *Plasmodium falciparum* that activates DCs. PLoS One 6(6), e20398. doi:10.1371/journal.pone.0020398
36. Hirako IC, Gallego-Marin C, Ataide MA, Andrade WA, Gravina H, Rocha BC, de Oliveira RB, Pereira DB, Vinetz J, Diamond B, Ram S, Golenbock DT, Gazzinelli RT (2015) DNA-containing immunocomplexes promote inflammasome assembly and release of pyrogenic

cytokines by CD14+ CD16+ CD64high CD32low Inflammatory Monocytes from Malaria Patients. MBio 6(6):e01605–e01615. doi:10.1128/mBio.01605-15
37. Sharma S, DeOliveira RB, Kalantari P, Parroche P, Goutagny N, Jiang Z, Chan J, Bartholomeu DC, Lauw F, Hall JP, Barber GN, Gazzinelli RT, Fitzgerald KA, Golenbock DT (2011) Innate immune recognition of an AT-rich stem-loop DNA motif in the *Plasmodium falciparum* genome. Immunity 35(2):194–207. doi:10.1016/j.immuni.2011.05.016
38. Lepenies B, Cramer JP, Burchard GD, Wagner H, Kirschning CJ, Jacobs T (2008) Induction of experimental cerebral malaria is independent of TLR2/4/9. Med Microbiol Immunol 197(1):39–44. doi:10.1007/s00430-007-0057-y
39. Baccarella A, Fontana MF, Chen EC, Kim CC (2013) Toll-like receptor 7 mediates early innate immune responses to malaria. Infect Immun 81(12):4431–4442. doi:10.1128/IAI.00923-13
40. Esposito S, Molteni CG, Zampiero A, Baggi E, Lavizzari A, Semino M, Daleno C, Groppo M, Scala A, Terranova L, Miozzo M, Pelucchi C, Principi N (2012) Role of polymorphisms of toll-like receptor (TLR) 4, TLR9, toll-interleukin 1 receptor domain containing adaptor protein (TIRAP) and FCGR2A genes in malaria susceptibility and severity in Burundian children. Malar J 11:196. doi:10.1186/1475-2875-11-196
41. Munde EO, Okeyo WA, Anyona SB, Raballah E, Konah S, Okumu W, Ogonda L, Vulule J, Ouma C (2012) Polymorphisms in the Fc gamma receptor IIIA and Toll-like receptor 9 are associated with protection against severe malarial anemia and changes in circulating gamma interferon levels. Infect Immun 80(12):4435–4443. doi:10.1128/IAI.00945-12
42. Campino S, Forton J, Auburn S, Fry A, Diakite M, Richardson A, Hull J, Jallow M, Sisay-Joof F, Pinder M, Molyneux ME, Taylor TE, Rockett K, Clark TG, Kwiatkowski DP (2009) TLR9 polymorphisms in African populations: no association with severe malaria, but evidence of cis-variants acting on gene expression. Malar J 8:44. doi:10.1186/1475-2875-8-44
43. Liehl P, Zuzarte-Luis V, Chan J, Zillinger T, Baptista F, Carapau D, Konert M, Hanson KK, Carret C, Lassnig C, Muller M, Kalinke U, Saeed M, Chora AF, Golenbock DT, Strobl B, Prudencio M, Coelho LP, Kappe SH, Superti-Furga G, Pichlmair A, Vigario AM, Rice CM, Fitzgerald KA, Barchet W, Mota MM (2014) Host-cell sensors for *Plasmodium* activate innate immunity against liver-stage infection. Nat Med 20(1):47–53. doi:10.1038/nm.3424
44. Orengo JM, Evans JE, Bettiol E, Leliwa-Sytek A, Day K, Rodriguez A (2008) *Plasmodium*-induced inflammation by uric acid. PLoS Pathog 4(3), e1000013
45. Orengo JM, Leliwa-Sytek A, Evans JE, Evans B, van de Hoef D, Nyako M, Day K, Rodriguez A (2009) Uric acid is a mediator of the *Plasmodium falciparum*-induced inflammatory response. PLoS One 4(4), e5194
46. van de Hoef DL, Coppens I, Holowka T, Ben Mamoun C, Branch O, Rodriguez A (2013) *Plasmodium falciparum*-derived uric acid precipitates induce maturation of dendritic cells. PLoS One 8(2), e55584. doi:10.1371/journal.pone.0055584
47. Martinon F, Petrilli V, Mayor A, Tardivel A, Tschopp J (2006) Gout-associated uric acid crystals activate the NALP3 inflammasome. Nature 440(7081):237–241
48. Ataide MA, Andrade WA, Zamboni DS, Wang D, Souza Mdo C, Franklin BS, Elian S, Martins FS, Pereira D, Reed G, Fitzgerald KA, Golenbock DT, Gazzinelli RT (2014) Malaria-induced NLRP12/NLRP3-dependent caspase-1 activation mediates inflammation and hypersensitivity to bacterial superinfection. PLoS Pathog 10(1), e1003885. doi:10.1371/journal.ppat.1003885
49. Guermonprez P, Helft J, Claser C, Deroubaix S, Karanje H, Gazumyan A, Darasse-Jeze G, Telerman SB, Breton G, Schreiber HA, Frias-Staheli N, Billerbeck E, Dorner M, Rice CM, Ploss A, Klein F, Swiecki M, Colonna M, Kamphorst AO, Meredith M, Niec R, Takacs C, Mikhail F, Hari A, Bosque D, Eisenreich T, Merad M, Shi Y, Ginhoux F, Renia L, Urban BC, Nussenzweig MC (2013) Inflammatory Flt3l is essential to mobilize dendritic cells and for T cell responses during *Plasmodium* infection. Nat Med 19(6):730–738. doi:10.1038/nm.3197
50. Sarma PS, Mandal AK, Khamis HJ (1998) Allopurinol as an additive to quinine in the treatment of acute complicated falciparum malaria. Am J Trop Med Hyg 58(4):454–457

51. Ismail N, Wang Y, Dakhlallah D, Moldovan L, Agarwal K, Batte K, Shah P, Wisler J, Eubank TD, Tridandapani S, Paulaitis ME, Piper MG, Marsh CB (2013) Macrophage microvesicles induce macrophage differentiation and miR-223 transfer. Blood 121(6):984–995. doi:10.1182/blood-2011-08-374793
52. Nantakomol D, Dondorp AM, Krudsood S, Udomsangpetch R, Pattanapanyasat K, Combes V, Grau GE, White NJ, Viriyavejakul P, Day NP, Chotivanich K (2011) Circulating red cell-derived microparticles in human malaria. J Infect Dis 203(5):700–706. doi:10.1093/infdis/jiq104
53. Couper KN, Barnes T, Hafalla JC, Combes V, Ryffel B, Secher T, Grau GE, Riley EM, de Souza JB (2010) Parasite-derived plasma microparticles contribute significantly to malaria infection-induced inflammation through potent macrophage stimulation. PLoS Pathog 6(1), e1000744. doi:10.1371/journal.ppat.1000744
54. Mantel PY, Hoang AN, Goldowitz I, Potashnikova D, Hamza B, Vorobjev I, Ghiran I, Toner M, Irimia D, Ivanov AR, Barteneva N, Marti M (2013) Malaria-infected erythrocyte-derived microvesicles mediate cellular communication within the parasite population and with the host immune system. Cell Host Microbe 13(5):521–534. doi:10.1016/j.chom.2013.04.009
55. Wheway J, Latham SL, Combes V, Grau GE (2014) Endothelial microparticles interact with and support the proliferation of T cells. J Immunol 193(7):3378–3387. doi:10.4049/jimmunol.1303431
56. Campos FM, Franklin BS, Teixeira-Carvalho A, Filho AL, de Paula SC, Fontes CJ, Brito CF, Carvalho LH (2010) Augmented plasma microparticles during acute *Plasmodium vivax* infection. Malar J 9:327. doi:10.1186/1475-2875-9-327
57. Combes V, Taylor TE, Juhan-Vague I, Mege JL, Mwenechanya J, Tembo M, Grau GE, Molyneux ME (2004) Circulating endothelial microparticles in malawian children with severe falciparum malaria complicated with coma. JAMA 291(21):2542–2544. doi:10.1001/jama.291.21.2542-b
58. Sahu U, Sahoo PK, Kar SK, Mohapatra BN, Ranjit M (2013) Association of TNF level with production of circulating cellular microparticles during clinical manifestation of human cerebral malaria. Hum Immunol 74(6):713–721. doi:10.1016/j.humimm.2013.02.006
59. McGinn CM, MacDonnell BF, Shan CX, Wallace R, Cummins PM, Murphy RP (2016) Microparticles: a pivotal nexus in vascular homeostasis and disease. Curr Clin Pharmacol 11(1):28–42
60. Francis SE, Sullivan DJ Jr, Goldberg DE (1997) Hemoglobin metabolism in the malaria parasite *Plasmodium falciparum*. Annu Rev Microbiol 51:97–123. doi:10.1146/annurev.micro.51.1.97
61. Liu M, Amodu AS, Pitts S, Patrickson J, Hibbert JM, Battle M, Ofori-Acquah SF, Stiles JK (2012) Heme mediated STAT3 activation in severe malaria. PLoS One 7(3), e34280. doi:10.1371/journal.pone.0034280
62. Liu M, Wilson NO, Hibbert JM, Stiles JK (2013) STAT3 regulates MMP3 in heme-induced endothelial cell apoptosis. PLoS One 8(8), e71366. doi:10.1371/journal.pone.0071366
63. Liu M, Dickinson-Copeland C, Hassana S, Stiles JK (2016) *Plasmodium*-infected erythrocytes (pRBC) induce endothelial cell apoptosis via a heme-mediated signaling pathway. Drug Des Devel Ther 10:1009–1018. doi:10.2147/DDDT.S96863
64. Dickinson-Copeland CM, Wilson NO, Liu M, Driss A, Salifu H, Adjei AA, Wilson M, Gyan B, Oduro D, Badu K, Botchway F, Anderson W, Bond V, Bacanamwo M, Singh S, Stiles JK (2015) Heme-mediated induction of CXCL10 and depletion of CD34^{+} progenitor cells is toll-like receptor 4 dependent. PLoS One 10(11), e0142328. doi:10.1371/journal.pone.0142328
65. Metzger A, Mukasa G, Shankar AH, Ndeezi G, Melikian G, Semba RD (2001) Antioxidant status and acute malaria in children in Kampala, Uganda. Am J Trop Med Hyg 65:115–119
66. Narsaria N, Mohanty C, Das BK, Mishra SP, Prasad R (2012) Oxidative stress in children with severe malaria. J Trop Pediatr 58:147–150. doi:10.1093/tropej/fmr043
67. Sohail M, Kaul A, Raziuddin M, Adak T (2007) Decreased glutathione-S-transferase activity: diagnostic and protective role in vivax malaria. Clin Biochem 40:377–382. doi:10.1016/j.clinbiochem.2007.01.005

68. Yazar S, Kilic E, Saraymen R, Ozbilge H (2004) Serum malondialdehyde levels in patients infected with *Plasmodium vivax*. West Indian Med J 53:147–149
69. Atamna H, Ginsburg H (1993) Origin of reactive oxygen species in erythrocytes infected with *Plasmodium falciparum*. Mol Biochem Parasitol 61:231–241
70. Dondorp AM, Omodeo-Sale F, Chotivanich K, Taramelli D, White NJ (2003) Oxidative stress and rheology in severe malaria. Redox Rep 8(5):292–294. doi:10.1179/135100003225002934
71. Huber SM, Uhlemann A-C, Gamper NL, Duranton C, Kremsner PG, Lang F (2002) *Plasmodium falciparum* activates endogenous Cl^- channels of human erythrocytes by membrane oxidation. EMBO J 21:22–30. doi:10.1093/emboj/21.1.22
72. Jaramillo M, Godbout M, Olivier M (2005) Hemozoin induces macrophage chemokine expression through oxidative stress-dependent and -independent mechanisms. J Immunol 174:475–484
73. Potter SM, Mitchell AJ, Cowden WB, Sanni LA, Dinauer M, de Haan JB, Hunt NH (2005) Phagocyte-derived reactive oxygen species do not influence the progression of murine blood-stage malaria infections. Infect Immun 73:4941–4947. doi:10.1128/IAI.73.8.4941-4947.2005
74. Iwalokun BA, Bamiro SB, Ogunledun A (2006) Levels and interactions of plasma xanthine oxidase, catalase and liver function parameters in Nigerian children with *Plasmodium falciparum* infection. APMIS 114(12):842–850
75. Das BS, Patnaik JK, Mohanty S, Mishra SK, Mohanty D, Satpathy SK, Bose TK (1993) Plasma antioxidants and lipid peroxidation products in falciparum malaria. Am J Trop Med Hyg 49(6):720–725
76. Das BS, Thurnham DI, Patnaik JK, Das DB, Satpathy R, Bose TK (1990) Increased plasma lipid peroxidation in riboflavin-deficient, malaria-infected children. Am J Clin Nutr 51(5):859–863
77. Isah MB, Ibrahim MA (2014) The role of antioxidants treatment on the pathogenesis of malarial infections: a review. Parasitol Res 113(3):801–809. doi:10.1007/s00436-014-3804-1
78. Lin JW, Spaccapelo R, Schwarzer E, Sajid M, Annoura T, Deroost K, Ravelli RB, Aime E, Capuccini B, Mommaas-Kienhuis AM, O'Toole T, Prins F, Franke-Fayard BM, Ramesar J, Chevalley-Maurel S, Kroeze H, Koster AJ, Tanke HJ, Crisanti A, Langhorne J, Arese P, Van den Steen PE, Janse CJ, Khan SM (2015) Replication of *Plasmodium* in reticulocytes can occur without hemozoin formation, resulting in chloroquine resistance. J Exp Med 212(6):893–903. doi:10.1084/jem.20141731
79. Pichyangkul S, Yongvanitchit K, Kum-arb U, Hemmi H, Akira S, Krieg AM, Heppner DG, Stewart VA, Hasegawa H, Looareesuwan S, Shanks GD, Miller RS (2004) Malaria blood stage parasites activate human plasmacytoid dendritic cells and murine dendritic cells through a Toll-like receptor 9-dependent pathway. J Immunol 172(8):4926–4933
80. Giusti P, Urban BC, Frascaroli G, Albrecht L, Tinti A, Troye-Blomberg M, Varani S (2011) *Plasmodium falciparum*-infected erythrocytes and beta-hematin induce partial maturation of human dendritic cells and increase their migratory ability in response to lymphoid chemokines. Infect Immun 79(7):2727–2736. doi:10.1128/IAI.00649-10
81. Walther M, Woodruff J, Edele F, Jeffries D, Tongren JE, King E, Andrews L, Bejon P, Gilbert SC, De Souza JB, Sinden R, Hill AV, Riley EM (2006) Innate immune responses to human malaria: heterogeneous cytokine responses to blood-stage *Plasmodium falciparum* correlate with parasitological and clinical outcomes. J Immunol 177(8):5736–5745
82. Franklin BS, Parroche P, Ataide MA, Lauw F, Ropert C, de Oliveira RB, Pereira D, Tada MS, Nogueira P, da Silva LH, Bjorkbacka H, Golenbock DT, Gazzinelli RT (2009) Malaria primes the innate immune response due to interferon-gamma induced enhancement of toll-like receptor expression and function. Proc Natl Acad Sci U S A 106(14):5789–5794. doi:10.1073/pnas.0809742106
83. Miller JL, Sack BK, Baldwin M, Vaughan AM, Kappe SH (2014) Interferon-mediated innate immune responses against malaria parasite liver stages. Cell Rep 7(2):436–447. doi:10.1016/j.celrep.2014.03.018

84. Schofield L, Ferreira A, Altszuler R, Nussenzweig V, Nussenzweig RS (1987) Interferon-gamma inhibits the intrahepatocytic development of malaria parasites in vitro. J Immunol 139(6):2020–2025
85. Vergara U, Ferreira A, Schellekens H, Nussenzweig V (1987) Mechanism of escape of exo-erythrocytic forms (EEF) of malaria parasites from the inhibitory effects of interferon-gamma. J Immunol 138(12):4447–4449
86. Abdalla SH (1988) Peripheral blood and bone marrow leucocytes in Gambian children with malaria: numerical changes and evaluation of phagocytosis. Ann Trop Paediatr 8(4):250–258
87. Mahanta A, Kar SK, Kakati S, Baruah S (2015) Heightened inflammation in severe malaria is associated with decreased IL-10 expression levels and neutrophils. Innate Immun 21(5):546–552. doi:10.1177/1753425914561277
88. Tangteerawatana P, Krudsood S, Kanchanakhan N, Troye-Blomberg M, Khusmith S (2014) Low monocyte to neutrophil ratio in peripheral blood associated with disease complication in primary *Plasmodium falciparum* infection. Southeast Asian J Trop Med Public Health 45(3):517–530
89. Pierrot C, Adam E, Hot D, Lafitte S, Capron M, George JD, Khalife J (2007) Contribution of T cells and neutrophils in protection of young susceptible rats from fatal experimental malaria. J Immunol 178(3):1713–1722
90. Ioannidis LJ, Nie CQ, Ly A, Ryg-Cornejo V, Chiu CY, Hansen DS (2016) Monocyte- and neutrophil-derived CXCL10 impairs efficient control of blood-stage malaria infection and promotes severe disease. J Immunol 196(3):1227–1238. doi:10.4049/jimmunol.1501562
91. Schumak B, Klocke K, Kuepper JM, Biswas A, Djie-Maletz A, Limmer A, van Rooijen N, Mack M, Hoerauf A, Dunay IR (2015) Specific depletion of Ly6C^{hi} inflammatory monocytes prevents immunopathology in experimental cerebral malaria. PLoS One 10(4), e0124080. doi:10.1371/journal.pone.0124080
92. Feintuch CM, Saidi A, Seydel K, Chen G, Goldman-Yassen A, Mita-Mendoza NK, Kim RS, Frenette PS, Taylor T, Daily JP (2015) Activated neutrophils are associated with pediatric cerebral malaria vasculopathy in Malawian children. MBio 7(1):e01300–e01315. doi:10.1128/mBio.01300-15
93. Rocha BC, Marques PE, Leoratti FM, Junqueira C, Pereira DB, Antonelli LR, Menezes GB, Golenbock DT, Gazzinelli RT (2015) Type I interferon transcriptional signature in neutrophils and low-density granulocytes are associated with tissue damage in malaria. Cell Rep 13(12):2829–2841. doi:10.1016/j.celrep.2015.11.055
94. Leoratti FM, Trevelin SC, Cunha FQ, Rocha BC, Costa PA, Gravina HD, Tada MS, Pereira DB, Golenbock DT, Antonelli LR, Gazzinelli RT (2012) Neutrophil paralysis in *Plasmodium vivax* malaria. PLoS Negl Trop Dis 6(6), e1710. doi:10.1371/journal.pntd.0001710
95. Furuta T, Kikuchi T, Iwakura Y, Watanabe N (2006) Protective roles of mast cells and mast cell-derived TNF in murine malaria. J Immunol 177(5):3294–3302
96. Stevenson MM, Ghadirian E, Phillips NC, Rae D, Podoba JE (1989) Role of mononuclear phagocytes in elimination of *Plasmodium chabaudi* AS infection. Parasite Immunol 11(5):529–544
97. Couper KN, Blount DG, Hafalla JC, van Rooijen N, de Souza JB, Riley EM (2007) Macrophage-mediated but gamma interferon-independent innate immune responses control the primary wave of *Plasmodium yoelii* parasitemia. Infect Immun 75(12):5806–5818. doi:10.1128/IAI.01005-07
98. Ayi K, Patel SN, Serghides L, Smith TG, Kain KC (2005) Nonopsonic phagocytosis of erythrocytes infected with ring-stage *Plasmodium falciparum*. Infect Immun 73(4):2559–2563. doi:10.1128/IAI.73.4.2559-2563.2005
99. Bettiol E, Van de Hoef DL, Carapau D, Rodriguez A (2010) Efficient phagosomal maturation and degradation of *Plasmodium*-infected erythrocytes by dendritic cells and macrophages. Parasite Immunol 32(6):389–398. doi:10.1111/j.1365-3024.2010.01198.x
100. Patel SN, Serghides L, Smith TG, Febbraio M, Silverstein RL, Kurtz TW, Pravenec M, Kain KC (2004) CD36 mediates the phagocytosis of *Plasmodium falciparum*-infected erythrocytes by rodent macrophages. J Infect Dis 189(2):204–213. doi:10.1086/380764

101. Su Z, Fortin A, Gros P, Stevenson MM (2002) Opsonin-independent phagocytosis: an effector mechanism against acute blood-stage *Plasmodium chabaudi* AS infection. J Infect Dis 186(9):1321–1329. doi:10.1086/344576
102. Fernandez-Arias C, Lopez JP, Hernandez-Perez JN, Bautista-Ojeda MD, Branch O, Rodriguez A (2013) Malaria inhibits surface expression of complement receptor 1 in monocytes/macrophages, causing decreased immune complex internalization. J Immunol 190(7):3363–3372. doi:10.4049/jimmunol.1103812
103. Yoneto T, Waki S, Takai T, Tagawa Y, Iwakura Y, Mizuguchi J, Nariuchi H, Yoshimoto T (2001) A critical role of Fc receptor-mediated antibody-dependent phagocytosis in the host resistance to blood-stage *Plasmodium berghei* XAT infection. J Immunol 166(10):6236–6241
104. Steinman RM (2012) Decisions about dendritic cells: past, present, and future. Annu Rev Immunol 30:1–22. doi:10.1146/annurev-immunol-100311-102839
105. Elliott SR, Spurck TP, Dodin JM, Maier AG, Voss TS, Yosaatmadja F, Payne PD, McFadden GI, Cowman AF, Rogerson SJ, Schofield L, Brown GV (2007) Inhibition of dendritic cell maturation by malaria is dose dependent and does not require *Plasmodium falciparum* erythrocyte membrane protein 1. Infect Immun 75(7):3621–3632. doi:10.1128/IAI.00095-07
106. Urban BC, Ferguson DJ, Pain A, Willcox N, Plebanski M, Austyn JM, Roberts DJ (1999) *Plasmodium falciparum*-infected erythrocytes modulate the maturation of dendritic cells. Nature 400(6739):73–77. doi:10.1038/21900
107. Teirlinck AC, McCall MB, Roestenberg M, Scholzen A, Woestenenk R, de Mast Q, van der Ven AJ, Hermsen CC, Luty AJ, Sauerwein RW (2011) Longevity and composition of cellular immune responses following experimental *Plasmodium falciparum* malaria infection in humans. PLoS Pathog 7(12), e1002389. doi:10.1371/journal.ppat.1002389
108. Kho S, Marfurt J, Noviyanti R, Kusuma A, Piera KA, Burdam FH, Kenangalem E, Lampah DA, Engwerda CR, Poespoprodjo JR, Price RN, Anstey NM, Minigo G, Woodberry T (2015) Preserved dendritic cell HLA-DR expression and reduced regulatory T cell activation in asymptomatic *Plasmodium falciparum* and *P. vivax* infection. Infect Immun 83(8):3224–3232. doi:10.1128/IAI.00226-15
109. Loughland JR, Minigo G, Burel J, Tipping PE, Piera KA, Amante FH, Engwerda CR, Good MF, Doolan DL, Anstey NM, McCarthy JS, Woodberry T (2016) Profoundly reduced $CD1c^+$ myeloid dendritic cell HLA-DR and CD86 expression and increased TNF production in experimental human blood-stage malaria infection. Infect Immun 84(5):1403–1412. doi:10.1128/IAI.01522-15
110. Urban BC, Mwangi T, Ross A, Kinyanjui S, Mosobo M, Kai O, Lowe B, Marsh K, Roberts DJ (2001) Peripheral blood dendritic cells in children with acute *Plasmodium falciparum* malaria. Blood 98(9):2859–2861
111. Mukherjee P, Chauhan VS (2008) *Plasmodium falciparum*-free merozoites and infected RBCs distinctly affect soluble CD40 ligand-mediated maturation of immature monocyte-derived dendritic cells. J Leukoc Biol 84(1):244–254. doi:10.1189/jlb.0807565
112. Gowda NM, Wu X, Kumar S, Febbraio M, Gowda DC (2013) CD36 contributes to malaria parasite-induced pro-inflammatory cytokine production and NK and T cell activation by dendritic cells. PLoS One 8(10), e77604. doi:10.1371/journal.pone.0077604
113. Woodberry T, Minigo G, Piera KA, Amante FH, Pinzon-Charry A, Good MF, Lopez JA, Engwerda CR, McCarthy JS, Anstey NM (2012) Low-level *Plasmodium falciparum* blood-stage infection causes dendritic cell apoptosis and dysfunction in healthy volunteers. J Infect Dis 206(3):333–340. doi:10.1093/infdis/jis366
114. Pinzon-Charry A, Woodberry T, Kienzle V, McPhun V, Minigo G, Lampah DA, Kenangalem E, Engwerda C, Lopez JA, Anstey NM, Good MF (2013) Apoptosis and dysfunction of blood dendritic cells in patients with *falciparum* and *vivax* malaria. J Exp Med 210(8):1635–1646. doi:10.1084/jem.20121972
115. Urban BC, Cordery D, Shafi MJ, Bull PC, Newbold CI, Williams TN, Marsh K (2006) The frequency of BDCA3-positive dendritic cells is increased in the peripheral circulation of Kenyan children with severe malaria. Infect Immun 74(12):6700–6706. doi:10.1128/IAI.00861-06

116. Teirlinck AC, Roestenberg M, Bijker EM, Hoffman SL, Sauerwein RW, Scholzen A (2015) *Plasmodium falciparum* infection of human volunteers activates monocytes and $CD16^+$ dendritic cells and induces upregulation of CD16 and CD1c expression. Infect Immun 83(9):3732–3739. doi:10.1128/IAI.00473-15
117. Artavanis-Tsakonas K, Eleme K, McQueen KL, Cheng NW, Parham P, Davis DM, Riley EM (2003) Activation of a subset of human NK cells upon contact with *Plasmodium falciparum*-infected erythrocytes. J Immunol 171(10):5396–5405
118. Horowitz A, Newman KC, Evans JH, Korbel DS, Davis DM, Riley EM (2010) Cross-talk between T cells and NK cells generates rapid effector responses to *Plasmodium falciparum*-infected erythrocytes. J Immunol 184(11):6043–6052. doi:10.4049/jimmunol.1000106
119. Stegmann KA, De Souza JB, Riley EM (2015) IL-18-induced expression of high-affinity IL-2R on murine NK cells is essential for NK-cell IFN-gamma production during murine *Plasmodium yoelii* infection. Eur J Immunol 45(12):3431–3440. doi:10.1002/eji.201546018
120. Newman KC, Korbel DS, Hafalla JC, Riley EM (2006) Cross-talk with myeloid accessory cells regulates human natural killer cell interferon-gamma responses to malaria. PLoS Pathog 2(12), e118. doi:10.1371/journal.ppat.0020118
121. Kitaguchi T, Nagoya M, Amano T, Suzuki M, Minami M (1996) Analysis of roles of natural killer cells in defense against *Plasmodium chabaudi* in mice. Parasitol Res 82(4):352–357
122. Mohan K, Moulin P, Stevenson MM (1997) Natural killer cell cytokine production, not cytotoxicity, contributes to resistance against blood-stage *Plasmodium chabaudi* AS infection. J Immunol 159(10):4990–4998
123. Roussilhon C, Agrapart M, Ballet JJ, Bensussan A (1990) T lymphocytes bearing the gamma delta T cell receptor in patients with acute *Plasmodium falciparum* malaria. J Infect Dis 162(1):283–285
124. Ho M, Webster HK, Tongtawe P, Pattanapanyasat K, Weidanz WP (1990) Increased gamma delta T cells in acute *Plasmodium falciparum* malaria. Immunol Lett 25(1-3):139–141
125. Behr C, Poupot R, Peyrat MA, Poquet Y, Constant P, Dubois P, Bonneville M, Fournie JJ (1996) *Plasmodium falciparum* stimuli for human gammadelta T cells are related to phosphorylated antigens of mycobacteria. Infect Immun 64(8):2892–2896
126. Costa G, Loizon S, Guenot M, Mocan I, Halary F, de Saint-Basile G, Pitard V, Dechanet-Merville J, Moreau JF, Troye-Blomberg M, Mercereau-Puijalon O, Behr C (2011) Control of *Plasmodium falciparum* erythrocytic cycle: $\gamma\delta$ T cells target the red blood cell-invasive merozoites. Blood 118(26):6952–6962. doi:10.1182/blood-2011-08-376111
127. D'Ombrain MC, Hansen DS, Simpson KM, Schofield L (2007) gammadelta-T cells expressing NK receptors predominate over NK cells and conventional T cells in the innate IFN-gamma response to *Plasmodium falciparum* malaria. Eur J Immunol 37(7):1864–1873. doi:10.1002/eji.200636889
128. Goodier MR, Lundqvist C, Hammarstrom ML, Troye-Blomberg M, Langhorne J (1995) Cytokine profiles for human V gamma 9^+ T cells stimulated by *Plasmodium falciparum*. Parasite Immunol 17(8):413–423
129. Stanisic DI, Cutts J, Eriksson E, Fowkes FJ, Rosanas-Urgell A, Siba P, Laman M, Davis TM, Manning L, Mueller I, Schofield L (2014) gammadelta T cells and $CD14^+$ monocytes are predominant cellular sources of cytokines and chemokines associated with severe malaria. J Infect Dis 210(2):295–305. doi:10.1093/infdis/jiu083
130. Jones SM, Goodier MR, Langhorne J (1996) The response of gamma delta T cells to *Plasmodium falciparum* is dependent on activated $CD4^+$ T cells and the recognition of MHC class I molecules. Immunology 89(3):405–412
131. Waterfall M, Black A, Riley E (1998) $Gammadelta^+$ T cells preferentially respond to live rather than killed malaria parasites. Infect Immun 66(5):2393–2398
132. Inoue S, Niikura M, Takeo S, Mineo S, Kawakami Y, Uchida A, Kamiya S, Kobayashi F (2012) Enhancement of dendritic cell activation via CD40 ligand-expressing gammadelta T cells is responsible for protective immunity to *Plasmodium* parasites. Proc Natl Acad Sci U S A 109(30):12129–12134. doi:10.1073/pnas.1204480109

133. Kobayashi F, Niikura M, Waki S, Matsui T, Fujino T, Tsuruhara T, Kamiya S (2007) *Plasmodium berghei* XAT: contribution of gammadelta T cells to host defense against infection with blood-stage nonlethal malaria parasite. Exp Parasitol 117(4):368–375. doi:10.1016/j.exppara.2007.05.002
134. Weidanz WP, LaFleur G, Brown A, Burns JM Jr, Gramaglia I, van der Heyde HC (2010) Gammadelta T cells but not NK cells are essential for cell-mediated immunity against *Plasmodium chabaudi* malaria. Infect Immun 78(10):4331–4340. doi:10.1128/IAI.00539-10
135. Obiero JM, Shekalaghe S, Hermsen CC, Mpina M, Bijker EM, Roestenberg M, Teelen K, Billingsley PF, Sim BK, James ER, Daubenberger CA, Hoffman SL, Abdulla S, Sauerwein RW, Scholzen A (2015) Impact of malaria preexposure on antiparasite cellular and humoral immune responses after controlled human malaria infection. Infect Immun 83(5):2185–2196. doi:10.1128/IAI.03069-14
136. Jagannathan P, Kim CC, Greenhouse B, Nankya F, Bowen K, Eccles-James I, Muhindo MK, Arinaitwe E, Tappero JW, Kamya MR, Dorsey G, Feeney ME (2014) Loss and dysfunction of Vdelta2^{+} gammadelta T cells are associated with clinical tolerance to malaria. Sci Transl Med 6(251):251ra117. doi:10.1126/scitranslmed.3009793
137. Druilhe P, Rhodes-Feuillette A, Canivet M, Gentilini M, Periês J (1982) Circulating interferon in patients with *Plasmodium falciparum*, *P. ovale* and *P. vivax* malaria. Trans R Soc Trop Med Hyg 76:422–423
138. Ojo-Amaize EA, Salimonu LS, Williams AI, Akinwolere OA, Shabo R, Alm GV, Wigzell H (1981) Positive correlation between degree of parasitemia, interferon titers, and natural killer cell activity in *Plasmodium falciparum*-infected children. J Immunol 127:2296–2300
139. Andrade BB, Reis-Filho A, Souza-Neto SM, Clarêncio J, Camargo LMA, Barral A, Barral-Netto M (2010) Severe *Plasmodium vivax* malaria exhibits marked inflammatory imbalance. Malar J 9:13. doi:10.1186/1475-2875-9-13
140. Angulo I, Fresno M (2002) Cytokines in the pathogenesis of and protection against malaria. Clin Vaccine Immunol 9:1145–1152. doi:10.1128/CDLI.9.6.1145-1152.2002
141. Grau GE, Taylor TE, Molyneux ME, Wirima JJ, Vassalli P, Hommel M, Lambert PH (1989) Tumor necrosis factor and disease severity in children with falciparum malaria. N Engl J Med 320:1586–1591. doi:10.1056/NEJM198906153202404
142. Kern P, Hemmer CJ, Van Damme J, Gruss HJ, Dietrich M (1989) Elevated tumor necrosis factor alpha and interleukin-6 serum levels as markers for complicated *Plasmodium falciparum* malaria. Am J Med 87:139–143
143. Kremsner PG, Winkler S, Brandts C, Wildling E, Jenne L, Graninger W, Prada J, Bienzle U, Juillard P, Grau GE (1995) Prediction of accelerated cure in *Plasmodium falciparum* malaria by the elevated capacity of tumor necrosis factor production. Am J Trop Med Hyg 53:532–538
144. Kwiatkowski D, Sambou I, Twumasi P, Greenwood BM, Hill AVS, Manogue KR, Cerami A, Castracane J, Brewster DR (1990) TNF concentration in fatal cerebral, non-fatal cerebral, and uncomplicated *Plasmodium falciparum* malaria. Lancet 336:1201–1204. doi:10.1016/0140-6736(90)92827-5
145. Lyke KE, Burges R, Cissoko Y, Sangare L, Dao M, Diarra I, Kone A, Harley R, Plowe CV, Doumbo OK, Sztein MB (2004) Serum levels of the proinflammatory cytokines interleukin-1 beta (IL-1beta), IL-6, IL-8, IL-10, tumor necrosis factor alpha, and IL-12(p70) in Malian children with severe *Plasmodium falciparum* malaria and matched uncomplicated malaria or healthy controls. Infect Immun 72:5630–5637. doi:10.1128/IAI.72.10.5630-5637.2004
146. Mordmüller BG, Metzger WG, Juillard P, Brinkman BM, Verweij CL, Grau GE, Kremsner PG (1997) Tumor necrosis factor in *Plasmodium falciparum* malaria: high plasma level is associated with fever, but high production capacity is associated with rapid fever clearance. Eur Cytokine Netw 8:29–35
147. Mshana RN, Boulandi J, Mshana NM, Mayombo J, Mendome G (1991) Cytokines in the pathogenesis of malaria: levels of IL-I beta, IL-4, IL-6, TNF-alpha and IFN-gamma in plasma of healthy individuals and malaria patients in a holoendemic area. J Clin Lab Immunol 34:131–139
148. Ockenhouse CF, Hu W-c, Kester KE, Cummings JF, Stewart A, Heppner DG, Jedlicka AE, Scott AL, Wolfe ND, Vahey M, Burke DS (2006) Common and divergent immune response

signaling pathways discovered in peripheral blood mononuclear cell gene expression patterns in presymptomatic and clinically apparent malaria. Infect Immun 74:5561–5573. doi:10.1128/IAI.00408-06
149. Peyron F, Burdin N, Ringwald P, Vuillez JP, Rousset F, Banchereau J (1994) High levels of circulating IL-10 in human malaria. Clin Exp Immunol 95:300–303
150. Ringwald P, Peyron F, Vuillez JP, Touze JE, Le Bras J, Deloron P (1991) Levels of cytokines in plasma during *Plasmodium falciparum* malaria attacks. J Clin Microbiol 29:2076–2078
151. Brown H, Turner G, Rogerson S, Tembo M, Mwenechanya J, Molyneux M, Taylor T (1999) Cytokine expression in the brain in human cerebral malaria. J Infect Dis 180:1742–1746
152. Maneerat Y, Pongponratn E, Viriyavejakul P, Punpoowong B, Looareesuwan S, Udomsangpetch R (1999) Cytokines associated with pathology in the brain tissue of fatal malaria. Southeast Asian J Trop Med Public Health 30:643–649
153. De Souza JB, Williamson KH, Otani T, Playfair JH (1997) Early gamma interferon responses in lethal and nonlethal murine blood-stage malaria. Infect Immun 65:1593–1598
154. Bate CA, Taverne J, Playfair JH (1988) Malarial parasites induce TNF production by macrophages. Immunology 64:227–231
155. Clark IA, Hunt NH, Butcher GA, Cowden WB (1987) Inhibition of murine malaria (*Plasmodium chabaudi*) in vivo by recombinant interferon-gamma or tumor necrosis factor, and its enhancement by butylated hydroxyanisole. J Immunol 139:3493–3496
156. Shear HL, Srinivasan R, Nolan T, Ng C (1989) Role of IFN-gamma in lethal and nonlethal malaria in susceptible and resistant murine hosts. J Immunol 143:2038–2044
157. Taverne J, Tavernier J, Fiers W, Playfair JH (1987) Recombinant tumour necrosis factor inhibits malaria parasites in vivo but not in vitro. Clin Exp Immunol 67:1–4
158. Rockett KA, Awburn MM, Aggarwal BB, Cowden WB, Clark IA (1992) In vivo induction of nitrite and nitrate by tumor necrosis factor, lymphotoxin, and interleukin-1: possible roles in malaria. Infect Immun 60:3725–3730
159. Knight JC, Udalova I, Hill AV, Greenwood BM, Peshu N, Marsh K, Kwiatkowski D (1999) A polymorphism that affects OCT-1 binding to the TNF promoter region is associated with severe malaria. Nat Genet 22:145–150. doi:10.1038/9649
160. McGuire W, Hill AV, Allsopp CE, Greenwood BM, Kwiatkowski D (1994) Variation in the TNF-alpha promoter region associated with susceptibility to cerebral malaria. Nature 371:508–510. doi:10.1038/371508a0
161. McGuire W, Knight JC, Hill AV, Allsopp CE, Greenwood BM, Kwiatkowski D (1999) Severe malarial anemia and cerebral malaria are associated with different tumor necrosis factor promoter alleles. J Infect Dis 179:287–290. doi:10.1086/314533
162. Ribeiro BP, Cassiano GC, de Souza RM, Cysne DN, Grisotto MAG, de Azevedo Dos Santos APS, Marinho CRF, Machado RLD, Nascimento FRF (2016) Polymorphisms in *Plasmodium vivax* circumsporozoite protein (CSP) influence parasite burden and cytokine balance in a pre-amazon endemic area from Brazil. PLoS Negl Trop Dis 10, e0004479. doi:10.1371/journal.pntd.0004479
163. Wattavidanage J, Carter R, Perera KL, Munasingha A, Bandara S, McGuinness D, Wickramasinghe AR, Alles HK, Mendis KN, Premawansa S (1999) TNFα*2 marks high risk of severe disease during *Plasmodium falciparum* malaria and other infections in Sri Lankans. Clin Exp Immunol 115:350–355
164. van Hensbroek MB, Palmer A, Onyiorah E, Schneider G, Jaffar S, Dolan G, Memming H, Frenkel J, Enwere G, Bennett S, Kwiatkowski D, Greenwood B (1996) The effect of a monoclonal antibody to tumor necrosis factor on survival from childhood cerebral malaria. J Infect Dis 174:1091–1097. doi:10.1093/infdis/174.5.1091
165. Deloron P, Chougnet C, Lepers JP, Tallet S, Coulanges P (1991) Protective value of elevated levels of gamma interferon in serum against exoerythrocytic stages of *Plasmodium falciparum*. J Clin Microbiol 29:1757–1760
166. Hoffman SL, Crutcher JM, Puri SK, Ansari AA, Villinger F, Franke ED, Singh PP, Finkelman F, Gately MK, Dutta GP, Sedegah M (1997) Sterile protection of monkeys against malaria after administration of interleukin-12. Nat Med 3:80–83

167. Bienzle U, Fritsch KG, Hoth G, Rozdzinski E, Köhler K, Kalinowski M, Kremsner P, Rosenkaimer F, Feldmeier H (1988) Inhibition of *Plasmodium vinckei*-malaria in mice by recombinant murine interferon-gamma. Acta Trop 45:289–290
168. Favre N, Ryffel B, Bordmann G, Rudin W (1997) The course of *Plasmodium chabaudi* chabaudi infections in interferon-gamma receptor deficient mice. Parasite Immunol 19:375–383
169. Huang KY, Schultz WW, Gordon FB (1968) Interferon induced by *Plasmodium berghei.* Science 162:123–124
170. Jahiel RI, Nussenzweig RS, Vilcek J, Vanderberg J (1969) Protective effect of interferon inducers on *Plasmodium berghei* malaria. Am J Trop Med Hyg 18:823–835
171. Kobayashi F, Ishida H, Matsui T, Tsuji M (2000) Effects of in vivo administration of anti-IL-10 or anti-IFN-gamma monoclonal antibody on the host defense mechanism against *Plasmodium yoelii* yoelii infection. J Vet Med Sci 62:583–587
172. Meding SJ, Cheng SC, Simon-Haarhaus B, Langhorne J (1990) Role of gamma interferon during infection with *Plasmodium chabaudi* chabaudi. Infect Immun 58:3671–3678
173. Schultz WW, Huang KY, Gordon FB (1968) Role of interferon in experimental mouse malaria. Nature 220:709–710
174. Stevenson MM, Tam MF, Nowotarski M (1990) Role of interferon-gamma and tumor necrosis factor in host resistance to *Plasmodium chabaudi* AS. Immunol Lett 25:115–121
175. Su Z, Stevenson MM (2000) Central role of endogenous gamma interferon in protective immunity against blood-stage *Plasmodium chabaudi* AS infection. Infect Immun 68:4399–4406
176. Sam H, Stevenson MM (1999) In vivo IL-12 production and IL-12 receptors beta1 and beta2 mRNA expression in the spleen are differentially up-regulated in resistant B6 and susceptible A/J mice during early blood-stage *Plasmodium chabaudi* AS malaria. J Immunol 162:1582–1589
177. Singh RP, S-i K, Rao P, Okamura H, Mukherjee A, Chauhan VS (2002) The role of IL-18 in blood-stage immunity against murine malaria *Plasmodium yoelii* 265 and *Plasmodium berghei* ANKA. J Immunol 168:4674–4681
178. Stevenson MM, Tam MF, Wolf SF, Sher A (1995) IL-12-induced protection against blood-stage *Plasmodium chabaudi* AS requires IFN-gamma and TNF-alpha and occurs via a nitric oxide-dependent mechanism. J Immunol 155:2545–2556
179. Adachi K, Tsutsui H, Kashiwamura S, Seki E, Nakano H, Takeuchi O, Takeda K, Okumura K, Van Kaer L, Okamura H, Akira S, Nakanishi K (2001) *Plasmodium berghei* infection in mice induces liver injury by an IL-12- and toll-like receptor/myeloid differentiation factor 88-dependent mechanism. J Immunol 167:5928–5934
180. Yoshimoto T, Takahama Y, Wang CR, Yoneto T, Waki S, Nariuchi H (1998) A pathogenic role of IL-12 in blood-stage murine malaria lethal strain *Plasmodium berghei* NK65 infection. J Immunol 160:5500–5505
181. Ho M, Sexton MM, Tongtawe P, Looareesuwan S, Suntharasamai P, Webster HK (1995) Interleukin-10 inhibits tumor necrosis factor production but not antigen-specific lymphoproliferation in acute *Plasmodium falciparum* malaria. J Infect Dis 172:838–844
182. Luty AJ, Perkins DJ, Lell B, Schmidt-Ott R, Lehman LG, Luckner D, Greve B, Matousek P, Herbich K, Schmid D, Weinberg JB, Kremsner PG (2000) Low interleukin-12 activity in severe *Plasmodium falciparum* malaria. Infect Immun 68:3909–3915
183. Day NP, Hien TT, Schollaardt T, Loc PP, Chuong LV, Chau TT, Mai NT, Phu NH, Sinh DX, White NJ, Ho M (1999) The prognostic and pathophysiologic role of pro- and antiinflammatory cytokines in severe malaria. J Infect Dis 180:1288–1297. doi:10.1086/315016
184. Perkins DJ, Weinberg JB, Kremsner PG (2000) Reduced interleukin-12 and transforming growth factor-beta1 in severe childhood malaria: relationship of cytokine balance with disease severity. J Infect Dis 182:988–992. doi:10.1086/315762
185. Kurtzhals JA, Adabayeri V, Goka BQ, Akanmori BD, Oliver-Commey JO, Nkrumah FK, Behr C, Hviid L (1998) Low plasma concentrations of interleukin 10 in severe malarial anaemia compared with cerebral and uncomplicated malaria. Lancet 351:1768–1772. doi:10.1016/S0140-6736(97)09439-7

186. May J, Lell B, Luty AJ, Meyer CG, Kremsner PG (2000) Plasma interleukin-10: tumor necrosis factor (TNF)-alpha ratio is associated with TNF promoter variants and predicts malarial complications. J Infect Dis 182:1570–1573. doi:10.1086/315857
187. Othoro C, Lal AA, Nahlen B, Koech D, Orago AS, Udhayakumar V (1999) A low interleukin-10 tumor necrosis factor-alpha ratio is associated with malaria anemia in children residing in a holoendemic malaria region in western Kenya. J Infect Dis 179:279–282. doi:10.1086/314548
188. Ouma C, Davenport GC, Were T, Otieno MF, Hittner JB, Vulule JM, Martinson J, Ong'echa JM, Ferrell RE, Perkins DJ (2008) Haplotypes of IL-10 promoter variants are associated with susceptibility to severe malarial anemia and functional changes in IL-10 production. Hum Genet 124:515–524. doi:10.1007/s00439-008-0578-5
189. Hugosson E, Montgomery SM, Premji Z, Troye-Blomberg M, Björkman A (2004) Higher IL-10 levels are associated with less effective clearance of *Plasmodium falciparum* parasites. Parasite Immunol 26:111–117. doi:10.1111/j.0141-9838.2004.00678.x
190. Zeyrek FY, Kurcer MA, Zeyrek D, Simsek Z (2006) Parasite density and serum cytokine levels in *Plasmodium vivax* malaria in Turkey. Parasite Immunol 28:201–207. doi:10.1111/j.1365-3024.2006.00822.x

Mechanisms of Adaptive Immunity to *Plasmodium* Liver-Stage Infection: The Known and Unknown

Stina L. Urban, Katherine L. Doll, and John T. Harty

Contents

1 Introduction 28
2 Humoral Responses to Liver-Stage Infection 28
2.1 Mechanisms of Antibody-Mediated Inhibition of Preerythrocytic Infection 30
2.2 Antibody and Specific B Cell Responses to Sporozoite Antigens 31
3 CD8 T Cells Are Potent Mediators of Protection Against *Plasmodium* Liver-Stage Infections 32
3.1 Quantitative and Qualitative Features of Protective Liver-Stage-Specific CD8 T Cells 32
3.2 Novel CD8 T Cell Epitopes Provide Additional Tools to Study Features of Protective *Plasmodium*-Specific CD8 T Cell Responses 34
3.3 Localization of Protective CD8 T Cell Responses 35
4 Role of CD4 T Cells to Liver-Stage Infection 36
4.1 Role of CD4 T Cell Help in Protective Immunity to Liver-Stage Infection 36
4.2 Role of Cytotoxic CD4 T Cells in Protective Immunity 37
5 Conclusion 38
References 39

S.L. Urban • K.L. Doll
Department of Microbiology, University of Iowa, 3-512 Bowen Science Building, 51 Newton Road, Iowa City, IA 52242, USA

J.T. Harty (✉)
Department of Microbiology, University of Iowa, 3-512 Bowen Science Building, 51 Newton Road, Iowa City, IA 52242, USA

Pathology, University of Iowa, 3-512 Bowen Science Building, 51 Newton Road, Iowa City, IA 52242, USA

Interdisciplinary Program in Immunology, University of Iowa, 3-512 Bowen Science Building, 51 Newton Road, Iowa City, IA 52242, USA
e-mail: john-harty@uiowa.edu

M.M. Mota, A. Rodriguez (eds.), *Malaria*, DOI 10.1007/978-3-319-45210-4_2

Abbreviations

CPS	Chemoprophylaxis sporozoites
CSP	Circumsporozoite protein
GAP	Genetically attenuated parasites
IVM	Intravital microscopy
RAS	Radiation-attenuated sporozoites
WSV	Whole sporozoite vaccination

1 Introduction

Malaria infections remain a global health concern with a mortality rate of ~500,000 individuals per year [1]. Therefore, the need to develop a vaccine that provides lifelong sterilizing immunity is of great importance. Sterilizing immunity to malaria infections involves preventing the liver-stage parasite from leaving the liver and initiating the symptomatic blood stage of infection. It should be noted this review focuses on memory responses and not the primary (effector) response following the initial exposure of a naïve individual to *Plasmodium* antigens, as this response, when assessed through physiological experiments, is incapable of controlling the parasite at the liver stage of infection. Whole sporozoite vaccination (WSV) approaches, such as radiation-attenuated sporozoites (RAS), viable sporozoites co-administered with the antimalarial drug chloroquine (chemoprophylaxis sporozoites, CPS), or liver-stage-arresting genetically attenuated parasites (GAP), have been most successful at providing sterilizing immunity relative to subunit, prime-boost vaccination strategies [2–5] through the actions of antiparasitic CD8 T cells, CD4 T cells, and antibodies (Fig. 1a). However, widespread application of WSV to human vaccination is complicated due to the high-dose requirement for RAS immunization, need for laboratory-reared mosquitoes, and logistical issues [6]. Application of WSV approaches to study the adaptive immune response against liver-stage infection may lead to the design of better subunit vaccines with easier deployment in the field.

Adaptive immunity against liver-stage infections is multifaceted, with contributions from the humoral and cellular arms. This review focuses on both arms of the adaptive immune response against preerythrocytic stage infection with a strong emphasis on the protective roles of antibodies and CD8 T cells. Lastly, we will highlight the caveats to our current understanding of what constitutes a protective memory anti-*Plasmodium* immune response and also describe major areas of research that would benefit from more attention.

2 Humoral Responses to Liver-Stage Infection

Antibodies have been shown to play a substantial role in providing sterilizing immunity to malaria infections. Importantly, antibodies against sporozoite antigens have been shown to inhibit infection via different mechanisms at distinct stages of

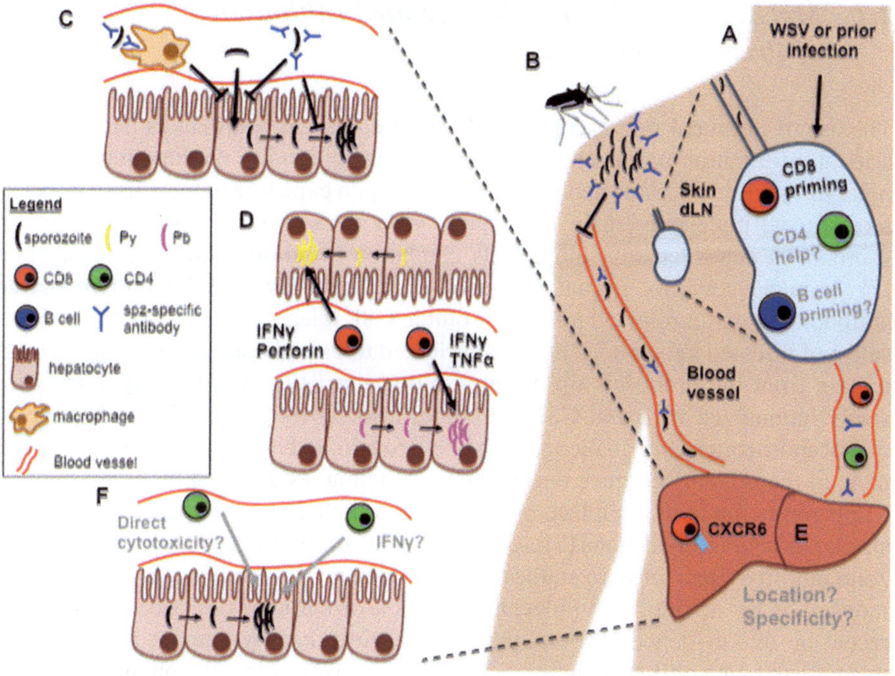

Fig. 1 Adaptive immune responses to preerythrocytic antigens. Black lines and text indicate direct evidence to support mechanisms of protection. Gray lines and text indicate more data are needed to support the possible mechanisms of protection. (**a**) Upon WSV or infection, priming of sporozoite-specific CD8 T cells occurs in skin-draining lymph nodes (dLNs). It is unclear if the skin dLN is also a site for B cell priming or a location for CD4 T cells to provide help to CD8 T cells and B cells. After WSV or infection, antibodies and antigen-specific T cells are released into the blood where they can traffic throughout the body to provide multiple levels of protection, as described below. (**b**) After bites from infected mosquitoes, sporozoite-specific antibodies can reduce sporozoite deposition into the dermis and inhibit motility and therefore reduce entry to the underlying blood vessels. (**c**) Sporozoites travel through the blood to the liver where sporozoite-specific antibodies can increase opsonization and reduce sporozoite motility contributing to inhibition of hepatocyte invasion and subsequent cell traversal. (**d**) CD8 T cell-mediated killing of infected hepatocytes uses differential effector mechanisms depending on the rodent *Plasmodium* species. It is unclear if these cells are located in the liver sinusoids or parenchyma during this killing event. (**e**) Liver-localized CD8 T cell populations express CXCR6. The exact location (parenchyma or liver sinusoids) and specificity of these CD8 T cells following vaccination and challenge are unclear. (**f**) A role for cytotoxic CD4 T cells has been described in multiple models, but the mechanism as to how these cells contribute to sterilizing protection needs further investigation. It may be possible that infected hepatocytes upregulate class II MHC and become direct targets of cytotoxic CD4 T cells. Alternatively, CD4 T cells may inhibit infection via IFNγ production

sporozoite infection. This section describes specific antibody and B cell response to sporozoite and liver-stage antigens and mechanisms of antibody-mediated inhibition of sporozoite infection.

2.1 Mechanisms of Antibody-Mediated Inhibition of Preerythrocytic Infection

The use of intravital microscopy (IVM) and fluorescent sporozoites has provided critical information to our understanding of how antibodies mediate inhibition of preerythrocytic infections depicted in Fig. 1b. Upon exposure to bites from infected mosquitoes, mice previously immunized with RAS showed significantly fewer sporozoites deposited into the dermis compared to nonimmunized control mice [7]. Immune complex formation between anti-circumsporozoite protein (CSP) antibodies from immunized mice and soluble CSP released by sporozoites into the saliva of infected mosquitoes likely contributed to partial obstruction of sporozoite release from the proboscis tip during a blood meal [7]. Additionally, mice passively immunized with anti-CSP antibodies also showed reduced dermal deposition of sporozoites after challenge with bites from infected mosquitoes. Importantly, none of the immunized mice developed parasitemia, as detected by blood smears, compared to the nonimmunized control mice, which developed parasitemia under similar infectious conditions [7]. Anti-sporozoite antibodies can also reduce sporozoite motility. Early in vitro studies showed that anti-CSP antibodies inhibited the motility of sporozoites and prevented invasion of cultured target cells [8]. More recent in vivo evidence supports the early in vitro data by demonstrating that in mice treated with anti-CSP antibodies, fewer sporozoites travel from the dermis to underlining blood vessels [9], a step which is necessary for trafficking to the liver for infection of hepatocytes.

Should sporozoites enter the bloodstream, antibodies may increase opsonization and phagocyte uptake, thus reducing the number of sporozoites capable of hepatocyte invasion (Fig. 1c). Anti-CSP antibodies can increase sporozoite opsonization [10], which has been shown to be a mechanism of protective immunity in response to vaccination in humans [11]. CSP expression and sporozoite motility are both required for productive infection of hepatocytes and cell traversal [12]. Importantly, CSP-specific antibodies have been shown to inhibit sporozoite infection of hepatocytes [13]. Therefore, sporozoites coated with antibodies show limited motility resulting in reduction of hepatocyte invasion and subsequent cell traversal (Fig. 1c). The capacity of anti-CSP antibodies to limit liver-stage infection is thought to be an important mechanism underlying the partial efficacy of the RTS,S vaccine, consisting of CSP fused to hepatitis B surface Ag, which was recently approved for use in humans by the EU [14].

By reducing the number of infected hepatocytes, antibody-mediated inhibition of liver-stage infections could substantially help a concurrent CD8 T cell response by limiting the number of infected hepatocytes that need to be targeted. The multiple mechanisms that anti-sporozoite antibodies use to inhibit infection explain why the antibody response targeting sporozoites is an essential component that contributes to sterilizing protective immunity in vaccinated individuals and will be an important feature in any new vaccines against malaria.

2.2 Antibody and Specific B Cell Responses to Sporozoite Antigens

Development of protective immunity after various immunization methods including RAS, CPS, and the subunit vaccine RTS,S has revealed a role for antibody-mediated protective immunity. The first monoclonal antibodies that mediated protective immunity were determined to be against CSP [15]. However, the role anti-CSP antibodies play in providing sterilizing protection in response to various vaccinations remains quite controversial [16–22]. Anti-CSP antibodies have been shown to be important for sterilizing immunity in response to RAS immunization RTS,S vaccination [17, 23–25]. However, anti-CSP antibodies not strongly correlate with protection after CPS [21]. This result with CPS vaccination is consistent with recent studies showing that blood-stage immunity contribute to protection in this model [26, 27]. Additional anti-sporozoite antibodies targeting antigens including TRAP and LSA-1 have also been associated with protection against infection [20], but the use of these antigens as targets in subunit vaccines did not result in protection [28, 29]. It is likely that antibodies to a variety of preerythrocytic antigens, and not just to a single specificity, contribute to sterilizing immunity in response to vaccination [19, 20].

To further understand the role that antibodies play in vaccine-induced sterilizing immunity, we first need a better idea of the spectrum of sporozoite and liver-stage antigenic targets and ways to evaluate the relevance of each target for protection. Having more tools including monoclonal antibodies and additional targets of protective epitopes in rodent models will be essential in determining the quantity and quality of antibodies required for a sterilizing immune response.

Although many studies have described a significant role of antibodies against liver-stage antigens in providing sterilizing immunity, the development and differentiation of liver-stage antigen-specific B cell populations have not been well described. Upon antigen encounter, naïve B cells can proliferate and differentiate into plasma cells or memory B cells [30]. However, the relative contribution of these distinct populations of B cells to liver-stage immunity has not been thoroughly investigated in rodent models of malaria, and the vast majority of information gathered on specific B cell responses to malaria infection has come from individuals who were naturally exposed or vaccinated. Of the studies conducted in humans in response to vaccination, an overwhelming majority of the work has been done studying blood-stage-specific B cell responses rather than liver-stage B cell responses [30]. One study that investigated the memory B cell response to a liver-stage antigen, CSP, in response to CPS immunization, determined that memory B cell responses increase with the number of immunizations but did not correlate with protection [21].

Because anti-sporozoite antibody responses are so important in contributing to sterilizing immunity, identifying how sporozoite-specific plasma and memory B cells are developed and maintained is of great importance. Blood-stage antigen-specific B cell populations have been identified using flow cytometry [31], but liver-stage antigen-specific B cell responses have not been described using this approach.

Capacity to track liver-stage antigen-specific B cells through various vaccinations and natural infection will be important in determining how antibody production changes over time and thus alters protection. A particularly interesting question that should be addressed using such approaches involves how blood-stage infection may potentially affect the preexisting B cell response to liver-stage antigens or to subsequent sporozoite infections. Indeed, increased apoptosis of memory B cells and plasma cells has been described after blood-stage infection, but the specificity of those B cells has not been determined [32, 33].

One outstanding question regarding B cell activation and differentiation involves the priming of B cells in response to sporozoite antigens (Fig. 1a). Where and how is this occurring? Sporozoites are initially injected into the dermis of mammalian hosts, but not all will reach the bloodstream, and therefore some sporozoites remain in the dermis. Additionally, some sporozoites travel to skin-draining lymph nodes [34], which have been shown to be particularly important for CD8 T cell priming [35]. Is this also the case for sporozoite-specific B cells? This is an important question to address in regard to vaccination strategies. With new IVM technology, it may be possible to track sporozoites from initial deposition and determine where antigen-specific B cells are primed.

3 CD8 T Cells Are Potent Mediators of Protection Against *Plasmodium* Liver-Stage Infections

Plasmodium-specific CD8 T cells targeting liver-stage-expressed antigens can provide sterilizing immunity in humans and rodents [36–41]. The importance of CD8 T cells as mediators of protection against *Plasmodium* has been appreciated as early as the 1980s from studies using rodents immunized with RAS [42, 43]. Because of the potent protection against *Plasmodium* induced by RAS vaccination, it has been considered the "gold standard" for vaccination. Consequently, WSV platforms are frequently used to study the generation of protective adaptive immunity against *Plasmodium* infection. In this section, we will highlight general features of what constitutes a protective CD8 T cell response, and also areas where more recently developed tools can increase our ability to study immunity mediated by *Plasmodium*-specific CD8 T cells.

3.1 Quantitative and Qualitative Features of Protective Liver-Stage-Specific CD8 T Cells

The degree of CD8 T cell-mediated control of *Plasmodium* infection is determined by the magnitude and the quality of the CD8 T cell response. Very large frequencies, >1 % of all peripheral blood lymphocytes, targeting the liver-stage antigen CSP were required to provide sterilizing immunity in a rodent model of *P. berghei* infection [44]. The superior protection afforded by immunization with late liver-stage-arresting GAP was dependent on a larger CD8 T cell response targeting a wider spectrum of liver-stage antigens, relative to RAS vaccination [45]. Thus, in rodent models, the magnitude of the *Plasmodium*-specific CD8 T cell response can be a predictive indicator of protection. Likewise, RAS immunization of humans demonstrated that individuals with larger CD8 T cell responses better protective outcomes [41]. However, in order to generate these responses, human subjects were exposed to the bites of large numbers of *Plasmodium falciparum*-infected mosquitoes through several exposures (~1000–3000 bites) [38] or through the delivery of 4–5 IV administrations of 135,000 *P. falciparum* sporozoites harvested from laboratory-reared irradiated mosquitoes [41]. Thus, only large RAS doses over multiple administrations were able to engender protective immunity of human volunteers. The need for large parasite-immunizing doses, multiple administrations, and laboratory-reared mosquitoes are just a few of the hurdles inherent to application of RAS vaccination in the field [6, 46]. Currently, subunit vaccination of humans, such as the recently licensed RTS,S vaccine [14], has not revealed robust sterilizing immunity [2–5, 47, 48]. In large part, this may be due to the failure of RTS,S to elicit detectable anti-CSP CD8 T cell response [49]. Therefore, it remains important to understand the superior immunity developed by WSV approaches, such as RAS, to lead to better design of subunit vaccines.

While it is known that large magnitude CD8 T cell responses generated through vaccination are required to provide sterilizing immunity to rodents and likely to human subjects [44], less is known about the qualitative features (phenotype, functionality, specificity, localization, etc.) that are important for CD8 T cell-mediated clearance of parasite-infected hepatocytes. In regard to phenotype (Fig. 1d), CD8 T cells exhibiting an effector memory phenotype ($CD62L^{lo}$) have correlated with better protection relative to central memory phenotype ($CD62L^{hi}$) CD8 T cells in two independent studies [50, 51]. Importantly, these studies used distinct vaccination methods (RAS versus heterologous prime boost) to arrive at a similar conclusion. In regard to functionality, such as cytokine production and effector capacity, it has been repeatedly reported that expression of IFNγ by CD8 T cells is required for a protective response [42, 52, 53]. Of interest, the cytolytic mechanism by which CD8 T cells mediate clearance of infection differs depending on the rodent *Plasmodium* infection [52]. For instance, when *P. berghei* CSP-specific CD8 T cells were induced using a prime-boost subunit vaccine approach in wild-type or various knockout mouse backgrounds, it was demonstrated that CSP-specific CD8 T cells depend on IFNγ and TNFα to mediate protection from challenge (Fig. 1d) [52]. In contrast, in a similar prime-boost vaccination model inducing *P. yoelii* CSP-specific CD8 T cells, it was shown that CSP-specific CD8 T cells largely mediate protection using IFNγ and perforin-mediated cytolysis following challenge. If these results extend into human *Plasmodium* species, it could have many implications. For example, it would be interesting to determine if a particular effector mechanism is more efficient at mediating parasite clearance and if this information can be applied to generating CD8 T cells via vaccination that preferentially utilize certain effector mechanisms. Collectively, details regarding the phenotype and functionality of *Plasmodium*-specific CD8 T cells have identified some important features that relate to protection, but much remains to be learned to enhance immunity to vaccination.

3.2 Novel CD8 T Cell Epitopes Provide Additional Tools to Study Features of Protective Plasmodium-Specific CD8 T Cell Responses

New CD8 T cell epitopes derived from liver-stage proteins expressed by rodent *Plasmodium* have been described enhancing the ability to study *Plasmodium*-specific CD8 T cell responses [54–57]. These novel epitopes will allow additional questions to be addressed such as how specificity of the CD8 T cell response may impact protective capacity. For instance, it is currently unclear whether all *Plasmodium*-specific CD8 T cell responses induced by WSV contribute to protective immunity—a question that has important implications for the identification of antigens for inclusion in subunit vaccines. To date, the majority of our understanding of the quantitative and qualitative features of protective CD8 T cell responses has tracked CD8 T cells directed against the immunodominant CSP epitopes: $CS_{252–260}$ in *P. berghei* and $CS_{280–288}$ in *P. yoelii* [44, 52, 58–64]. However, CD8 T cell-mediated protection following RAS is possible even in the absence of CSP-specific CD8 T cells [61], suggesting that currently undefined *Plasmodium*-specific CD8 T cells can mediate protection following challenge.

To date, subunit vaccination using prime-boost strategies to generate CSP- or TRAP-specific CD8 T cells has had limited success in protecting human subjects [2–5]. Thus, it remains necessary to continue to define and study *Plasmodium* CD8 T cell epitopes to identify candidate antigens for inclusion in subunit vaccines. Fortunately, with the description of novel rodent *Plasmodium* CD8 T cell epitopes, studies can expand beyond tracking the immunodominant CSP response. Since the magnitude of endogenous CD8 T cells primed following WSV is generally small ([54, 56] and unpublished data), additional tools such as TCR transgenic [65] or retrogenic mice [66] may be necessary to enhance the small numbers of endogenous precursor CD8 T cells, which limit the resolution in which these responses can be tracked. Alternatively, tools to generate *Plasmodium*-specific CD8 T cells via heterologous prime-boost methods could help overcome CD8 T cell numerical limitations typically inherent to the WSV approach. Prime-boost vaccination strategies can help determine the protective capacity of these new CD8 T cell epitopes through examining individual CD8 T cell specificities in the absence of any other anti-*Plasmodial* response, which can ultimately help in the design of a successful subunit vaccine.

In addition to characterizing the protective capacity of single CD8 T cell epitopes, general features of protective CD8 T cell epitopes can be identified to help in predictive epitope screens of the *Plasmodium* proteome. The *Plasmodium* parasite encodes over 5000 open reading frames [67, 68], which consequently present a challenge in screening for new CD8 T cell epitopes for inclusion for a subunit vaccine. As CD8 T cell epitopes are described and studied, general features (antigen localization, abundance, expression patterns, etc.) of protective CD8 T cell epitopes be revealed to help in future screens for additional protective epitopes.

3.3 Localization of Protective CD8 T Cell Responses

Several in vitro and in vivo studies have demonstrated CD8 T cell-mediated killing of parasite-infected hepatocytes, but increased technological advances in cellular imaging, particularly IVM, have the potential to reveal information regarding the location of CD8 T cell responses following vaccination or challenge. Multiple studies have provided evidence that protective *Plasmodium*-specific CD8 T cells target and kill liver-stage-infected hepatocytes [69–71]. More recently, IVM was applied to study the mechanism in which CD8 T cells target *Plasmodium*-infected hepatocytes. Using GFP-expressing sporozoites to infect mice, a loss of GFP fluorescence was observed in hepatocytes surrounded by clusters of CSP-specific in vitro-generated effector CD8 T cells, suggesting the direct killing of *Plasmodium*-infected hepatocytes via a mechanism requiring multiple antigen-specific CD8 T cells [72]. These observations help provide an explanation regarding the large CD8 T cell numerical requirements for protection since several CD8 T cells were associated with killing of a single infected hepatocyte [44]. However, it is still unclear where protective *Plasmodium*-specific CD8 T cells are localized following vaccination and the movements of these cells upon challenge. There is an increasing interest in the role of tissue-resident memory CD8 T cell populations generated following infection or vaccination in multiple models (reviewed elsewhere [73, 74]). However, to date it remains unclear how the resident memory populations identified in the skin, brain, and mucosal tissues compare phenotypically and functionally to populations of *Plasmodium*-specific CD8 T cells localized in the liver of vaccinated mice. It will be important to thoroughly describe *Plasmodium*-specific CD8 T cells within the liver, particularly in regard to whether these cells are resident within the parenchymal tissue, or alternatively, whether they are associated with the endothelial barrier of the liver sinusoids. Recent IVM data suggests that hepatitis B virus-specific in vitro-generated effector CD8 T cells in the liver are localized in the vasculature and do not require migration into liver parenchymal tissue to kill infected hepatocytes [75]. While this is a different infection setting, it is possible that *Plasmodium*-specific CD8 T cells in the liver exhibit a similar location in the vasculature during killing of parasite-infected hepatocytes (Fig. 1e). This result has important implications as most studies of liver-resident memory CD8 T cells in *Plasmodium* have utilized perfusion techniques to eliminate circulating cells, but it is possible perfusion techniques may dissociate important "resident" CD8 T cell populations, closely associated with the vasculature, from analysis.

To date, liver-resident memory populations generated by WSV have been described as CD8 T cells that remain in the liver following perfusion [76, 77], but their contribution to protective immunity is unclear. CXCR6 expression has also been described as an important molecule involved in CD8 T cell liver homing and residence [78]. Expression of chemokine receptor CXCR6 may be a marker to identify these liver-resident *Plasmodium*-specific CD8 T cell populations (Fig. 1e) [76, 77]. For example, CXCR6 expression on CD8 T cells was shown to be required for long-term maintenance of *Plasmodium*-specific CD8 T cell populations in the liver [76].

Further studies need to define these liver-resident CD8 T cells, their protective capacity, and how they differ from circulating CD8 T cell populations in addition to their differences from the more strict definitions of resident T cell populations in other tissues and model systems [73]. Comparisons of these populations will be helpful in determining the characteristics of liver-resident CD8 T cells exhibit, their importance in vaccine-induced protection, and how we create or modify liver-localized CD8 T cell responses against *Plasmodium* to foster better liver-stage immunity.

4 Role of CD4 T Cells to Liver-Stage Infection

The role CD8 T cells play in sterilizing immunity to liver-stage infection in rodent models of malaria is well characterized, but the role of CD4 T cells is mouse strain dependent. CD4 T cell depletion studies revealed that the two major mouse strains used in rodent malaria models, C57BL/6 and BALB/c, showed differential requirements for CD4 T cells in protection against *P. yoelii* sporozoite challenge [39]. While depletion of CD4 T cells had no impact on protection of RAS-immunized BALB/c mice, CD4 T cell-depleted C57BL/6 mice previously immunized with RAS were not protected [39]. How CD4 T cells mediate protection in these mouse strains needs further investigation, but based on the role CD4 T cells play in other infection models, these cells may play a cytotoxic role or provide help to B cells and CD8 T cells, both of which have been shown to contribute to sterilizing immunity. This section focuses on the roles that CD4 T cells may be playing in response to liver-stage infection and highlights remaining questions that still need to be addressed.

4.1 Role of CD4 T Cell Help in Protective Immunity to Liver-Stage Infection

CD4 T cells have the capacity to differentiate into various subsets including Th1, Th2, Tfh, Treg, and ThCTLs [79]. However, CD4 T cell differentiation in response to malaria infections has not been widely investigated in part due to lack of identifiable epitopes that induce detectable responses. Nevertheless, it is likely that Tfh plays a strong role in antibody response to liver-stage antigens. Given the fact that antibody responses to sporozoites can mediate sterilizing protection after vaccination, Tfhs are likely playing a role in helping B cells in terms of memory B cell formation and antibody production. CD4 T cell help for B cells is an area that requires further investigation, and information gathered may be applied to enhance specific components of a protective vaccine.

A few studies have identified a strong role for CD4 T cell help of CD8 T cells in malaria infections. CD4 T cells were found to be important for the expansion and survival of CD8 T cell effector and memory responses after sporozoite infection, indicating that the size of the CD8 T cell memory pool after WSV or RAS immunization was highly dependent upon helper T cells [80]. Interestingly, the memory CD8 T cells that did form in the absence of CD4 T cells exhibited normal effector functions but were unable to protect against sporozoite challenge. The size of the memory CD8 T cell response is especially important in mediating sterilizing protection as discussed in aforementioned Sect. 3.1 [81, 82]. Thus, the absence of CD4 T cells produced functional but significantly fewer antigen-specific CD8 T cells, resulting in an inability to protect against liver-stage infection. Specifically, IL-4 production by CD4 T cells was shown to contribute to the expansion of malaria-specific CD8 T cells [83]. IL-4 production from CD4 T cells may also promote antibody production from B cells during malaria infections, but this has yet to be described.

To date, only a few studies have addressed the role CD4 T cells play in providing B cell and CD8 T cell help in response to liver-stage antigens. Given the fact that both antibodies and CD8 T cells play such an important role in providing protective sterilizing immunity against liver-stage infections, more work on how CD4 T cells contribute to helping both B cells and CD8 T cells is needed.

4.2 Role of Cytotoxic CD4 T Cells in Protective Immunity

Several studies have identified a role for cytotoxic CD4 T cells in protection against liver-stage infections. Some of the first studies to describe cytotoxic CD4 T cells in sterilizing protection were performed in murine models using CD4 T cell clones specific for CSP and non-CSP epitopes [84, 85]. More recent studies identified a role for cytotoxic CD4 T cells following RAS immunization in β2M knockout mice, which lack endogenous CD8 T cells [86]. Liver-stage-specific cytotoxic CD4 T cells have also been described in humans after various immunization methods [87–89]. However, despite the numerous reports describing cytotoxic CD4 T cells, the mechanisms of cytolytic action remain quite controversial and require further investigation (Fig. 1f). This is in part due to the variability in direct cytolytic capacity of described CD4 T cell populations and the means in which such cytotoxic T cell populations were identified [84–88]. Only some specific CD4 T cell clones showed direct cytolytic capability, whereas others did not. Moreover, CD4 T cells that did show cytolytic potential were in response to peptide-pulsed autologous cells or parasitized RBC-stimulated cells [85, 87, 88]. Other studies showed CD4 T cells increased degranulation markers (CD107a/b) after parasitized RBC stimulation, suggesting cytolytic activity [88]. However, direct cytolytic activity of CD4 T cells against infected hepatocytes was not measured. This may call into question if CD4 T cells can directly lyse infected cells via similar mechanisms as CD8 T cells (i.e., perforin/granzymes). Combined, these studies highlight the many unknowns about the actual role of cytotoxic CD4 T cells in response against liver-stage *Plasmodium* infections, especially in regard to the recognition of infected hepatocytes. Upregulation of class II MHC on hepatocytes has been described in some disease states [90], but it has yet to be determined during *Plasmodium* infection.

Many questions still need to be addressed to determine the actual role cytolytic CD4 T cells play in sterilizing immunity against liver-stage infections. How do CD4 T cells mediate cytotoxicity if not by direct recognition of infected hepatocytes? Neutralization of IFNγ in β2M knockout hosts reduced the protective capacity, indicating IFNγ may play a partial role in protection against liver stage [86]. CD4 T cells may, however, be mediating cytotoxicity indirectly via IFNγ-induced NO production [91]. Do cytotoxic CD4 T cells also play a role in the presence of CD8 T cells, which have been shown to be a major contributor to protective immunity in most animal models, whereas CD4 T cells have only been shown to contribute to protection in a few mouse models [39]? The role cytotoxic CD4 T cells play in sterilizing immunity to liver-stage infection may not be as straightforward as described in some studies, and more work could help address some of these underlying questions.

5 Conclusion

Adaptive immune responses against liver-stage infections are critical for mediating protection against malarial disease. Highlighted in this review and depicted in Fig. 1 are mechanisms of the adaptive immune response known to contribute to protective immunity (black lines/text). Moreover, we have identified certain holes in our current understanding of the adaptive immune response to liver-stage antigens that will be important areas of future studies that will enable the development of more effective vaccines (gray lines/text). A large portion of the current literature has applied WSV approaches in rodent models of malaria to arrive at an understanding of the critical importance of antibodies and CD8 T cells that recognize sporozoite and liver-stage antigens. Although general features of these protective antibody and CD8 T cell responses are understood, there remains a need to continue to define these responses since the majority of the antigens targeted by CD8 T cells, and likely antibodies, have not been characterized. Further, the helpers of these responses, namely, CD4 T cells, require attention as these responses may be critical in manipulating CD8 T cells and antibodies qualitatively following subunit vaccination into responses capable of mediating livelong sterilizing immunity. Whether CD4 T cells can contribute in the direct killing of hepatocytes will be important to determine as it may provide critical assistance to antibodies and CD8 T cells in clearing the infected liver before symptomatic blood stage. Further, the impact on CD8 T cell-mediated protection due to specificity and location is important area for further research as enhance the quality of the CD8 T cell response may help overcome issues in vaccination approaches that are incapable of eliciting quantitatively large responses. Taken together, despite the advances in understanding of the role of antibodies and CD8 T cells in the adaptive immune response against liver stage, what qualitative features impact protection and how can we manipulate vaccine-induced responses to provide better protective immunity is an important area of research that may dictate the design of a successful human subunit vaccine.

References

1. WMR (2015) World Malaria Report 2015. December, 2015. 280 pages. SBN: 978 92 4 156515 8
2. Ewer KJ, O'Hara GA, Duncan CJ, Collins KA, Sheehy SH, Reyes-Sandoval A, Goodman AL, Edwards NJ, Elias SC, Halstead FD, Longley RJ, Rowland R, Poulton ID, Draper SJ, Blagborough AM, Berrie E, Moyle S, Williams N, Siani L, Folgori A, Colloca S, Sinden RE, Lawrie AM, Cortese R, Gilbert SC, Nicosia A, Hill AV (2013) Protective CD8+ T-cell immunity to human malaria induced by chimpanzee adenovirus-MVA immunisation. Nat Commun 4:2836. doi:10.1038/ncomms3836
3. Sedegah M, Hollingdale MR, Farooq F, Ganeshan H, Belmonte M, Kim Y, Peters B, Sette A, Huang J, McGrath S, Abot E, Limbach K, Shi M, Soisson L, Diggs C, Chuang I, Tamminga C, Epstein JE, Villasante E, Richie TL (2014) Sterile immunity to malaria after DNA prime/adenovirus boost immunization is associated with effector memory CD8+ T cells targeting AMA1 class I epitopes. PLoS One 9(9), e106241. doi:10.1371/journal.pone.0106241
4. Ogwang C, Kimani D, Edwards NJ, Roberts R, Mwacharo J, Bowyer G, Bliss C, Hodgson SH, Njuguna P, Viebig NK, Nicosia A, Gitau E, Douglas S, Illingworth J, Marsh K, Lawrie A, Imoukhuede EB, Ewer K, Urban BC, S Hill AV, Bejon P, MVVC Group (2015) Prime-boost vaccination with chimpanzee adenovirus and modified vaccinia Ankara encoding TRAP provides partial protection against *Plasmodium falciparum* infection in Kenyan adults. Sci Transl Med 7(286):e286re5. doi:10.1126/scitranslmed.aaa2373
5. Chuang I, Sedegah M, Cicatelli S, Spring M, Polhemus M, Tamminga C, Patterson N, Guerrero M, Bennett JW, McGrath S, Ganeshan H, Belmonte M, Farooq F, Abot E, Banania JG, Huang J, Newcomer R, Rein L, Litilit D, Richie NO, Wood C, Murphy J, Sauerwein R, Hermsen CC, McCoy AJ, Kamau E, Cummings J, Komisar J, Sutamihardja A, Shi M, Epstein JE, Maiolatesi S, Tosh D, Limbach K, Angov E, Bergmann-Leitner E, Bruder JT, Doolan DL, King CR, Carucci D, Dutta S, Soisson L, Diggs C, Hollingdale MR, Ockenhouse CF, Richie TL (2013) DNA prime/Adenovirus boost malaria vaccine encoding *P. falciparum* CSP and AMA1 induces sterile protection associated with cell-mediated immunity. PLoS One 8(2), e55571. doi:10.1371/journal.pone.0055571
6. Hoffman SL, Billingsley PF, James E, Richman A, Loyevsky M, Li T, Chakravarty S, Gunasekera A, Chattopadhyay R, Li M, Stafford R, Ahumada A, Epstein JE, Sedegah M, Reyes S, Richie TL, Lyke KE, Edelman R, Laurens MB, Plowe CV, Sim BK (2010) Development of a metabolically active, non-replicating sporozoite vaccine to prevent *Plasmodium falciparum* malaria. Hum Vaccin 6(1):97–106
7. Kebaier C, Voza T, Vanderberg J (2009) Kinetics of mosquito-injected *Plasmodium* sporozoites in mice: fewer sporozoites are injected into sporozoite-immunized mice. PLoS Pathog 5(4), e1000399
8. Stewart MJ, Nawrot RJ, Schulman S, Vanderberg JP (1986) *Plasmodium berghei* sporozoite invasion is blocked in vitro by sporozoite-immobilizing antibodies. Infect Immun 51(3): 859–864
9. Vanderberg JP, Frevert U (2004) Intravital microscopy demonstrating antibody-mediated immobilisation of *Plasmodium berghei* sporozoites injected into skin by mosquitoes. Int J Parasitol 34(9):991–996. doi:10.1016/j.ijpara.2004.05.005
10. Seguin MC, Ballou WR, Nacy CA (1989) Interactions of *Plasmodium berghei* sporozoites and murine Kupffer cells in vitro. J Immunol 143(5):1716–1722
11. Schwenk R, Asher LV, Chalom I, Lanar D, Sun P, White K, Keil D, Kester KE, Stoute J, Heppner DG, Krzych U (2003) Opsonization by antigen-specific antibodies as a mechanism of protective immunity induced by *Plasmodium falciparum* circumsporozoite protein-based vaccine. Parasite Immunol 25(1):17–25. doi:10.1046/j.1365-3024.2003.00495.x
12. Mota MM, Rodriguez A (2004) Migration through host cells: the first steps of *Plasmodium* sporozoites in the mammalian host. Cell Microbiol 6(12):1113–1118. doi:10.1111/j.1462-5822.2004.00460.x

13. Finney OC, Keitany GJ, Smithers H, Kaushansky A, Kappe S, Wang R (2014) Immunization with genetically attenuated *P. falciparum* parasites induces long-lived antibodies that efficiently block hepatocyte invasion by sporozoites. Vaccine 32(19):2135–2138. doi:10.1016/j.vaccine.2014.02.055
14. Morrison C (2015) Landmark green light for Mosquirix malaria vaccine. Nat Biotechnol 33(10):1015–1016. doi:10.1038/nbt1015-1015
15. Zavala F, Cochrane AH, Nardin EH, Nussenzweig RS, Nussenzweig V (1983) Circumsporozoite proteins of malaria parasites contain a single immunodominant region with two or more identical epitopes. J Exp Med 157(6):1947–1957
16. Grüner AC, Mauduit M, Tewari R, Romero JF, Depinay N, Kayibanda M, Lallemand E, Chavatte J-M, Crisanti A, Sinnis P, Mazier D, Corradin G, Snounou G, Rénia L (2007) Sterile protection against malaria is independent of immune responses to the circumsporozoite protein. PLoS One 2(12), e1371. doi:10.1371/journal.pone.0001371
17. Arun Kumar K, Sano G, Boscardin S, Nussenzweig RS, Nussenzweig MC, Zavala F, Nussenzweig V (2006) The circumsporozoite protein is an immunodominant protective antigen in irradiated sporozoites. Nature 444(7121):937–940, http://www.nature.com/nature/journal/v444/n7121/suppinfo/nature05361_S1.html
18. Trieu A, Kayala MA, Burk C, Molina DM, Freilich DA, Richie TL, Baldi P, Felgner PL, Doolan DL (2011) Sterile protective immunity to malaria is associated with a panel of novel *P falciparum* antigens. Mol Cell Proteomics 10(9), M111.007948. doi:10.1074/mcp.M111.007948
19. Doolan DL, Mu Y, Unal B, Sundaresh S, Hirst S, Valdez C, Randall A, Molina D, Liang X, Freilich DA, Oloo JA, Blair PL, Aguiar JC, Baldi P, Davies DH, Felgner PL (2008) Profiling humoral immune responses to *P. falciparum* infection with protein microarrays. Proteomics 8(22):4680–4694. doi:10.1002/pmic.200800194
20. John C, Moormann A, Pregibon D, Sumba P, McHugh M, Narum D, Lanar D, Schluchter M, Kazura J (2005) Correlation of high levels of antibodies to multiple pre-erythrocytic *Plasmodium falciparum* antigens and protection from infection. AmJTrop Med Hyg 73(1):222–228
21. Nahrendorf W, Scholzen A, Bijker EM, Teirlinck AC, Bastiaens GJH, Schats R, Hermsen CC, Visser LG, Langhorne J, Sauerwein RW (2014) Memory B-cell and antibody responses induced by *Plasmodium falciparum* sporozoite immunization. J Infect Dis 210(12): 1981–1990. doi:10.1093/infdis/jiu354
22. Felgner PL, Roestenberg M, Liang L, Hung C, Jain A, Pablo J, Nakajima-Sasaki R, Molina D, Teelen K, Hermsen CC, Sauerwein R (2013) Pre-erythrocytic antibody profiles induced by controlled human malaria infections in healthy volunteers under chloroquine prophylaxis. Sci Rep 3:3549. doi:10.1038/srep03549, http://www.nature.com/articles/srep03549 - supplementary-information
23. Kester K, Cummings J, Ofori Anyinam O, Ockenhouse C, Krzych U, Moris P, Schwenk R, Nielsen R, Debebe Z, Pinelis E, Juompan L, Williams J, Dowler M, Stewart VA, Wirtz R, Dubois M-C, Lievens M, Cohen J, Ballou WR, Heppner DG (2009) Randomized, double-blind, phase 2a trial of falciparum malaria vaccines RTS, S/AS01B and RTS, S/AS02A in malaria-naive adults: safety, efficacy, and immunologic associates of protection. J Infect Dis 200(3):337–346
24. White MT, Bejon P, Olotu A, Griffin JT, Riley EM, Kester KE, Ockenhouse CF, Ghani AC (2013) The relationship between RTS, S vaccine-induced antibodies, $CD4^+$ T cell responses and protection against *Plasmodium falciparum* infection. PLoS One 8(4), e61395. doi:10.1371/journal.pone.0061395
25. Foquet L, Hermsen CC, van Gemert G-J, Van Braeckel E, Weening KE, Sauerwein R, Meuleman P, Leroux-Roels G (2014) Vaccine-induced monoclonal antibodies targeting circumsporozoite protein prevent *Plasmodium falciparum* infection. J Clin Invest 124(1): 140–144. doi:10.1172/JCI70349
26. Doll KL, Butler NS, Harty JT (2014) CD8 T cell independent immunity after single dose infection-treatment-vaccination (ITV) against *Plasmodium yoelii*. Vaccine 32(4):483–491. doi:10.1016/j.vaccine.2013.11.058

27. Nahrendorf W, Spence PJ, Tumwine I, Levy P, Jarra W, Sauerwein RW, Langhorne J (2015) Blood-stage immunity to *Plasmodium chabaudi* malaria following chemoprophylaxis and sporozoite immunization. Elife 4, e05165. doi:10.7554/eLife.05165
28. Kester K, Gray Heppner D, Moris P, Ofori Anyinam O, Krzych U, Tornieporth N, McKinney D, Delchambre M, Ockenhouse C, Voss G, Holland C, Beckey J, Ballou WR, Cohen J (2014) Sequential Phase 1 and Phase 2 randomized, controlled trials of the safety, immunogenicity and efficacy of combined pre-erythrocytic vaccine antigens RTS, S and TRAP formulated with AS02 Adjuvant System in healthy, malaria naïve adults. Vaccine 32(49):6683–6691
29. Cummings J, Spring M, Schwenk R, Ockenhouse C, Kester K, Polhemus M, Walsh D, Yoon I-K, Prosperi C, Juompan L, Lanar D, Krzych U, Hall BT, Ware L, Stewart VA, Williams J, Dowler M, Nielsen R, Hillier C, Giersing B, Dubovsky F, Malkin E, Tucker K, Dubois M-C, Cohen J, Ballou WR, Heppner DG (2010) Recombinant Liver Stage Antigen-1 (LSA-1) formulated with AS01 or AS02 is safe, elicits high titer antibody and induces IFN-gamma/IL-2 $CD4^+$ T cells but does not protect against experimental *Plasmodium falciparum* infection. Vaccine 28(31):5135–5144
30. Dups JN, Pepper M, Cockburn IA (2014) Antibody and B cell responses to *Plasmodium* sporozoites. Front Microbiol 5:625. doi:10.3389/fmicb.2014.00625
31. Muellenbeck MF, Ueberheide B, Amulic B, Epp A, Fenyo D, Busse CE, Esen M, Theisen M, Mordmüller B, Wardemann H (2013) Atypical and classical memory B cells produce *Plasmodium falciparum* neutralizing antibodies. J Exp Med 210(2):389–399. doi:10.1084/jem.20121970
32. Wykes MN, Zhou Y-H, Liu XQ, Good MF (2005) *Plasmodium yoelii* can ablate vaccine-induced long-term protection in mice. J Immunol 175(4):2510–2516. doi:10.4049/jimmunol.175.4.2510
33. Banga S, Coursen J, Portugal S, Tran T, Hancox L, Ongoiba A, Traore B, Doumbo O, Huang C-Y, Harty J, Crompton P (2015) Impact of acute malaria on pre-existing antibodies to viral and vaccine antigens in mice and humans. PLoS One 10(4), e0125090
34. Amino R, Thiberge S, Martin B, Celli S, Shorte S, Frischknecht F, Ménard R (2006) Quantitative imaging of *Plasmodium* transmission from mosquito to mammal. Nat Med 12(2):220–224
35. Chakravarty S, Cockburn IA, Kuk S, Overstreet MG, Sacci JB, Zavala F (2007) $CD8^+$ T lymphocytes protective against malaria liver stages are primed in skin-draining lymph nodes. Nat Med 13(9):1035–1041, http://www.nature.com/nm/journal/v13/n9/suppinfo/nm1628_S1.html
36. Nussenzweig RS, Vanderberg J, Most H, Orton C (1967) Protective immunity produced by the injection of x-irradiated sporozoites of *Plasmodium berghei*. Nature 216(5111):160–162
37. Clyde DF (1975) Immunization of man against *falciparum* and *vivax* malaria by use of attenuated sporozoites. Am J Trop Med Hyg 24(3):397–401
38. Hoffman SL, Goh LM, Luke TC, Schneider I, Le TP, Doolan DL, Sacci J, de la Vega P, Dowler M, Paul C, Gordon DM, Stoute JA, Church LW, Sedegah M, Heppner DG, Ballou WR, Richie TL (2002) Protection of humans against malaria by immunization with radiation-attenuated *Plasmodium falciparum* sporozoites. J Infect Dis 185(8):1155–1164. doi:10.1086/339409
39. Doolan DL, Hoffman SL (2000) The complexity of protective immunity against liver-stage malaria. J Immunol 165(3):1453–1462
40. Epstein JE, Tewari K, Lyke KE, Sim BK, Billingsley PF, Laurens MB, Gunasekera A, Chakravarty S, James ER, Sedegah M, Richman A, Velmurugan S, Reyes S, Li M, Tucker K, Ahumada A, Ruben AJ, Li T, Stafford R, Eappen AG, Tamminga C, Bennett JW, Ockenhouse CF, Murphy JR, Komisar J, Thomas N, Loyevsky M, Birkett A, Plowe CV, Loucq C, Edelman R, Richie TL, Seder RA, Hoffman SL (2011) Live attenuated malaria vaccine designed to protect through hepatic $CD8^+$ T cell immunity. Science 334(6055):475–480. doi:10.1126/science.1211548
41. Seder RA, Chang LJ, Enama ME, Zephir KL, Sarwar UN, Gordon IJ, Holman LA, James ER, Billingsley PF, Gunasekera A, Richman A, Chakravarty S, Manoj A, Velmurugan S, Li M, Ruben AJ, Li T, Eappen AG, Stafford RE, Plummer SH, Hendel CS, Novik L, Costner PJ, Mendoza FH, Saunders JG, Nason MC, Richardson JH, Murphy J, Davidson SA, Richie TL, Sedegah M, Sutamihardja A, Fahle GA, Lyke KE, Laurens MB, Roederer M, Tewari K,

Epstein JE, Sim BK, Ledgerwood JE, Graham BS, Hoffman SL (2013) Protection against malaria by intravenous immunization with a nonreplicating sporozoite vaccine. Science 341(6152):1359–1365. doi:10.1126/science.1241800

42. Schofield L, Villaquiran J, Ferreira A, Schellekens H, Nussenzweig R, Nussenzweig V (1987) Gamma interferon, $CD8^+$ T cells and antibodies required for immunity to malaria sporozoites. Nature 330(6149):664–666. doi:10.1038/330664a0
43. Weiss WR, Sedegah M, Beaudoin RL, Miller LH, Good MF (1988) $CD8^+$ T cells (cytotoxic/suppressors) are required for protection in mice immunized with malaria sporozoites. Proc Natl Acad Sci U S A 85(2):573–576
44. Schmidt NW, Podyminogin RL, Butler NS, Badovinac VP, Tucker BJ, Bahjat KS, Lauer P, Reyes-Sandoval A, Hutchings CL, Moore AC, Gilbert SC, Hill AV, Bartholomay LC, Harty JT (2008) Memory CD8 T cell responses exceeding a large but definable threshold provide long-term immunity to malaria. Proc Natl Acad Sci U S A 105(37):14017–14022. doi:10.1073/pnas.0805452105
45. Butler NS, Schmidt NW, Vaughan AM, Aly AS, Kappe SH, Harty JT (2011) Superior antimalarial immunity after vaccination with late liver stage-arresting genetically attenuated parasites. Cell Host Microbe 9(6):451–462. doi:10.1016/j.chom.2011.05.008
46. Sheehy SH, Spencer AJ, Douglas AD, Sim BK, Longley RJ, Edwards NJ, Poulton ID, Kimani D, Williams AR, Anagnostou NA, Roberts R, Kerridge S, Voysey M, James ER, Billingsley PF, Gunasekera A, Lawrie AM, Hoffman SL, Hill AV (2013) Optimising controlled human malaria infection studies using cryopreserved parasites administered by needle and syringe. PLoS One 8(6), e65960. doi:10.1371/journal.pone.0065960
47. Olotu A, Fegan G, Wambua J, Nyangweso G, Awuondo KO, Leach A, Lievens M, Leboulleux D, Njuguna P, Peshu N, Marsh K, Bejon P (2013) Four-year efficacy of RTS, S/AS01E and its interaction with malaria exposure. N Engl J Med 368(12):1111–1120. doi:10.1056/NEJMoa1207564
48. Agnandji ST, Lell B, Fernandes JF, Abossolo BP, Methogo BG, Kabwende AL, Adegnika AA, Mordmuller B, Issifou S, Kremsner PG, Sacarlal J, Aide P, Lanaspa M, Aponte JJ, Machevo S, Acacio S, Bulo H, Sigauque B, Macete E, Alonso P, Abdulla S, Salim N, Minja R, Mpina M, Ahmed S, Ali AM, Mtoro AT, Hamad AS, Mutani P, Tanner M, Tinto H, D'Alessandro U, Sorgho H, Valea I, Bihoun B, Guiraud I, Kabore B, Sombie O, Guiguemde RT, Ouedraogo JB, Hamel MJ, Kariuki S, Oneko M, Odero C, Otieno K, Awino N, McMorrow M, Muturi-Kioi V, Laserson KF, Slutsker L, Otieno W, Otieno L, Otsyula N, Gondi S, Otieno A, Owira V, Oguk E, Odongo G, Woods JB, Ogutu B, Njuguna P, Chilengi R, Akoo P, Kerubo C, Maingi C, Lang T, Olotu A, Bejon P, Marsh K, Mwambingu G, Owusu-Agyei S, Asante KP, Osei-Kwakye K, Boahen O, Dosoo D, Asante I, Adjei G, Kwara E, Chandramohan D, Greenwood B, Lusingu J, Gesase S, Malabeja A, Abdul O, Mahende C, Liheluka E, Malle L, Lemnge M, Theander TG, Drakeley C, Ansong D, Agbenyega T, Adjei S, Boateng HO, Rettig T, Bawa J, Sylverken J, Sambian D, Sarfo A, Agyekum A, Martinson F, Hoffman I, Mvalo T, Kamthunzi P, Nkomo R, Tembo T, Tegha G, Tsidya M, Kilembe J, Chawinga C, Ballou WR, Cohen J, Guerra Y, Jongert E, Lapierre D, Leach A, Lievens M, Ofori-Anyinam O, Olivier A, Vekemans J, Carter T, Kaslow D, Leboulleux D, Loucq C, Radford A, Savarese B, Schellenberg D, Sillman M, Vansadia P (2012) A phase 3 trial of RTS, S/AS01 malaria vaccine in African infants. N Engl J Med 367(24):2284–2295. doi:10.1056/NEJMoa1208394
49. Lalvani A, Moris P, Voss G, Pathan AA, Kester KE, Brookes R, Lee E, Koutsoukos M, Plebanski M, Delchambre M, Flanagan KL, Carton C, Slaoui M, Van Hoecke C, Ballou WR, Hill AV, Cohen J (1999) Potent induction of focused Th1-type cellular and humoral immune responses by RTS, S/SBAS2, a recombinant *Plasmodium falciparum* malaria vaccine. J Infect Dis 180(5):1656–1664. doi:10.1086/315074
50. Schmidt NW, Butler NS, Badovinac VP, Harty JT (2010) Extreme CD8 T cell requirements for anti-malarial liver-stage immunity following immunization with radiation attenuated sporozoites. PLoS Pathog 6(7), e1000998. doi:10.1371/journal.ppat.1000998
51. Reyes-Sandoval A, Wyllie DH, Bauza K, Milicic A, Forbes EK, Rollier CS, Hill AV (2011) $CD8^+$ T effector memory cells protect against liver-stage malaria. J Immunol 187(3):1347–1357. doi:10.4049/jimmunol.1100302

52. Butler NS, Schmidt NW, Harty JT (2010) Differential effector pathways regulate memory CD8 T cell immunity against *Plasmodium berghei* versus *P. yoelii* sporozoites. J Immunol 184(5):2528–2538. doi:10.4049/jimmunol.0903529
53. McCall MB, Sauerwein RW (2010) Interferon-gamma—central mediator of protective immune responses against the pre-erythrocytic and blood stage of malaria. J Leukoc Biol 88(6):1131–1143. doi:10.1189/jlb.0310137
54. Hafalla JC, Bauza K, Friesen J, Gonzalez-Aseguinolaza G, Hill AV, Matuschewski K (2013) Identification of targets of CD8$^+$ T cell responses to malaria liver stages by genome-wide epitope profiling. PLoS Pathog 9(5), e1003303. doi:10.1371/journal.ppat.1003303
55. Howland SW, Poh CM, Gun SY, Claser C, Malleret B, Shastri N, Ginhoux F, Grotenbreg GM, Renia L (2013) Brain microvessel cross-presentation is a hallmark of experimental cerebral malaria. EMBO Mol Med 5(7):916–931. doi:10.1002/emmm.201202273
56. Lau LS, Fernandez-Ruiz D, Mollard V, Sturm A, Neller MA, Cozijnsen A, Gregory JL, Davey GM, Jones CM, Lin YH, Haque A, Engwerda CR, Nie CQ, Hansen DS, Murphy KM, Papenfuss AT, Miles JJ, Burrows SR, de Koning-Ward T, McFadden GI, Carbone FR, Crabb BS, Heath WR (2014) CD8$^+$ T cells from a novel T cell receptor transgenic mouse induce liver-stage immunity that can be boosted by blood-stage infection in rodent malaria. PLoS Pathog 10(5), e1004135. doi:10.1371/journal.ppat.1004135
57. Murphy SC, Kas A, Stone BC, Bevan MJ (2013) A T-cell response to a liver-stage *Plasmodium* antigen is not boosted by repeated sporozoite immunizations. Proc Natl Acad Sci U S A 110(15):6055–6060. doi:10.1073/pnas.1303834110
58. Cockburn IA, Tse SW, Zavala F (2014) CD8$^+$ T cells eliminate liver-stage *Plasmodium berghei* parasites without detectable bystander effect. Infect Immun 82(4):1460–1464. doi:10.1128/IAI.01500-13
59. Cockburn IA, Chen YC, Overstreet MG, Lees JR, van Rooijen N, Farber DL, Zavala F (2010) Prolonged antigen presentation is required for optimal CD8$^+$ T cell responses against malaria liver stage parasites. PLoS Pathog 6(5), e1000877. doi:10.1371/journal.ppat.1000877
60. Chakravarty S, Cockburn IA, Kuk S, Overstreet MG, Sacci JB, Zavala F (2007) CD8$^+$ T lymphocytes protective against malaria liver stages are primed in skin-draining lymph nodes. Nat Med 13(9):1035–1041. doi:10.1038/nm1628
61. Kumar KA, Sano G, Boscardin S, Nussenzweig RS, Nussenzweig MC, Zavala F, Nussenzweig V (2006) The circumsporozoite protein is an immunodominant protective antigen in irradiated sporozoites. Nature 444(7121):937–940. doi:10.1038/nature05361
62. Rodrigues MM, Cordey AS, Arreaza G, Corradin G, Romero P, Maryanski JL, Nussenzweig RS, Zavala F (1991) CD8$^+$ cytolytic T cell clones derived against the *Plasmodium yoelii* circumsporozoite protein protect against malaria. Int Immunol 3(6):579–585
63. Romero P, Maryanski JL, Corradin G, Nussenzweig RS, Nussenzweig V, Zavala F (1989) Cloned cytotoxic T cells recognize an epitope in the circumsporozoite protein and protect against malaria. Nature 341(6240):323–326. doi:10.1038/341323a0
64. Cockburn IA, Tse SW, Radtke AJ, Srinivasan P, Chen YC, Sinnis P, Zavala F (2011) Dendritic cells and hepatocytes use distinct pathways to process protective antigen from *Plasmodium* in vivo. PLoS Pathog 7(3), e1001318. doi:10.1371/journal.ppat.1001318
65. Chen YC, Zavala F (2013) Development and use of TCR transgenic mice for malaria immunology research. Methods Mol Biol 923:481–491. doi:10.1007/978-1-62703-026-7_33
66. Holst J, Szymczak-Workman AL, Vignali KM, Burton AR, Workman CJ, Vignali DA (2006) Generation of T-cell receptor retrogenic mice. Nat Protoc 1(1):406–417. doi:10.1038/nprot.2006.61
67. Florens L, Washburn MP, Raine JD, Anthony RM, Grainger M, Haynes JD, Moch JK, Muster N, Sacci JB, Tabb DL, Witney AA, Wolters D, Wu Y, Gardner MJ, Holder AA, Sinden RE, Yates JR, Carucci DJ (2002) A proteomic view of the *Plasmodium falciparum* life cycle. Nature 419(6906):520–526. doi:10.1038/nature01107
68. Doolan DL, Southwood S, Freilich DA, Sidney J, Graber NL, Shatney L, Bebris L, Florens L, Dobano C, Witney AA, Appella E, Hoffman SL, Yates JR 3rd, Carucci DJ, Sette A (2003) Identification of *Plasmodium falciparum* antigens by antigenic analysis of genomic and proteomic data. Proc Natl Acad Sci U S A 100(17):9952–9957. doi:10.1073/pnas.1633254100

69. Trimnell A, Takagi A, Gupta M, Richie TL, Kappe SH, Wang R (2009) Genetically attenuated parasite vaccines induce contact-dependent $CD8^+$ T cell killing of *Plasmodium yoelii* liver stage-infected hepatocytes. J Immunol 183(9):5870–5878. doi:10.4049/jimmunol.0900302
70. Bongfen SE, Torgler R, Romero JF, Renia L, Corradin G (2007) *Plasmodium berghei*-infected primary hepatocytes process and present the circumsporozoite protein to specific $CD8^+$ T cells in vitro. J Immunol 178(11):7054–7063
71. Renia L, Marussig MS, Grillot D, Pied S, Corradin G, Miltgen F, Del Giudice G, Mazier D (1991) In vitro activity of $CD4^+$ and $CD8^+$ T lymphocytes from mice immunized with a synthetic malaria peptide. Proc Natl Acad Sci U S A 88(18):7963–7967
72. Cockburn IA, Amino R, Kelemen RK, Kuo SC, Tse SW, Radtke A, Mac-Daniel L, Ganusov VV, Zavala F, Menard R (2013) In vivo imaging of $CD8^+$ T cell-mediated elimination of malaria liver stages. Proc Natl Acad Sci U S A 110(22):9090–9095. doi:10.1073/pnas.1303858110
73. Schenkel JM, Masopust D (2014) Tissue-resident memory T cells. Immunity 41(6):886–897. doi:10.1016/j.immuni.2014.12.007
74. Carbone FR (2015) Tissue-resident memory T cells and fixed immune surveillance in nonlymphoid organs. J Immunol 195(1):17–22. doi:10.4049/jimmunol.1500515
75. Guidotti LG, Inverso D, Sironi L, Di Lucia P, Fioravanti J, Ganzer L, Fiocchi A, Vacca M, Aiolfi R, Sammicheli S, Mainetti M, Cataudella T, Raimondi A, Gonzalez-Aseguinolaza G, Protzer U, Ruggeri ZM, Chisari FV, Isogawa M, Sitia G, Iannacone M (2015) Immunosurveillance of the liver by intravascular effector $CD8^+$ T cells. Cell 161(3):486–500. doi:10.1016/j.cell.2015.03.005
76. Tse SW, Radtke AJ, Espinosa DA, Cockburn IA, Zavala F (2014) The chemokine receptor CXCR6 is required for the maintenance of liver memory $CD8^+$ T cells specific for infectious pathogens. J Infect Dis 210(9):1508–1516. doi:10.1093/infdis/jiu281
77. Tse SW, Cockburn IA, Zhang H, Scott AL, Zavala F (2013) Unique transcriptional profile of liver-resident memory $CD8^+$ T cells induced by immunization with malaria sporozoites. Genes Immun 14(5):302–309. doi:10.1038/gene.2013.20
78. Sato T, Thorlacius H, Johnston B, Staton TL, Xiang W, Littman DR, Butcher EC (2005) Role for CXCR6 in recruitment of activated $CD8^+$ lymphocytes to inflamed liver. J Immunol 174(1):277–283
79. Swain SL, McKinstry KK, Strutt TM (2012) Expanding roles for $CD4^+$ T cells in immunity to viruses. Nat Rev Immunol 12(2):136–148
80. Overstreet MG, Chen Y-C, Cockburn IA, Tse S-W, Zavala F (2011) $CD4^+$ T cells modulate expansion and survival but not functional properties of effector and memory $CD8^+$ T cells induced by malaria sporozoites. PLoS One 6(1), e15948. doi:10.1371/journal.pone.0015948
81. Van Braeckel-Budimir N, Harty JT (2014) CD8 T-cell-mediated protection against liver-stage malaria: lessons from a mouse model. Front Microbiol 5:272. doi:10.3389/fmicb.2014.00272
82. Doll KL, Harty JT (2014) Correlates of protective immunity following whole sporozoite vaccination against malaria. Immunol Res 59:166–176. doi:10.1007/s12026-014-8525-0
83. Carvalho L, Sano G-I, Hafalla JCR, Morrot A, Curotto de Lafaille MA, Zavala F (2002) IL-4-secreting $CD4^+$ T cells are crucial to the development of $CD8^+$ T-cell responses against malaria liver stages. Nat Med 8(2):166–170
84. Rénia L, Grillot D, Marussig M, Corradin G, Miltgen F, Lambert PH, Mazier D, Del Giudice G (1993) Effector functions of circumsporozoite peptide-primed $CD4^+$ T cell clones against *Plasmodium yoelii* liver stages. J Immunol 150(4):1471–1478
85. Tsuji M, Romero P, Nussenzweig RS, Zavala F (1990) $CD4^+$ cytolytic T cell clone confers protection against murine malaria. J Exp Med 172(5):1353–1357
86. Oliveira GA, Kumar KA, Calvo-Calle JM, Othoro C, Altszuler D, Nussenzweig V, Nardin EH (2008) Class II-restricted protective immunity induced by malaria sporozoites. Infect Immun 76(3):1200–1206. doi:10.1128/iai.00566-07
87. Moreno A, Clavijo P, Edelman R, Davis J, Sztein M, Herrington D, Nardin E (1991) Cytotoxic $CD4^+$ T cells from a sporozoite-immunized volunteer recognize the *Plasmodium falciparum* CS protein. Int Immunol 3(10):997–1003

88. Bijker EM, Teirlinck AC, Schats R, van Gemert G-J, van de Vegte-Bolmer M, van Lieshout L, IntHout J, Hermsen CC, Scholzen A, Visser LG, Sauerwein RW (2014) Cytotoxic markers associate with protection against malaria in human volunteers immunized with *Plasmodium falciparum* sporozoites. J Infect Dis 210(10):1605–1615. doi:10.1093/infdis/jiu293
89. Frevert U, Moreno A, Calvo-Calle JM, Klotz C, Nardin E (2009) Imaging effector functions of human cytotoxic CD4$^+$ T cells specific for *Plasmodium falciparum* circumsporozoite protein. Int J Parasitol 39(1):119–132. doi:10.1016/j.ijpara.2008.06.014
90. Herkel J, Jagemann B, Wiegard C, Lazaro JFG, Lueth S, Kanzler S, Blessing M, Schmitt E, Lohse A (2003) MHC class II-expressing hepatocytes function as antigen-presenting cells and activate specific CD4 T lymphocyutes. Hepatology 37(5):1079–1085
91. Seguin MC, Klotz FW, Schneider I, Weir JP, Goodbary M, Slayter M, Raney JJ, Aniagolu JU, Green SJ (1994) Induction of nitric oxide synthase protects against malaria in mice exposed to irradiated *Plasmodium berghei* infected mosquitoes: involvement of interferon gamma and CD8$^+$ T cells. J Exp Med 180(1):353–358

Adaptive Immunity to *Plasmodium* Blood Stages

Michelle N. Wykes, Robin Stephens, and Ian A. Cockburn

Contents

1 Introduction: Lessons from the Field and Controlled Infection Studies 48
2 Mechanisms of Protection 49
2.1 Antibody and B Cell-Mediated Protection 49
2.2 T Cell-Mediated Protection 52
3 Why Does Better Adaptive Immunity to Blood Stages Not Develop? 54
3.1 B Cell Memory 54
3.2 T Cell Memory and Exhaustion 56
4 Concluding Remarks 57
References 57

M.N. Wykes
QIMR Berghofer Medical Research Institute,
300 Herston Road, Brisbane, QLD 4029, Australia
e-mail: michelle.wykes@qimrberghofer.edu.au

R. Stephens
Division of Infectious Diseases, Departments of Internal Medicine and Microbiology and Immunology, University of Texas Medical Branch,
301 University Drive, Galveston, TX 77555-0435, USA
e-mail: rostephe@utmb.edu

I.A. Cockburn (✉)
Department of Immunology and Infectious Disease, John Curtin School of Medical Research, The Australian National University, Canberra, ACT 2601, Australia
e-mail: ian.cockburn@anu.edu.au

M.M. Mota, A. Rodriguez (eds.), *Malaria*, DOI 10.1007/978-3-319-45210-4_3

1 Introduction: Lessons from the Field and Controlled Infection Studies

Adaptive immune responses to *Plasmodium* blood stages provide three kinds of immunity that evolve at different rates. Over time and with exposure, immunity reduces lethal pathology and mild malaria disease and finally reduces peak parasitemia; however, unlike many other infections, there is incomplete protection from re-infection [1–3]. Moreover, while emigrants out of endemic areas maintain some protection from severe malaria and high parasite loads, protection from malaria disease is lost in the absence of exposure [4, 5]. Nonetheless, one malaria vaccine strategy would be to mimic natural immunity to blood stages thereby reducing morbidity and mortality due to infection. However, in order to develop these strategies, we will need to fully understand the immune effector mechanisms involved and develop accurate correlates of protective immunity.

Much fundamental information about blood-stage immunity comes from studies of the development of immunity among individuals in endemic areas and data collected from the use of deliberate *Plasmodium* infection to treat tertiary syphilis [6–8]. Epidemiological studies show that peak susceptibility to severe disease occurs in infants and young children, with neonates (up to 6 months) protected by maternally transmitted antibodies [3]. Indeed it has been suggested that only one or two infections are required for protection against severe disease [1]. Once children in endemic areas reach beyond the age of 5, *Plasmodium* infection typically results in a debilitating, but not life-threatening, illness termed mild malaria. By the time exposed individuals reach their teens, most malaria infections are asymptomatic, and average parasitemias are lower [2, 3, 9]. Naturally acquired protection is almost entirely directed at the blood-stages with no strong evidence in field studies of infection-blocking immunity [10]. This was recently demonstrated in a recent study in Kalifabougou, Mali, where all individuals in the village were treated with antimalarials to clear residual subclinical infections in the weeks prior to the onset of the wet season. The time to seropositivity was then intensively monitored from the start of the transmission. Strikingly, the time to first parasitemia (as measured by PCR) was the same in adults as infants, indicating that there is no sterilizing immunity to infection. However, adults were less likely to develop symptoms and their peak parasitemia was lower, indicating that their immunity to disease had developed over years of exposure [10, 11]. Epidemiological studies also provide strong evidence that *Plasmodium* infections can be very long-lived, as parasites can persist through the dry season to establish chronic infections in the community once the rains and mosquito vectors return [12].

Findings from the field are generally supported by data from controlled infections of individuals with *Plasmodium*. Much of this data comes from the use of malaria to limit syphilis infection and pathology [6–8]. Monitoring of infection in these individuals showed a pattern of recrudescent parasitemia [6], which has been shown to be due to sequential expression of variant surface antigens on the infected RBC [13, 14]. With each recrudescence, the level of parasitemia typically became lower, while symptoms waned after the initial stages of infection [6]. Eventually infections resolved even without drug treatment, with a mean time to resolution of ~200 days [8]. It was also shown that homologous reinfection generally resulted in lower parasitemia than primary infections, especially when controlling for each recrudescent peak of parasitemia [6, 7]. Collectively these observations from the field and controlled human infection show that adaptive immunity to blood-stage parasites plays a critical role in limiting pathology and ultimately resolving infection.

2 Mechanisms of Protection

2.1 Antibody and B Cell-Mediated Protection

Seminal passive transfer studies in the 1960s demonstrated a critical role for antibodies in the clearance of parasites [15]. In these studies, IgG from immune adults was transferred to children with clinical malaria in the Gambia resulting in a 3–4 log reduction of parasitemia. Similar experiments were subsequently performed in which West African sera were transferred to naturally infected Thai adults [16, 17]. In addition to demonstrating that antibodies are important, these data show that sera from one part of the world can kill parasites in another region and suggest that there is a significant degree of antibody cross-reactivity to genetically distinct parasites. Mouse models have also shown that B cells are required for protection and more specifically for full clearance of the parasite [18–21]. Furthermore, malaria antigen-specific B cells can be detected using a cultured ELISpot in both mice and humans long after a single infection showing that malaria infection can induce B cell memory [22–26].

The targets of protective antibodies are still unclear. To identify whether a candidate antigen is a target of protective immunity, two major approaches have been taken. One approach is to determine if the presence of antibodies in exposed individuals correlates with protection, ideally in a longitudinal prospective study. The other is to determine if antibodies targeting that antigen can inhibit parasite expansion using some kind of growth inhibition assay (GIA). It has been shown that individuals who have high overall levels of growth-inhibiting antibodies are protected against malaria, linking these approaches [27]. In general, two classes of antigen have been considered as likely targets of protective antibodies. One class of molecules is variant surface antigens (VSAs), which are exported to the surface of the infected red blood cells (RBCs) [28]. Other major targets of protective immunity are those on the surface of the merozoite, which are involved in the attachment and invasion of parasites into RBCs [29–31].

A range of VSAs are exported to the RBC surface, and there is robust evidence that these can be the targets of protective antibodies (reviewed in [28]). In *P. falciparum* malaria, four classes of VSAs have been identified: *P. falciparum* erythrocyte membrane protein 1 (PfEMP1; ~50 members/parasite), repetitive interspersed family proteins (RIFIN; ~150 members/parasite), sub-telomeric variable open reading frame proteins (STEVOR: ~30 members/parasite), and surface-associated interspersed gene family proteins (SURFIN; 10 members/parasite). Mouse models have similar multigene families; the largest, related to RIFINs and present in at least five species, is termed *Plasmodium* interspersed repeats (PIR), which are just being characterized for mechanistic studies [32, 33]. Classic studies showed that immune sera can drive the switching of VSAs in *P. knowlesi* and *P. chabaudi* infections [13, 14, 34], highlighting the importance of antibodies targeting these molecules. Moreover, the presence of antibodies capable of recognizing the surface antigens of a broad range of parasite isolates has been associated with protection, with children in endemic areas generally developing cross-reactivity to an increasing percentage of isolates over time [35]. Compellingly, in a prospective study of Kenyan children, it was found that parasites that caused infections were often not recognized by pre-infection sera; i.e., they appeared to be exploiting holes in the antibody repertoire. However, those same parasite variants were subsequently recognized by convalescent sera as the B cells caught up to the parasite diversity [36].

While the association between antibodies to VSAs in general with protection is robust, identifying which particular molecules are the targets of protective antibodies has been harder. The bulk of VSA-specific antibodies appear to recognize variants of PfEMP1 as shown by experiments using parasites that had been engineered to suppress the expression of PfEMP1 [37]. In these studies, the binding of immune sera to infected RBCs was found to be significantly reduced in the absence of PfEMP1, while the presence of serum antibodies specifically capable of binding PfEMP1 was found to be significantly associated with protection [38]. Protection against severe disease has also been suggested to be associated with antibodies targeting specific families of PfEMP1 molecules. The *var* genes, which encode PfEMP1 molecules, are generally classified into three groups (A, B, and C) based on upstream sequences [39, 40]. The expression of group-A and group-B *var* genes has generally been associated with severe and symptomatic infections [41–43], while the expression of group-C *var* genes is more often associated with asymptomatic infections [42]. Consistent with antibodies to PfEMP1 being important for protection against symptomatic infection, children first develop antibodies to Group A PfEMP1 molecules and only later acquire antibodies to other subtypes [44, 45].

RIFIN proteins may also be targets of protective broadly neutralizing antibodies. An older study associated higher levels of anti-RIFIN antibodies with rapid parasite clearance and asymptomatic infection [46]. More recently, a recent screen for monoclonal antibodies capable of agglutinating multiple parasite variants identified two RIFIN-specific antibodies [47]. These antibodies derived from different donors nonetheless shared a highly unusual structure, having incorporated a ~100 amino acid insert derived from the LAIR1 protein between the V and D regions of the antibodies. LAIR1 is a collagen-binding inhibitory receptor; however, the insert from this protein contained somatic mutations that rendered the insert incapable of binding collagen, but conferred the ability to bind a broad range of RIFIN proteins [47].

Antibodies targeting various molecules involved in invasion have also been implicated in protection. Longitudinal studies have examined the association between antibodies to various merozoite surface proteins and protection against malaria [30]. A recent meta-analysis of these studies showed that antibodies to apical membrane antigen 1 (AMA1), glutamine-rich protein (GLURP), merozoite surface protein (MSP)-3, and MSP-1_{19}—a 19KDa fragment of MSP1 retained after the proteolytic cleavage of the remaining molecule from the surface—have been consistently associated with protection [30]. Many of these have been subsequently proposed as vaccine candidates based on the fact that antisera generated against these antigens have been shown to inhibit parasite growth in GIAs [48, 49]. The potential importance of antibodies targeting MSP-1_{19}, in naturally acquired immunity, was further demonstrated in elegant studies in which transgenic *P. falciparum* parasites were generated with the endogenous MSP-1_{19} fragment replaced with *P. chabaudi* ortholog (which is antigenically distinct) [50]. It was found that the sera from immune individuals were much more effective in blocking the growth of control parasites compared to those without the *P. falciparum* MSP-1_{19}. Thus, the authors were able to specifically dissect the importance of antibodies targeting a single antigen of interest from whole human sera.

Other proteins involved in the invasion process that are believed to be targets of protective antibodies are the two invasion ligand families: the erythrocyte-binding antigens (EBA175/EBA 140/EBA 181) and the reticulocyte-binding homologue proteins (PfRh1, −2a, −2b, −4–5). These molecules invade either by a sialic acid-dependent pathway (EBA175/EBA140/EBA181 and Rh1), or by using complement receptor 1 (PfRh4) or basigin (PfRh5). EBA-175 antibodies and PfRh5 antibodies have recently been associated with protection against malaria [29, 31, 51]. However, the ability of the parasite to switch between multiple invasion pathways may enable it to evade antibodies targeting one or other invasion ligand [52].

The above approaches to defining the targets of protective immunity are essentially "candidate approaches," where highly expressed surface antigens were explored for immunogenicity and protection. The development of protein arrays carrying ~1200 of the 5400 or so malaria proteins has allowed more unbiased approached to be attempted to understand the targets of immunity in naturally exposed individuals. A prospective study examined the antibodies present in the sera of ~200 individuals from a village in Mali before and after the transmission season [53]. Antibody reactivity to this broad panel of antigens was then compared between individuals who suffered a bout of clinical malaria and those who did not. Forty-nine proteins were found to be significantly differentially recognized in this analysis suggesting that these molecules may be the targets of protective antibodies. Most of these 49 proteins were not previously considered possible vaccine antigens; conversely many leading vaccine candidates were not differentially recognized, suggesting that the traditional approaches may not be selecting the optimal immunogens [53, 54].

The mechanisms of antibody action are also unclear. For simplicity and standardization, most GIAs are performed with purified heat-inactivated sera and in the absence of lymphocytes and monocytes. The fact that growth inhibition occurs in these circumstances suggests that the inhibition of invasion or neutralization may be sufficient, in some cases, to block infection. However, GIAs have also been performed with other immune system components added to the culture. One study found that the addition of monocytes augmented growth inhibition by West African sera suggesting that cytophilic antibodies may be critical for protection [16]. More recently, a study showed that non-heat-inactivated immune sera containing complement components had significantly enhanced growth inhibition compared to heat-inactivated sera [55]. In support of the role of complement, the presence of antibodies capable of fixing C1q on the surface of merozoites correlated with protection from clinical malaria [55]. On the other hand, *P. falciparum* has recently been shown to have mechanisms to evade elimination by complement [56, 57].

2.2 T Cell-Mediated Protection

While the role of antibodies in protection against malaria is clear, our understanding of the contribution of T cells has been relatively slow to develop. Mouse models of malaria have provided the foundation of our understanding of T cell immunity. $CD4^+$ T cells are required in control of malaria both for their ability to help B cells [58, 59] and their promotion of phagocytosis [60]. Early studies with a model of chronic malaria (*P. chabaudi* (AS)) conclusively showed that $CD4^+$ T cells control the peak of parasitemia in the primary acute phase of blood-stage infections via the production of high levels of interferon-γ (IFN-γ) during the first week of infection [61–63]. In fact, IFN-γ contributes to a vast network of protective responses against malaria, recently summarized in [64]. However, $CD4^+$ T cells were shown to be the key source of both IFN-γ and tumor necrosis factor (TNF) during malaria in mice [65, 66]. Studies in mice infected with *P. chabaudi* malaria have also shown that IFN-γ and TNF cooperate to induce nitric oxide synthase expression in the spleen to control peak parasite burden [67]. $CD4^+$ T cells consist of several subtypes, which shape the nature of immunity against malaria. The use of mice with MSP-1-specific transgenic $CD4^+$ T cells (B5 TCR transgenic) identified effector T cells (characterized as IL-7Rα$^-$), which developed during acute infection and $CD4^+$ memory T cells ($CD44^{hi}$; IL-7Rα^{hi}) which formed the majority of malaria-specific T cells by day 45 [68]. As in other chronic infections, the memory cells were primarily effector memory cells ($CD62L^{lo}$; $CD44^{hi}$; IL-7Rα^{hi}) [68]. During the effector phase, the (IL-7Rα$^-$; $CD62L^{lo}CD27^+$) intermediate effector subset includes the most multicytokine-producing T cells [69]. Interestingly, chronic infection improves maintenance of IFN-γ$^+$ TNF$^+$ interleukin-2$^-$ T cells suggesting a mechanism for the maintenance of protection by continued exposure [70], commonly called premunition [71]. In addition to IFN-γ and TNF, IL-21 has recently been shown to be produced by $CD4^+$ T cells in humans [72], to correlate with parasite density in Gambian children [73], and to be required in mice for complete clearance of parasite [57].

Controlled human malaria infections (CHMI) have recently provided insights into malaria immunity independent of coinfections, malnutrition, and factors associated with repeated malarial infections. One of the earliest CHMI gave naïve volunteers repeated low-dose blood-stage parasite infections followed by drug cure with atovaquone. This protocol induced protective parasite-specific T cell responses and nitric oxide synthase activity of mononuclear cells, but not antibodies [74].

Unfortunately, the interpretation was confounded by the prolonged effects of atovaquone in vivo [75]. More recent CHMI studies in which individuals are immunized multiple times with live sporozoites under drug cover have shown that this protocol efficiently induces both sporozoite and blood-stage-specific T cells which were polyfunctional [76]. However, while immunized individuals were protected against sporozoite challenge, they were not protected when inoculated directly with blood stages, suggesting a longer infection may be required to establish blood-stage immunity [77].

Although malaria challenges in mice suggest that T cells are critical for immunity to malaria, reliable T cell correlates of exposure to and protection from malaria in endemic areas are relatively limited. In humans, early IFN-γ responses to *P. falciparum* correlate with better anti-parasite immunity [64, 78]. It has been more challenging to show this at the cellular level using intracellular cytokine staining of T cells. A longitudinal study in Uganda found that malaria-specific $CD4^+$ T cell responses were measurable in nearly all children, with the majority of children having $CD4^+$ T cells producing both IFN-γ and interleukin-10 (IL-10) in response to malaria-infected RBCs. Frequencies of IFN-γ/IL-10 co-producing $CD4^+$ T cells, which express the Th1 transcription factor T-bet, inversely correlated with duration since infection [79]. In a larger longitudinal study, IFN-γ responses to blood-stage antigens, especially MSP-1, were common and associated with recent exposure to malaria, but still not with protection from subsequent malaria infection, while responses to pre-erythrocytic antigens were uncommon, but were associated with protection from subsequent infection [80]. Finally, another study compared T cell responses to *P. falciparum* between children and adults in high or low malaria transmission areas [81]. In high-transmission areas, most *P. falciparum*-specific $CD4^+$ T cells in children produced IL-10, while responses in adults were dominated by IFN-γ and TNF which could explain better immunity seen in adults. In contrast, in the low-transmission setting, responses in both children and adults were dominated by IFN-γ and TNF [81]. The increase in IL-10 in T cells on repeated infection may be the basis for protection from severe pathology from T cells, though this has not yet been definitively proven [20, 79]. Overall, it would seem that $CD4^+$ T cell cytokines do contribute to protection, and more work needs to be done to determine the relative contribution to antibody production versus cellular immunity.

Perhaps most confounding has been the contribution of $CD8^+$ T cell-mediated immunity against blood-stage malaria. Research on these cells was initially limited to protection against liver-stage infection, the pathogenesis of cerebral malaria, and damage to splenic architecture [82, 83]. Protection by these cells was largely overlooked, because parasites and infected erythrocytes have no antigen presentation machinery, and therefore T cells cannot interact directly with the pathogen [9]. However, previous studies in experimental animal models found that depletion of $CD8^+$ T lymphocytes during blood-stage *P. chabaudi* infections significantly delayed clearance of the infection [62, 84]. Interestingly, naïve mice, transfused with $CD8^+$ T cells derived from mice infected twice with *P. yoelii* survived lethal blood-stage malaria challenge [85]. Elegant studies in mouse models have now shown that *Plasmodia* can parasitize erythroblasts, immature RBCs that still express MHCI, and therefore have the capacity to activate CD8⁺ T cells [86]. There is also evidence in rats that severe malarial anemia is caused by CD8⁺ T cell-dependent parasite clearance and erythrocyte removal in the spleen [87]. Finally, CD8⁺ T cells in mouse models have been shown to contribute to completely clearing parasites during chronic malaria [88]. Overall, the contribution of these cells to protection against blood-stage malaria in the field requires further investigation.

3 Why Does Better Adaptive Immunity to Blood Stages Not Develop?

Fundamental questions that remain unresolved are why adaptive immunity to malaria is not sterilizing and why immunity wanes in the absence of exposure. This may be partly explained by the variant or polymorphic nature of many malaria antigens as outlined above. It has also been suggested that there may be defects in dendritic cell function during blood stages (previously reviewed elsewhere [89, 90]). A role for regulatory T cells in limiting the effectiveness of immune responses to malaria has also been proposed. The presence of $FOXP3^+$ $CD4^+CD25^+$ regulatory T cells has been found to correlate with more rapid parasite growth in CHMI studies [91], while elevated numbers of a highly suppressive subset of regulatory T cells have been observed in patients with severe malaria [92]. More recently, there have been more systematic investigations of the fates of memory B and T cells in *Plasmodium* infection with the finding that these key cells of the adaptive immune system can appear "dysregulated" [93]. The unusual T and B cell response likely represents the détente between the parasite and the host where the parasite maximizes its ability to transmit by surviving as a chronic infection, and the host minimizes the pathological damage done by an excessive immune response.

3.1 B Cell Memory

The clearest example of unusual immune responses in malaria is the observation that polyclonal B cells in the blood of individuals in malaria-endemic areas include a high level of "atypical" memory B cells [93, 94]. Atypical memory B cells express FCRL5 and lack expression of classical memory B cell markers such as CD21 and CD27 [95, 96] and have been found to be expanded in a variety of chronic infections [97–99]. Most studies characterize these cells as anergic, as unlike classical memory B cells, they do not respond to polyclonal stimuli by secreting antibody [95]. Atypical B cells isolated from individuals in malaria-endemic areas have been shown in one study to have reduced B cell receptor signaling and effector function [95]. Another study looking at antigen-specific atypical and classical memory B cells isolated from symptomatic individuals suggested that atypical B cells might be proliferating and producing antibody [100]; thus, the exact significance of the presence of these cells remains unclear.

More generally there is strong evidence that the levels of many malaria-specific antibodies decay rapidly, as previously reviewed [101]. Protective memory B cell and presumably long-lived plasma cell (LLPC) populations specific for malaria take many years to develop [22, 102]. One study in Mali found that while boosting with tetanus toxoid induced a rapid and sustained increase in the number of TT-specific memory B cells, malaria infection only resulted in a short-lived increase in memory B cells specific for a variety of blood-stage antigens [102]. This short-lived B cell expansion was associated with a transient increase in blood-stage-specific antibodies with short half-lives (<10 days). These data are consistent with *Plasmodium* infection inducing a transient plasmablast response to a large number of parasite antigens. These B cells are likely derived from the marginal zone and appear to include cross-reactive specificities from this memory B cell containing zone, which is the first point of contact for this blood-borne infection [103, 104]. Due to their generation outside of the germinal center, which forms much later than in other infections, the plasma cells formed are not long-lived, and the number of malaria-specific LLPCs in the bone marrow does not appear to increase dramatically [23, 105]. Consistent with this, memory B cells specific for blood-stage antigens increased in number only incrementally with age and, even in adults, are relatively few in number [102]. It was therefore proposed that the acquisition of immunity correlates with the development of sufficient memory B cells and LLPCs to provide a level of antibodies above a certain protective threshold, though this may take years to reach [106].

One reason that has been proposed for the slow acquisition of memory B cells is that malaria infection induces an immune response that at least initially is skewed toward a Th1 response and away from the generation of T follicular helper cells (Tfh) that are crucial for B cell memory [107, 108]. Mouse studies show that Tfh cells are inhibited by high levels of the pro-inflammatory cytokines TNF and IFN-γ during fulminant blood-stage infection [108, 109]. Pre-Tfh-like cells were found to express Bcl-6^{lo} and IL-21, but also the Th1 associated molecules T-bet^{lo} and CXCR3 during blood-stage infection [107, 108]. The blockade or knockout of the Th1 cytokines IFN-γ and TNF was found to restore Tfh differentiation and germinal center formation [108]. These Th1/Tfh cells survive into the memory phase with the mixed Th1/Tfh phenotype suggesting that they will also play a role in suboptimal antibody responses in subsequent infections [107]. Interestingly, while CD4$^+$ T cells in *P. chabaudi*-infected mice express ICOS in response to infection, ICOS$^{-/-}$ mice accumulated fewer splenic Tfh compared with ICOS-sufficient mice, leading to substantially fewer GC B cells and a decrease in affinity, but not the production of parasite-specific isotype-switched Abs. These mice also had an enhanced Th1 immune response that reduced peak parasitemia but at the expense of the quality of the antibody [110]. These findings have been corroborated in a recent study examining Tfh cells in naturally exposed children [111]. In human PBMCs, CD4$^+$ T cells expressing CXCR5 and PD1 are generally assumed to be the circulating counterparts of germinal center Tfh cells; within this population, there is a fraction that expresses CXCR3 and provides suboptimal help to B cells [112]. At baseline, children in a malaria-endemic region in Mali were found to have circulating Tfh cells that were phenotypically similar to those found in US adults; however, during malaria infection, only the CXCR3$^+$ Tfh-like cells expanded. Notably, the expansion of this subset with characteristics of both Th1 and Tfh cells did not correlate with increased levels of circulating antibodies [111].

3.2 T Cell Memory and Exhaustion

Development of T cell memory during chronic infections is a controversial topic, as memory cells are not thought to coexist with ongoing infection. However, CD4$^+$ T cells to the blood stages of *P. chabaudi* infection with the phenotypic hallmarks of memory cells have been identified in mice and humans [68, 113, 114]. As in other chronic infections, these are predominantly effector memory T cells [115–118]. However, very little is actually known about the functionality of effector memory or the differences with acute effector cells. In chronic *Leishmania major* infection of resistant C57Bl/6 mice, CD44$^+$; CD62L^{lo}; T-bet$^+$; Ly6C$^+$ effector CD4$^+$ T cells that are short-lived in the absence of infection and are not derived from memory cells reactivated by secondary challenge were found to be the main mediators of protection [119].

The role of continued infection in maintaining *Plasmodium*-specific T cell memory has been studied. A longitudinal study in mice, over a period of 200 days, reported a progressive decline in the T cell response to *P. chabaudi* parasites, which occurs similarly in untreated and drug-treated mice with time after infection [120]. In contrast, it has also been reported that effector memory cells (CD62L^{lo}; CD44^{hi}; IL-7Rα^{hi}) were maintained and protective [68]. Finally, an analysis of malaria-specific CD4$^+$ T cell responses in individuals living in an area of low malaria transmission, with documented clinical attack of *P. falciparum* and/or *P. vivax* in the past 6 years, found that the number of IFN-γ-producing effector memory T cells declined significantly over the 12 months of the study; in sharp contrast, IL-10 responses were sustained for many years after the last known malaria infection [121]. Therefore, there are many unanswered questions about how the combination of effector memory T cells and effector T cells that are promoted by chronic infection may explain the decay of disease immunity in mice and humans and/or provide clues about how to induce a well-regulated T cell response by vaccination.

Cellular exhaustion is another potential mechanism for reduction of a long-term protective immune response that clears infection. Programmed cell death-1 (PD-1) is the best studied molecule that reduces effector T cell functions. PD-1 has two known ligands, PD-L1 (B7-H1) [122, 123] and PD-L2 (B7-DC) [124, 125], and when PD-1 is engaged simultaneously with T cell receptor signals, it can trigger an inhibitory signal in lymphocytes [126]. One of the first studies to examine PD-1 expression during malaria used a mouse model to show PD-1 expression on IL-7R^{lo}-expressing CD4$^+$ and CD8$^+$ T cells [127, 128]. Similarly, subsequent studies showed that PD-1 was also expressed on CD4$^+$ [93, 129] and CD8$^+$ T cells [93] in blood of *Pf*-infected individuals in Mali and Kenya, but no functional evidence of exhaustion was provided. Subsequent studies used a murine model of blood-stage malaria to show that the combined blockade of PD-L1 and LAG-3 inhibitory molecules with antibodies, during *P. yoelii* malaria in mice, dramatically reduced parasitemia, while in *P. chabaudi*, it reduced the recrudescence [129]. These studies showed that lymphocyte exhaustion modulated immunity against malaria. Ensuing studies used mice with a deletion of PD-1 (PD-1KO) to conclusively show that PD-1 mediated a reduction in the capacity of parasite-specific $CD4^+$ T cells to proliferate and secrete IFN-γ and TNF-α during the late phase (Day 35) of *P. chabaudi* infection indicating exhaustion of these cells [88]. Further, while the $CD8^+$ T cell contribution to protection from *Plasmodia* has been challenging to detect, studies in PD-1KO mice showed that full activation of parasite-specific $CD8^+$ T cells leads to a dramatically reduced recrudescence in these animals. PD-1 mediates a 95 % loss in the numbers and functional capacity of $CD8^+$ T cells during the acute phase of malaria, which was shown to exacerbate the infection and lead to chronic malaria [88]. The role of $CD8^+$ T cells was dramatically revealed in these mutant animals, explaining why these cells have escaped past scrutiny. Furthermore, ongoing studies in humans are anticipated to determine the degree of the role of exhaustion in the chronicity of *P. falciparum* and *vivax* malaria.

4 Concluding Remarks

In recent years the emphasis in the malaria vaccine field has shifted to vaccines targeting the infectious preerythrocytic life cycle stages of the *Plasmodium* parasite. Nonetheless while our most advanced vaccine candidate confers some protection against malaria, it does not provide an absolute block to infection, and so individuals remain exposed to the disease causing blood stages and thus at risk of death [130, 131]. Recent work has continued to identify novel potential targets of protective immunity and provided insights into the mechanisms of immune (dys)regulation in malaria. It is clear that continued research (1) into the immune responses that are required for naturally acquired immunity and (2) the factors that prevent better immunity from developing are required if we are to significantly limit malaria mortality via vaccination.

References

1. Gupta S, Snow RW, Donnelly CA, Marsh K, Newbold C (1999) Immunity to non-cerebral severe malaria is acquired after one or two infections. Nat Med 5(3):340–343. doi:10.1038/6560
2. McGregor IA (1964) Studies in the acquisition of immunity of *Plasmodium falciparum* infections in Africa. Trans R Soc Trop Med Hyg 58:80–92
3. Snow RW, Nahlen B, Palmer A, Donnelly CA, Gupta S, Marsh K (1998) Risk of severe malaria among African infants: direct evidence of clinical protection during early infancy. J Infect Dis 177(3):819–822

4. Bouchaud O, Cot M, Kony S, Durand R, Schiemann R, Ralaimazava P, Coulaud JP, Le Bras J, Deloron P (2005) Do African immigrants living in France have long-term malarial immunity? Am J Trop Med Hyg 72(1):21–25
5. Pistone T, Diallo A, Mechain M, Receveur MC, Malvy D (2014) Epidemiology of imported malaria give support to the hypothesis of 'long-term' semi-immunity to malaria in sub-Saharan African migrants living in France. Travel Med Infect Dis 12(1):48–53. doi:10.1016/j.tmaid.2013.08.006
6. Collins WE, Jeffery GM (1999) A retrospective examination of the patterns of recrudescence in patients infected with *Plasmodium falciparum*. Am J Trop Med Hyg 61(1 Suppl):44–48
7. Collins WE, Jeffery GM (1999) A retrospective examination of secondary sporozoite- and trophozoite-induced infections with *Plasmodium falciparum*: development of parasitologic and clinical immunity following secondary infection. Am J Trop Med Hyg 61(1 Suppl):20–35
8. Collins WE, Jeffery GM (1999) A retrospective examination of sporozoite- and trophozoite-induced infections with *Plasmodium falciparum*: development of parasitologic and clinical immunity during primary infection. Am J Trop Med Hyg 61(1 Suppl):4–19
9. Langhorne J, Ndungu FM, Sponaas AM, Marsh K (2008) Immunity to malaria: more questions than answers. Nat Immunol 9(7):725–732. doi:10.1038/ni.f.205
10. Tran TM, Li S, Doumbo S, Doumtabe D, Huang CY, Dia S, Bathily A, Sangala J, Kone Y, Traore A, Niangaly M, Dara C, Kayentao K, Ongoiba A, Doumbo OK, Traore B, Crompton PD (2013) An intensive longitudinal cohort study of Malian children and adults reveals no evidence of acquired immunity to *Plasmodium falciparum* infection. Clin Infect Dis 57(1):40–47. doi:10.1093/cid/cit174
11. Portugal S, Moebius J, Skinner J, Doumbo S, Doumtabe D, Kone Y, Dia S, Kanakabandi K, Sturdevant DE, Virtaneva K, Porcella SF, Li S, Doumbo OK, Kayentao K, Ongoiba A, Traore B, Crompton PD (2014) Exposure-dependent control of malaria-induced inflammation in children. PLoS Pathog 10(4), e1004079. doi:10.1371/journal.ppat.1004079
12. Sonden K, Doumbo S, Hammar U, Vafa Homann M, Ongoiba A, Traore B, Bottai M, Crompton PD, Farnert A (2015) Asymptomatic multiclonal *Plasmodium falciparum* infections carried through the dry season predict protection against subsequent clinical malaria. J Infect Dis 212(4):608–616. doi:10.1093/infdis/jiv088
13. Brown IN, Brown KN, Hills LA (1968) Immunity to malaria: the antibody response to antigenic variation by *Plasmodium knowlesi*. Immunology 14(1):127–138
14. McLean SA, Pearson CD, Phillips RS (1982) *Plasmodium chabaudi*: antigenic variation during recrudescent parasitaemias in mice. Exp Parasitol 54(3):296–302
15. Cohen S, Mc GI, Carrington S (1961) Gamma-globulin and acquired immunity to human malaria. Nature 192:733–737
16. Bouharoun-Tayoun H, Attanath P, Sabchareon A, Chongsuphajaisiddhi T, Druilhe P (1990) Antibodies that protect humans against *Plasmodium falciparum* blood stages do not on their own inhibit parasite growth and invasion in vitro, but act in cooperation with monocytes. J Exp Med 172(6):1633–1641
17. Sabchareon A, Burnouf T, Ouattara D, Attanath P, Bouharoun-Tayoun H, Chantavanich P, Foucault C, Chongsuphajaisiddhi T, Druilhe P (1991) Parasitologic and clinical human response to immunoglobulin administration in falciparum malaria. Am J Trop Med Hyg 45(3):297–308
18. Hirunpetcharat C, Vukovic P, Liu XQ, Kaslow DC, Miller LH, Good MF (1999) Absolute requirement for an active immune response involving B cells and Th cells in immunity to *Plasmodium yoelii* passively acquired with antibodies to the 19-kDa carboxyl-terminal fragment of merozoite surface protein-1. J Immunol 162(12):7309–7314
19. Meding SJ, Langhorne J (1991) $CD4^+$ T cells and B cells are necessary for the transfer of protective immunity to *Plasmodium chabaudi chabaudi*. Eur J Immunol 21(6):1433–1438. doi:10.1002/eji.1830210616
20. Stephens R, Albano FR, Quin S, Pascal BJ, Harrison V, Stockinger B, Kioussis D, Weltzien HU, Langhorne J (2005) Malaria-specific transgenic $CD4^+$ T cells protect immunodeficient mice from lethal infection and demonstrate requirement for a protective threshold of antibody

production for parasite clearance. Blood 106(5):1676–1684. doi:10.1182/blood-2004-10-4047
21. Yap GS, Stevenson MM (1994) Differential requirements for an intact spleen in induction and expression of B-cell-dependent immunity to *Plasmodium chabaudi* AS. Infect Immun 62(10):4219–4225
22. Dorfman JR, Bejon P, Ndungu FM, Langhorne J, Kortok MM, Lowe BS, Mwangi TW, Williams TN, Marsh K (2005) B cell memory to 3 *Plasmodium falciparum* blood-stage antigens in a malaria-endemic area. J Infect Dis 191(10):1623–1630. doi:10.1086/429671
23. Ndungu FM, Cadman ET, Coulcher J, Nduati E, Couper E, Macdonald DW, Ng D, Langhorne J (2009) Functional memory B cells and long-lived plasma cells are generated after a single *Plasmodium chabaudi* infection in mice. PLoS Pathog 5(12), e1000690. doi:10.1371/journal.ppat.1000690
24. Ndungu FM, Lundblom K, Rono J, Illingworth J, Eriksson S, Farnert A (2013) Long-lived *Plasmodium falciparum* specific memory B cells in naturally exposed Swedish travelers. Eur J Immunol 43(11):2919–2929. doi:10.1002/eji.201343630
25. Ndungu FM, Olotu A, Mwacharo J, Nyonda M, Apfeld J, Mramba LK, Fegan GW, Bejon P, Marsh K (2012) Memory B cells are a more reliable archive for historical antimalarial responses than plasma antibodies in no-longer exposed children. Proc Natl Acad Sci U S A 109(21):8247–8252. doi:10.1073/pnas.1200472109
26. Wykes MN, Zhou YH, Liu XQ, Good MF (2005) *Plasmodium yoelii* can ablate vaccine-induced long-term protection in mice. J Immunol 175(4):2510–2516
27. Crompton PD, Miura K, Traore B, Kayentao K, Ongoiba A, Weiss G, Doumbo S, Doumtabe D, Kone Y, Huang CY, Doumbo OK, Miller LH, Long CA, Pierce SK (2010) In vitro growth-inhibitory activity and malaria risk in a cohort study in mali. Infect Immun 78(2):737–745. doi:10.1128/IAI.00960-09
28. Chan JA, Fowkes FJ, Beeson JG (2014) Surface antigens of *Plasmodium falciparum*-infected erythrocytes as immune targets and malaria vaccine candidates. Cell Mol Life Sci 71(19):3633–3657. doi:10.1007/s00018-014-1614-3
29. Chiu CY, Healer J, Thompson JK, Chen L, Kaul A, Savergave L, Raghuwanshi A, Li Wai Suen CS, Siba PM, Schofield L, Mueller I, Cowman AF, Hansen DS (2014) Association of antibodies to *Plasmodium falciparum* reticulocyte binding protein homolog 5 with protection from clinical malaria. Front Microbiol 5:314. doi:10.3389/fmicb.2014.00314
30. Fowkes FJ, Richards JS, Simpson JA, Beeson JG (2010) The relationship between anti-merozoite antibodies and incidence of *Plasmodium falciparum* malaria: a systematic review and meta-analysis. PLoS Med 7(1), e1000218. doi:10.1371/journal.pmed.1000218
31. Tran TM, Ongoiba A, Coursen J, Crosnier C, Diouf A, Huang CY, Li S, Doumbo S, Doumtabe D, Kone Y, Bathily A, Dia S, Niangaly M, Dara C, Sangala J, Miller LH, Doumbo OK, Kayentao K, Long CA, Miura K, Wright GJ, Traore B, Crompton PD (2014) Naturally acquired antibodies specific for *Plasmodium falciparum* reticulocyte-binding protein homologue 5 inhibit parasite growth and predict protection from malaria. J Infect Dis 209(5):789–798. doi:10.1093/infdis/jit553
32. Lawton J, Brugat T, Yan YX, Reid AJ, Bohme U, Otto TD, Pain A, Jackson A, Berriman M, Cunningham D, Preiser P, Langhorne J (2012) Characterization and gene expression analysis of the cir multi-gene family of *Plasmodium chabaudi chabaudi* (AS). BMC Genomics 13:125. doi:10.1186/1471-2164-13-125
33. Yam XY, Brugat T, Siau A, Lawton J, Wong DS, Farah A, Twang JS, Gao X, Langhorne J, Preiser PR (2016) Characterization of the *Plasmodium* interspersed repeats (PIR) proteins of *Plasmodium chabaudi* indicates functional diversity. Sci Rep 6:23449. doi:10.1038/srep23449
34. Gilks CF, Walliker D, Newbold CI (1990) Relationships between sequestration, antigenic variation and chronic parasitism in *Plasmodium chabaudi chabaudi*—a rodent malaria model. Parasite Immunol 12(1):45–64
35. Bull PC, Lowe BS, Kortok M, Molyneux CS, Newbold CI, Marsh K (1998) Parasite antigens on the infected red cell surface are targets for naturally acquired immunity to malaria. Nat Med 4(3):358–360

36. Bull PC, Lowe BS, Kortok M, Marsh K (1999) Antibody recognition of *Plasmodium falciparum* erythrocyte surface antigens in Kenya: evidence for rare and prevalent variants. Infect Immun 67(2):733–739
37. Voss TS, Healer J, Marty AJ, Duffy MF, Thompson JK, Beeson JG, Reeder JC, Crabb BS, Cowman AF (2006) A var gene promoter controls allelic exclusion of virulence genes in *Plasmodium falciparum* malaria. Nature 439(7079):1004–1008. doi:10.1038/nature04407
38. Chan JA, Howell KB, Reiling L, Ataide R, Mackintosh CL, Fowkes FJ, Petter M, Chesson JM, Langer C, Warimwe GM, Duffy MF, Rogerson SJ, Bull PC, Cowman AF, Marsh K, Beeson JG (2012) Targets of antibodies against *Plasmodium falciparum*-infected erythrocytes in malaria immunity. J Clin Invest 122(9):3227–3238. doi:10.1172/JCI62182
39. Gardner MJ, Hall N, Fung E, White O, Berriman M, Hyman RW, Carlton JM, Pain A, Nelson KE, Bowman S, Paulsen IT, James K, Eisen JA, Rutherford K, Salzberg SL, Craig A, Kyes S, Chan MS, Nene V, Shallom SJ, Suh B, Peterson J, Angiuoli S, Pertea M, Allen J, Selengut J, Haft D, Mather MW, Vaidya AB, Martin DM, Fairlamb AH, Fraunholz MJ, Roos DS, Ralph SA, McFadden GI, Cummings LM, Subramanian GM, Mungall C, Venter JC, Carucci DJ, Hoffman SL, Newbold C, Davis RW, Fraser CM, Barrell B (2002) Genome sequence of the human malaria parasite *Plasmodium falciparum*. Nature 419(6906):498–511. doi:10.1038/nature01097
40. Kraemer SM, Smith JD (2003) Evidence for the importance of genetic structuring to the structural and functional specialization of the *Plasmodium falciparum* var gene family. Mol Microbiol 50(5):1527–1538
41. Jensen AT, Magistrado P, Sharp S, Joergensen L, Lavstsen T, Chiucchiuini A, Salanti A, Vestergaard LS, Lusingu JP, Hermsen R, Sauerwein R, Christensen J, Nielsen MA, Hviid L, Sutherland C, Staalsoe T, Theander TG (2004) *Plasmodium falciparum* associated with severe childhood malaria preferentially expresses PfEMP1 encoded by group A var genes. J Exp Med 199(9):1179–1190. doi:10.1084/jem.20040274
42. Kaestli M, Cockburn IA, Cortes A, Baea K, Rowe JA, Beck HP (2006) Virulence of malaria is associated with differential expression of *Plasmodium falciparum* var gene subgroups in a case–control study. J Infect Dis 193(11):1567–1574. doi:10.1086/503776
43. Kyriacou HM, Stone GN, Challis RJ, Raza A, Lyke KE, Thera MA, Kone AK, Doumbo OK, Plowe CV, Rowe JA (2006) Differential var gene transcription in *Plasmodium falciparum* isolates from patients with cerebral malaria compared to hyperparasitaemia. Mol Biochem Parasitol 150(2):211–218. doi:10.1016/j.molbiopara.2006.08.005
44. Cham GK, Turner L, Kurtis JD, Mutabingwa T, Fried M, Jensen AT, Lavstsen T, Hviid L, Duffy PE, Theander TG (2010) Hierarchical, domain type-specific acquisition of antibodies to *Plasmodium falciparum* erythrocyte membrane protein 1 in Tanzanian children. Infect Immun 78(11):4653–4659. doi:10.1128/IAI.00593-10
45. Cham GK, Turner L, Lusingu J, Vestergaard L, Mmbando BP, Kurtis JD, Jensen AT, Salanti A, Lavstsen T, Theander TG (2009) Sequential, ordered acquisition of antibodies to *Plasmodium falciparum* erythrocyte membrane protein 1 domains. J Immunol 183(5):3356–3363. doi:10.4049/jimmunol.0901331
46. Abdel-Latif MS, Dietz K, Issifou S, Kremsner PG, Klinkert MQ (2003) Antibodies to *Plasmodium falciparum* rifin proteins are associated with rapid parasite clearance and asymptomatic infections. Infect Immun 71(11):6229–6233
47. Tan J, Pieper K, Piccoli L, Abdi A, Foglierini M, Geiger R, Tully CM, Jarrossay D, Ndungu FM, Wambua J, Bejon P, Fregni CS, Fernandez-Rodriguez B, Barbieri S, Bianchi S, Marsh K, Thathy V, Corti D, Sallusto F, Bull P, Lanzavecchia A (2016) A LAIR1 insertion generates broadly reactive antibodies against malaria variant antigens. Nature 529(7584):105–109. doi:10.1038/nature16450
48. Blackman MJ, Scott-Finnigan TJ, Shai S, Holder AA (1994) Antibodies inhibit the protease-mediated processing of a malaria merozoite surface protein. J Exp Med 180(1):389–393
49. Kocken CH, Narum DL, Massougbodji A, Ayivi B, Dubbeld MA, van der Wel A, Conway DJ, Sanni A, Thomas AW (2000) Molecular characterisation of *Plasmodium reichenowi* api-

cal membrane antigen-1 (AMA-1), comparison with *P. falciparum* AMA-1, and antibody-mediated inhibition of red cell invasion. Mol Biochem Parasitol 109(2):147–156
50. O'Donnell RA, de Koning-Ward TF, Burt RA, Bockarie M, Reeder JC, Cowman AF, Crabb BS (2001) Antibodies against merozoite surface protein (MSP)-1_{19} are a major component of the invasion-inhibitory response in individuals immune to malaria. J Exp Med 193(12):1403–1412
51. Irani V, Ramsland PA, Guy AJ, Siba PM, Mueller I, Richards JS, Beeson JG (2015) Acquisition of functional antibodies that block the binding of erythrocyte-binding antigen 175 and protection against *Plasmodium falciparum* malaria in children. Clin Infect Dis 61(8):1244–1252. doi:10.1093/cid/civ525
52. Persson KE, McCallum FJ, Reiling L, Lister NA, Stubbs J, Cowman AF, Marsh K, Beeson JG (2008) Variation in use of erythrocyte invasion pathways by *Plasmodium falciparum* mediates evasion of human inhibitory antibodies. J Clin Invest 118(1):342–351. doi:10.1172/JCI32138
53. Crompton PD, Kayala MA, Traore B, Kayentao K, Ongoiba A, Weiss GE, Molina DM, Burk CR, Waisberg M, Jasinskas A, Tan X, Doumbo S, Doumtabe D, Kone Y, Narum DL, Liang X, Doumbo OK, Miller LH, Doolan DL, Baldi P, Felgner PL, Pierce SK (2010) A prospective analysis of the Ab response to *Plasmodium falciparum* before and after a malaria season by protein microarray. Proc Natl Acad Sci U S A 107(15):6958–6963. doi:10.1073/pnas.1001323107
54. Davies DH, Duffy P, Bodmer JL, Felgner PL, Doolan DL (2015) Large screen approaches to identify novel malaria vaccine candidates. Vaccine 33(52):7496–7505. doi:10.1016/j.vaccine.2015.09.059
55. Boyle MJ, Reiling L, Feng G, Langer C, Osier FH, Aspeling-Jones H, Cheng YS, Stubbs J, Tetteh KK, Conway DJ, McCarthy JS, Muller I, Marsh K, Anders RF, Beeson JG (2015) Human antibodies fix complement to inhibit *Plasmodium falciparum* invasion of erythrocytes and are associated with protection against malaria. Immunity 42(3):580–590. doi:10.1016/j.immuni.2015.02.012
56. Kennedy AT, Schmidt CQ, Thompson JK, Weiss GE, Taechalertpaisarn T, Gilson PR, Barlow PN, Crabb BS, Cowman AF, Tham WH (2016) Recruitment of factor H as a novel complement evasion strategy for blood-stage *Plasmodium falciparum* infection. J Immunol 196(3):1239–1248. doi:10.4049/jimmunol.1501581
57. Rosa TF, Flammersfeld A, Ngwa CJ, Kiesow M, Fischer R, Zipfel PF, Skerka C, Pradel G (2016) The *Plasmodium falciparum* blood stages acquire factor H family proteins to evade destruction by human complement. Cell Microbiol 18(4):573–590. doi:10.1111/cmi.12535
58. Perez-Mazliah D, Ng DH, Freitas do Rosario AP, McLaughlin S, Mastelic-Gavillet B, Sodenkamp J, Kushinga G, Langhorne J (2015) Disruption of IL-21 signaling affects T cell-B cell interactions and abrogates protective humoral immunity to malaria. PLoS Pathog 11(3), e1004715. doi:10.1371/journal.ppat.1004715
59. Su Z, Stevenson MM (2002) IL-12 is required for antibody-mediated protective immunity against blood-stage *Plasmodium chabaudi* AS malaria infection in mice. J Immunol 168(3):1348–1355
60. Mota MM, Brown KN, Holder AA, Jarra W (1998) Acute *Plasmodium chabaudi chabaudi* malaria infection induces antibodies which bind to the surfaces of parasitized erythrocytes and promote their phagocytosis by macrophages in vitro. Infect Immun 66(9):4080–4086
61. Langhorne J, Meding SJ, Eichmann K, Gillard SS (1989) The response of $CD4^+$ T cells to *Plasmodium chabaudi chabaudi*. Immunol Rev 112:71–94
62. Podoba JE, Stevenson MM (1991) $CD4^+$ and $CD8^+$ T lymphocytes both contribute to acquired immunity to blood-stage *Plasmodium chabaudi* AS. Infect Immun 59(1):51–58
63. Stevenson MM, Tam MF (1993) Differential induction of helper T cell subsets during blood-stage *Plasmodium chabaudi* AS infection in resistant and susceptible mice. Clin Exp Immunol 92(1):77–83
64. McCall MB, Sauerwein RW (2010) Interferon-gamma—central mediator of protective immune responses against the pre-erythrocytic and blood stage of malaria. J Leukoc Biol 88(6):1131–1143. doi:10.1189/jlb.0310137

65. Amante FH, Good MF (1997) Prolonged Th1-like response generated by a *Plasmodium yoelii*-specific T cell clone allows complete clearance of infection in reconstituted mice. Parasite Immunol 19(3):111–126
66. Muxel SM, Freitas do Rosario AP, Zago CA, Castillo-Mendez SI, Sardinha LR, Rodriguez-Malaga SM, Camara NO, Alvarez JM, Lima MR (2011) The spleen $CD4^{+}$ T cell response to blood-stage *Plasmodium chabaudi* malaria develops in two phases characterized by different properties. PLoS One 6(7), e22434. doi:10.1371/journal.pone.0022434
67. Jacobs P, Radzioch D, Stevenson MM (1996) In vivo regulation of nitric oxide production by tumor necrosis factor alpha and gamma interferon, but not by interleukin-4, during blood stage malaria in mice. Infect Immun 64(1):44–49
68. Stephens R, Langhorne J (2010) Effector memory Th1 CD4 T cells are maintained in a mouse model of chronic malaria. PLoS Pathog 6(11), e1001208. doi:10.1371/journal.ppat.1001208
69. Opata MM, Carpio VH, Ibitokou SA, Dillon BE, Obiero JM, Stephens R (2015) Early effector cells survive the contraction phase in malaria infection and generate both central and effector memory T cells. J Immunol 194(11):5346–5354. doi:10.4049/jimmunol.1403216
70. Achtman AH, Stephens R, Cadman ET, Harrison V, Langhorne J (2007) Malaria-specific antibody responses and parasite persistence after infection of mice with *Plasmodium chabaudi chabaudi*. Parasite Immunol 29(9):435–444. doi:10.1111/j.1365-3024.2007.00960.x
71. Perignon JL, Druilhe P (1994) Immune mechanisms underlying the premunition against *Plasmodium falciparum* malaria. Mem Inst Oswaldo Cruz 89(Suppl 2):51–53
72. Roetynck S, Olotu A, Simam J, Marsh K, Stockinger B, Urban B, Langhorne J (2013) Phenotypic and functional profiling of CD4 T cell compartment in distinct populations of healthy adults with different antigenic exposure. PLoS One 8(1), e55195. doi:10.1371/journal.pone.0055195
73. Mewono L, Matondo Maya DW, Matsiegui PB, Agnandji ST, Kendjo E, Barondi F, Issifou S, Kremsner PG, Mavoungou E (2008) Interleukin-21 is associated with IgG1 and IgG3 antibodies to erythrocyte-binding antigen-175 peptide 4 of *Plasmodium falciparum* in Gabonese children with acute falciparum malaria. Eur Cytokine Netw 19(1):30–36. doi:10.1684/ecn.2008.0114
74. Pombo DJ, Lawrence G, Hirunpetcharat C, Rzepczyk C, Bryden M, Cloonan N, Anderson K, Mahakunkijcharoen Y, Martin LB, Wilson D, Elliott S, Elliott S, Eisen DP, Weinberg JB, Saul A, Good MF (2002) Immunity to malaria after administration of ultra-low doses of red cells infected with *Plasmodium falciparum*. Lancet 360(9333):610–617. doi:10.1016/S0140-6736(02)09784-2
75. Edstein MD, Kotecka BM, Anderson KL, Pombo DJ, Kyle DE, Rieckmann KH, Good MF (2005) Lengthy antimalarial activity of atovaquone in human plasma following atovaquone-proguanil administration. Antimicrob Agents Chemother 49(10):4421–4422. doi:10.1128/AAC.49.10.4421-4422.2005
76. Roestenberg M, McCall M, Hopman J, Wiersma J, Luty AJ, van Gemert GJ, van de Vegte-Bolmer M, van Schaijk B, Teelen K, Arens T, Spaarman L, de Mast Q, Roeffen W, Snounou G, Renia L, van der Ven A, Hermsen CC, Sauerwein R (2009) Protection against a malaria challenge by sporozoite inoculation. N Engl J Med 361(5):468–477. doi:10.1056/NEJMoa0805832
77. Bijker EM, Bastiaens GJ, Teirlinck AC, van Gemert GJ, Graumans W, van de Vegte-Bolmer M, Siebelink-Stoter R, Arens T, Teelen K, Nahrendorf W, Remarque EJ, Roeffen W, Jansens A, Zimmerman D, Vos M, van Schaijk BC, Wiersma J, van der Ven AJ, de Mast Q, van Lieshout L, Verweij JJ, Hermsen CC, Scholzen A, Sauerwein RW (2013) Protection against malaria after immunization by chloroquine prophylaxis and sporozoites is mediated by preerythrocytic immunity. Proc Natl Acad Sci U S A 110(19):7862–7867. doi:10.1073/pnas.1220360110
78. Luty AJ, Lell B, Schmidt-Ott R, Lehman LG, Luckner D, Greve B, Matousek P, Herbich K, Schmid D, Migot-Nabias F, Deloron P, Nussenzweig RS, Kremsner PG (1999) Interferon-

gamma responses are associated with resistance to reinfection with *Plasmodium falciparum* in young African children. J Infect Dis 179(4):980–988. doi:10.1086/314689
79. Jagannathan P, Eccles-James I, Bowen K, Nankya F, Auma A, Wamala S, Ebusu C, Muhindo MK, Arinaitwe E, Briggs J, Greenhouse B, Tappero JW, Kamya MR, Dorsey G, Feeney ME (2014) IFNgamma/IL-10 co-producing cells dominate the CD4 response to malaria in highly exposed children. PLoS Pathog 10(1), e1003864. doi:10.1371/journal.ppat.1003864
80. Jagannathan P, Nankya F, Stoyanov C, Eccles-James I, Sikyomu E, Naluwu K, Wamala S, Nalubega M, Briggs J, Bowen K, Bigira V, Kapisi J, Kamya MR, Dorsey G, Feeney ME (2015) IFNgamma responses to pre-erythrocytic and blood-stage malaria antigens exhibit differential associations with past exposure and subsequent protection. J Infect Dis 211(12):1987–1996. doi:10.1093/infdis/jiu814
81. Boyle MJ, Jagannathan P, Bowen K, McIntyre TI, Vance HM, Farrington LA, Greenhouse B, Nankya F, Rek J, Katureebe A, Arinaitwe E, Dorsey G, Kamya MR, Feeney ME (2015) Effector phenotype of *Plasmodium falciparum*-specific $CD4^+$ T cells is influenced by both age and transmission intensity in naturally exposed populations. J Infect Dis 212(3):416–425. doi:10.1093/infdis/jiv054
82. Beattie L, Engwerda CR, Wykes M, Good MF (2006) $CD8^+$ T lymphocyte-mediated loss of marginal metallophilic macrophages following infection with *Plasmodium chabaudi chabaudi* AS. J Immunol 177(4):2518–2526
83. Hafalla JC, Cockburn IA, Zavala F (2006) Protective and pathogenic roles of $CD8^+$ T cells during malaria infection. Parasite Immunol 28(1–2):15–24. doi:10.1111/j.1365-3024.2006.00777.x
84. Suss G, Eichmann K, Kury E, Linke A, Langhorne J (1988) Roles of CD4- and CD8-bearing T lymphocytes in the immune response to the erythrocytic stages of *Plasmodium chabaudi*. Infect Immun 56(12):3081–3088
85. Imai T, Shen J, Chou B, Duan X, Tu L, Tetsutani K, Moriya C, Ishida H, Hamano S, Shimokawa C, Hisaeda H, Himeno K (2010) Involvement of $CD8^+$ T cells in protective immunity against murine blood-stage infection with *Plasmodium yoelii* 17XL strain. Eur J Immunol 40(4):1053–1061. doi:10.1002/eji.200939525
86. Imai T, Ishida H, Suzue K, Hirai M, Taniguchi T, Okada H, Suzuki T, Shimokawa C, Hisaeda H (2013) $CD8^+$ T cell activation by murine erythroblasts infected with malaria parasites. Sci Rep 3:1572. doi:10.1038/srep01572
87. Safeukui I, Gomez ND, Adelani AA, Burte F, Afolabi NK, Akondy R, Velazquez P, Holder A, Tewari R, Buffet P, Brown BJ, Shokunbi WA, Olaleye D, Sodeinde O, Kazura J, Ahmed R, Mohandas N, Fernandez-Reyes D, Haldar K (2015) Malaria induces anemia through $CD8^+$ T cell-dependent parasite clearance and erythrocyte removal in the spleen. MBio 6(1), e02493-14. doi:10.1128/mBio.02493-14
88. Horne-Debets JM, Faleiro R, Karunarathne DS, Liu XQ, Lineburg KE, Poh CM, Grotenbreg GM, Hill GR, MacDonald KP, Good MF, Renia L, Ahmed R, Sharpe AH, Wykes MN (2013) PD-1 dependent exhaustion of $CD8^+$ T cells drives chronic malaria. Cell Rep 5(5):1204–1213. doi:10.1016/j.celrep.2013.11.002
89. Cockburn IA, Zavala F (2016) Dendritic cell function and antigen presentation in malaria. Curr Opin Immunol 40:1–6. doi:10.1016/j.coi.2016.01.010
90. Wykes MN, Good MF (2008) What really happens to dendritic cells during malaria? Nat Rev Microbiol 6(11):864–870. doi:10.1038/nrmicro1988
91. Walther M, Tongren JE, Andrews L, Korbel D, King E, Fletcher H, Andersen RF, Bejon P, Thompson F, Dunachie SJ, Edele F, de Souza JB, Sinden RE, Gilbert SC, Riley EM, Hill AV (2005) Upregulation of TGF-beta, FOXP3, and $CD4^+CD25^+$ regulatory T cells correlates with more rapid parasite growth in human malaria infection. Immunity 23(3):287–296. doi:10.1016/j.immuni.2005.08.006
92. Minigo G, Woodberry T, Piera KA, Salwati E, Tjitra E, Kenangalem E, Price RN, Engwerda CR, Anstey NM, Plebanski M (2009) Parasite-dependent expansion of TNF receptor

II-positive regulatory T cells with enhanced suppressive activity in adults with severe malaria. PLoS Pathog 5(4), e1000402. doi:10.1371/journal.ppat.1000402
93. Illingworth J, Butler NS, Roetynck S, Mwacharo J, Pierce SK, Bejon P, Crompton PD, Marsh K, Ndungu FM (2013) Chronic exposure to *Plasmodium falciparum* is associated with phenotypic evidence of B and T cell exhaustion. J Immunol 190(3):1038–1047. doi:10.4049/jimmunol.1202438
94. Weiss GE, Crompton PD, Li S, Walsh LA, Moir S, Traore B, Kayentao K, Ongoiba A, Doumbo OK, Pierce SK (2009) Atypical memory B cells are greatly expanded in individuals living in a malaria-endemic area. J Immunol 183(3):2176–2182. doi:10.4049/jimmunol.0901297
95. Portugal S, Tipton CM, Sohn H, Kone Y, Wang J, Li S, Skinner J, Virtaneva K, Sturdevant DE, Porcella SF, Doumbo OK, Doumbo S, Kayentao K, Ongoiba A, Traore B, Sanz I, Pierce SK, Crompton PD (2015) Malaria-associated atypical memory B cells exhibit markedly reduced B cell receptor signaling and effector function. Elife 4, e07218. doi:10.7554/eLife.07218
96. Sullivan RT, Kim CC, Fontana MF, Feeney ME, Jagannathan P, Boyle MJ, Drakeley CJ, Ssewanyana I, Nankya F, Mayanja-Kizza H, Dorsey G, Greenhouse B (2015) FCRL5 delineates functionally impaired memory B cells associated with *Plasmodium falciparum* exposure. PLoS Pathog 11(5), e1004894. doi:10.1371/journal.ppat.1004894
97. Dauby N, Kummert C, Lecomte S, Liesnard C, Delforge ML, Donner C, Marchant A (2014) Primary human cytomegalovirus infection induces the expansion of virus-specific activated and atypical memory B cells. J Infect Dis 210(8):1275–1285. doi:10.1093/infdis/jiu255
98. Doi H, Tanoue S, Kaplan DE (2014) Peripheral CD27-CD21- B-cells represent an exhausted lymphocyte population in hepatitis C cirrhosis. Clin Immunol 150(2):184–191. doi:10.1016/j.clim.2013.12.001
99. Moir S, Ho J, Malaspina A, Wang W, DiPoto AC, O'Shea MA, Roby G, Kottilil S, Arthos J, Proschan MA, Chun TW, Fauci AS (2008) Evidence for HIV-associated B cell exhaustion in a dysfunctional memory B cell compartment in HIV-infected viremic individuals. J Exp Med 205(8):1797–1805. doi:10.1084/jem.20072683
100. Muellenbeck MF, Ueberheide B, Amulic B, Epp A, Fenyo D, Busse CE, Esen M, Theisen M, Mordmuller B, Wardemann H (2013) Atypical and classical memory B cells produce *Plasmodium falciparum* neutralizing antibodies. J Exp Med 210(2):389–399. doi:10.1084/jem.20121970
101. Achtman AH, Bull PC, Stephens R, Langhorne J (2005) Longevity of the immune response and memory to blood-stage malaria infection. Curr Top Microbiol Immunol 297:71–102
102. Weiss GE, Traore B, Kayentao K, Ongoiba A, Doumbo S, Doumtabe D, Kone Y, Dia S, Guindo A, Traore A, Huang CY, Miura K, Mircetic M, Li S, Baughman A, Narum DL, Miller LH, Doumbo OK, Pierce SK, Crompton PD (2010) The *Plasmodium falciparum*-specific human memory B cell compartment expands gradually with repeated malaria infections. PLoS Pathog 6(5), e1000912. doi:10.1371/journal.ppat.1000912
103. Achtman AH, Khan M, MacLennan IC, Langhorne J (2003) *Plasmodium chabaudi chabaudi* infection in mice induces strong B cell responses and striking but temporary changes in splenic cell distribution. J Immunol 171(1):317–324
104. Urban BC, Hien TT, Day NP, Phu NH, Roberts R, Pongponratn E, Jones M, Mai NT, Bethell D, Turner GD, Ferguson D, White NJ, Roberts DJ (2005) Fatal *Plasmodium falciparum* malaria causes specific patterns of splenic architectural disorganization. Infect Immun 73(4):1986–1994. doi:10.1128/IAI.73.4.1986-1994.2005
105. Stephens R, Ndungu FM, Langhorne J (2009) Germinal centre and marginal zone B cells expand quickly in a second *Plasmodium chabaudi* malaria infection producing mature plasma cells. Parasite Immunol 31(1):20–31. doi:10.1111/j.1365-3024.2008.01066.x
106. Portugal S, Pierce SK, Crompton PD (2013) Young lives lost as B cells falter: what we are learning about antibody responses in malaria. J Immunol 190(7):3039–3046. doi:10.4049/jimmunol.1203067
107. Carpio VH, Opata MM, Montanez ME, Banerjee PP, Dent AL, Stephens R (2015) IFN-gamma and IL-21 double producing T cells are Bcl6-independent and survive into the mem-

ory phase in *Plasmodium chabaudi* infection. PLoS One 10(12), e0144654. doi:10.1371/journal.pone.0144654

108. Ryg-Cornejo V, Ioannidis LJ, Ly A, Chiu CY, Tellier J, Hill DL, Preston SP, Pellegrini M, Yu D, Nutt SL, Kallies A, Hansen DS (2016) Severe malaria infections impair germinal center responses by inhibiting T follicular helper cell differentiation. Cell Rep 14(1):68–81. doi:10.1016/j.celrep.2015.12.006
109. Zander RA, Obeng-Adjei N, Guthmiller JJ, Kulu DI, Li J, Ongoiba A, Traore B, Crompton PD, Butler NS (2015) PD-1 co-inhibitory and OX40 co-stimulatory crosstalk regulates helper T cell differentiation and anti-*Plasmodium* humoral immunity. Cell Host Microbe 17(5):628–641. doi:10.1016/j.chom.2015.03.007
110. Wikenheiser DJ, Ghosh D, Kennedy B, Stumhofer JS (2016) The costimulatory molecule ICOS regulates host Th1 and follicular Th cell differentiation in response to *Plasmodium chabaudi chabaudi* AS infection. J Immunol 196(2):778–791. doi:10.4049/jimmunol.1403206
111. Obeng-Adjei N, Portugal S, Tran TM, Yazew TB, Skinner J, Li S, Jain A, Felgner PL, Doumbo OK, Kayentao K, Ongoiba A, Traore B, Crompton PD (2015) Circulating Th1-cell-type Tfh cells that exhibit impaired B cell help are preferentially activated during acute malaria in children. Cell Rep 13(2):425–439. doi:10.1016/j.celrep.2015.09.004
112. Morita R, Schmitt N, Bentebibel SE, Ranganathan R, Bourdery L, Zurawski G, Foucat E, Dullaers M, Oh S, Sabzghabaei N, Lavecchio EM, Punaro M, Pascual V, Banchereau J, Ueno H (2011) Human blood $CXCR5^{+}CD4^{+}$ T cells are counterparts of T follicular cells and contain specific subsets that differentially support antibody secretion. Immunity 34(1):108–121. doi:10.1016/j.immuni.2010.12.012
113. Chelimo K, Sumba PO, Kazura JW, Ofula AV, John CC (2003) Interferon-gamma responses to *Plasmodium falciparum* liver-stage antigen-1 and merozoite-surface protein-1 increase with age in children in a malaria holoendemic area of western Kenya. Malar J 2(1):37. doi:10.1186/1475-2875-2-37
114. Dent AE, Chelimo K, Sumba PO, Spring MD, Crabb BS, Moormann AM, Tisch DJ, Kazura JW (2009) Temporal stability of naturally acquired immunity to Merozoite Surface Protein-1 in Kenyan adults. Malar J 8:162. doi:10.1186/1475-2875-8-162
115. Bixby LM, Tarleton RL (2008) Stable $CD8^{+}$ T cell memory during persistent *Trypanosoma cruzi* infection. J Immunol 181(4):2644–2650
116. Colpitts SL, Dalton NM, Scott P (2009) IL-7 receptor expression provides the potential for long-term survival of both CD62Lhigh central memory T cells and Th1 effector cells during *Leishmania major* infection. J Immunol 182(9):5702–5711. doi:10.4049/jimmunol.0803450
117. Martin DL, Tarleton RL (2005) Antigen-specific T cells maintain an effector memory phenotype during persistent *Trypanosoma cruzi* infection. J Immunol 174(3):1594–1601
118. Zaph C, Uzonna J, Beverley SM, Scott P (2004) Central memory T cells mediate long-term immunity to *Leishmania major* in the absence of persistent parasites. Nat Med 10(10):1104–1110. doi:10.1038/nm1108
119. Peters NC, Pagan AJ, Lawyer PG, Hand TW, Henrique Roma E, Stamper LW, Romano A, Sacks DL (2014) Chronic parasitic infection maintains high frequencies of short-lived $Ly6C^{+}CD4^{+}$ effector T cells that are required for protection against re-infection. PLoS Pathog 10(12), e1004538. doi:10.1371/journal.ppat.1004538
120. Freitas do Rosario AP, Muxel SM, Rodriguez-Malaga SM, Sardinha LR, Zago CA, Castillo-Mendez SI, Alvarez JM, D'Imperio Lima MR (2008) Gradual decline in malaria-specific memory T cell responses leads to failure to maintain long-term protective immunity to *Plasmodium chabaudi* AS despite persistence of B cell memory and circulating antibody. J Immunol 181(12):8344–8355
121. Wipasa J, Okell L, Sakkhachornphop S, Suphavilai C, Chawansuntati K, Liewsaree W, Hafalla JC, Riley EM (2011) Short-lived IFN-gamma effector responses, but long-lived

IL-10 memory responses, to malaria in an area of low malaria endemicity. PLoS Pathog 7(2), e1001281. doi:10.1371/journal.ppat.1001281
122. Dong H, Zhu G, Tamada K, Chen L (1999) B7-H1, a third member of the B7 family, co-stimulates T-cell proliferation and interleukin-10 secretion. Nat Med 5(12):1365–1369. doi:10.1038/70932
123. Freeman GJ, Long AJ, Iwai Y, Bourque K, Chernova T, Nishimura H, Fitz LJ, Malenkovich N, Okazaki T, Byrne MC, Horton HF, Fouser L, Carter L, Ling V, Bowman MR, Carreno BM, Collins M, Wood CR, Honjo T (2000) Engagement of the PD-1 immunoinhibitory receptor by a novel B7 family member leads to negative regulation of lymphocyte activation. J Exp Med 192(7):1027–1034
124. Latchman Y, Wood CR, Chernova T, Chaudhary D, Borde M, Chernova I, Iwai Y, Long AJ, Brown JA, Nunes R, Greenfield EA, Bourque K, Boussiotis VA, Carter LL, Carreno BM, Malenkovich N, Nishimura H, Okazaki T, Honjo T, Sharpe AH, Freeman GJ (2001) PD-L2 is a second ligand for PD-1 and inhibits T cell activation. Nat Immunol 2(3):261–268. doi:10.1038/85330
125. Tseng SY, Otsuji M, Gorski K, Huang X, Slansky JE, Pai SI, Shalabi A, Shin T, Pardoll DM, Tsuchiya H (2001) B7-DC, a new dendritic cell molecule with potent costimulatory properties for T cells. J Exp Med 193(7):839–846
126. Sharpe AH, Wherry EJ, Ahmed R, Freeman GJ (2007) The function of programmed cell death 1 and its ligands in regulating autoimmunity and infection. Nat Immunol 8(3):239–245. doi:10.1038/ni1443
127. Chandele A, Mukerjee P, Das G, Ahmed R, Chauhan VS (2011) Phenotypic and functional profiling of malaria-induced CD8 and CD4 T cells during blood-stage infection with *Plasmodium yoelii*. Immunology 132(2):273–286. doi:10.1111/j.1365-2567.2010.03363.x
128. Stephens R, Seddon B, Langhorne J (2011) Homeostatic proliferation and IL-7R alpha expression do not correlate with enhanced T cell proliferation and protection in chronic mouse malaria. PLoS One 6(10), e26686. doi:10.1371/journal.pone.0026686
129. Butler NS, Moebius J, Pewe LL, Traore B, Doumbo OK, Tygrett LT, Waldschmidt TJ, Crompton PD, Harty JT (2012) Therapeutic blockade of PD-L1 and LAG-3 rapidly clears established blood-stage *Plasmodium* infection. Nat Immunol 13(2):188–195. doi:10.1038/ni.2180
130. Rts SCTP (2015) Efficacy and safety of RTS, S/AS01 malaria vaccine with or without a booster dose in infants and children in Africa: final results of a phase 3, individually randomised, controlled trial. Lancet 386(9988):31–45. doi:10.1016/S0140-6736(15)60721-8
131. Rts SCTP, Agnandji ST, Lell B, Fernandes JF, Abossolo BP, Methogo BG, Kabwende AL, Adegnika AA, Mordmuller B, Issifou S, Kremsner PG, Sacarlal J, Aide P, Lanaspa M, Aponte JJ, Machevo S, Acacio S, Bulo H, Sigauque B, Macete E, Alonso P, Abdulla S, Salim N, Minja R, Mpina M, Ahmed S, Ali AM, Mtoro AT, Hamad AS, Mutani P, Tanner M, Tinto H, D'Alessandro U, Sorgho H, Valea I, Bihoun B, Guiraud I, Kabore B, Sombie O, Guiguemde RT, Ouedraogo JB, Hamel MJ, Kariuki S, Oneko M, Odero C, Otieno K, Awino N, McMorrow M, Muturi-Kioi V, Laserson KF, Slutsker L, Otieno W, Otieno L, Otsyula N, Gondi S, Otieno A, Owira V, Oguk E, Odongo G, Woods JB, Ogutu B, Njuguna P, Chilengi R, Akoo P, Kerubo C, Maingi C, Lang T, Olotu A, Bejon P, Marsh K, Mwambingu G, Owusu-Agyei S, Asante KP, Osei-Kwakye K, Boahen O, Dosoo D, Asante I, Adjei G, Kwara E, Chandramohan D, Greenwood B, Lusingu J, Gesase S, Malabeja A, Abdul O, Mahende C, Liheluka E, Malle L, Lemnge M, Theander TG, Drakeley C, Ansong D, Agbenyega T, Adjei S, Boateng HO, Rettig T, Bawa J, Sylverken J, Sambian D, Sarfo A, Agyekum A, Martinson F, Hoffman I, Mvalo T, Kamthunzi P, Nkomo R, Tembo T, Tegha G, Tsidya M, Kilembe J, Chawinga C, Ballou WR, Cohen J, Guerra Y, Jongert E, Lapierre D, Leach A, Lievens M, Ofori-Anyinam O, Olivier A, Vekemans J, Carter T, Kaslow D, Leboulleux D, Loucq C, Radford A, Savarese B, Schellenberg D, Sillman M, Vansadia P (2012) A phase 3 trial of RTS, S/AS01 malaria vaccine in African infants. N Engl J Med 367(24):2284–2295. doi:10.1056/NEJMoa1208394

Pathogenetic Immune Responses in Cerebral Malaria

Georges Emile Raymond Grau and Samuel Crocodile Wassmer

Contents

1 Introduction 67
2 Innate Immune Responses and CM 68
3 Adaptive Immunity: T Cell Dependency of CM 70
4 Antigen-Presenting Cells (APCs): Monocytes, DC, DC Subsets 72
5 Antigen Processing, Co-stimulation and Cross Presentation 73
6 Endothelial Cells as APC 74
7 MPs as Amplifiers of Pathology 76
8 Concluding Remarks 76
References 77

1 Introduction

In addition to parasite-induced pathology, a large body of evidence indicates that the host immune response to parasitic infection can also play an essential role in cerebral malaria (CM) pathogenesis [1, 2]. Involvement of the cells and soluble mediators of the immune system has been widely recognised as contributing to the complications of viral, bacterial, fungal and parasitic infections. It would be extraordinary if malaria did not conform to this general pattern [3]. Activation of both

G.E.R. Grau (✉)
Vascular Immunology Unit, Department of Pathology, School of Medical Sciences and Marie Bashir Institute, University of Sydney, Camperdown, NSW, Australia
e-mail: ggrau@med.usyd.edu.au

S.C. Wassmer
Vascular Immunology Unit, Department of Pathology, School of Medical Sciences and Marie Bashir Institute, University of Sydney, Camperdown, NSW, Australia

Department of Immunology and Infection, London School of Hygiene and Tropical Medicine, London, UK

M.M. Mota, A. Rodriguez (eds.), *Malaria*, DOI 10.1007/978-3-319-45210-4_4

innate and adaptive immune responses has long been suspected to play a deleterious role in the development of CM. Notably for the latter, the activation of both CD4+ and CD8+ T lymphocytes is essential for the disease process in experimental CM, with CD8+ T cells accumulating in the cerebral microcirculation [4].

Numerous factors make it challenging to identify the essential steps in the pathogenic process. For example, in malaria-endemic areas, it may be next to impossible to discriminate the effects of co-morbidities. Furthermore, CM may not be a single entity but a group of similar syndromes [5]. Lastly, the variation in clinical presentation between adults from Southeast Asia and African children with CM is likely to be caused by a different immune status, potentially resulting from different exposure levels [6]. The pathogenesis of CM is thus multifactorial, which has made understanding the mechanisms underpinning this syndrome difficult and has contributed to our lack of development of effective adjunct treatments [7].

In this chapter, we review the evidence of immune responses that have pathogenetic consequences in malaria, with particular attention to the neurological syndrome. Several features of experimental models for CM have been critically reviewed, notably the model of *P. berghei* ANKA (PbA) infection in CBA or C57BL/6 mice, referred to as experimental cerebral malaria (ECM) below [8]. Among these features, the existence of sequestration [9], and the complexity of effector mechanisms, has been addressed [10, 11].

2 Innate Immune Responses and CM

The activation of innate immune cells and consequent systemic inflammation lead to the early signs and symptoms in malaria infection and contribute to the development of more severe forms of the disease, including CM. During schizogony, the simultaneous rupture of *P. falciparum*-infected erythrocytes (IEs) leads to the release of parasite-derived components, which in turn trigger a deleterious activation of the innate immune system. This activation involves pathogen-associated molecular patterns (PAMPs) and host damage-associated molecular patterns (DAMPs). In recent years, considerable advances have been made in the identification of molecules belonging to both patterns, which are reviewed in [12]. PAMPs are microbial structures that are abnormally abundant in specific pathogens and are detected by pattern recognition receptors (PRRs) of innate immune cells. PRRs are a primitive part of the innate immune system and include the large families of membrane-bound Toll-like receptors [13] as well as cytoplasmic nucleotide-binding oligomerisation domain (NOD)-like receptors [14]. The main PAMPs in *P. falciparum* are glycophosphatidylinositol (GPI) anchors, haemozoin and immune stimulatory nucleic acid motifs. GPI anchors have been shown to induce a strong response from macrophages, leading to the production of pro-inflammatory mediators, including tumour necrosis factor (TNF) [15] and nitric oxide [16]. Haemozoin, a by-product crystal of the parasite metabolism, elicits a similar effect in dendritic cells (DCs) and macrophages through an activation of the inflammasome, as well as the cleavage of pro-IL-1beta and the activation of caspase-1 [17, 18]. Lastly, released plasmodial DNA

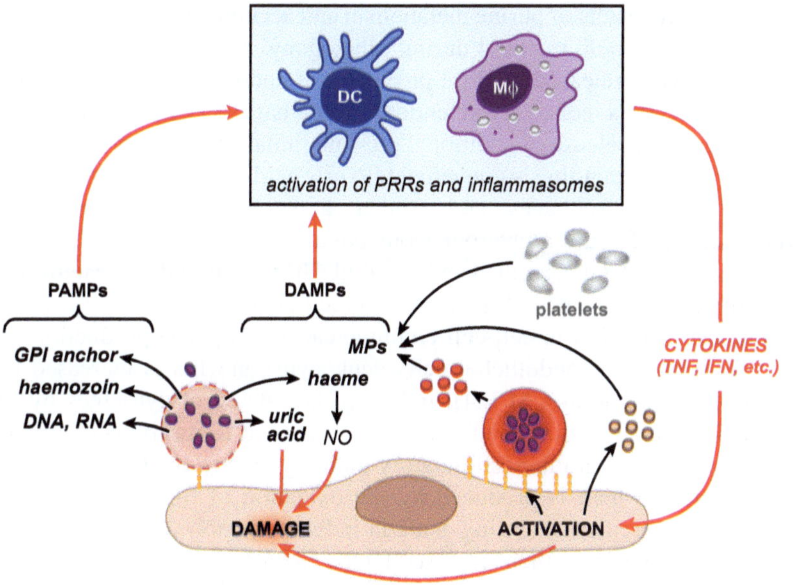

Fig. 1 Innate immune response processes potentially contributing to CM lesions. During schizogony, the plasma membrane of *Plasmodium falciparum*-infected erythrocytes (IEs) ruptures to liberate merozoites in the bloodstream. This process leads to the release of both parasite-derived factors (pathogen-associated molecular patterns or PAMPs), which include GPI anchor, haemozoin and nucleic acids, and host-derived factors (host damage-associated molecular patterns or DAMPs), such as haem and uric acid. When released in close proximity to the endothelium, the latter products can have a direct and deleterious effect on endothelial cells, participating in the microvascular dysfunction in CM. After phagocytosis, both PAMPs and DAMPs can elicit a strong stimulation of dendritic cells (DCs) and macrophages (Mϕ) through the activation of their pattern recognition receptors (PRRs) and inflammasome, resulting in the secretion of pro-inflammatory cytokines such as TNF and IFNs. Microvascular endothelial cells are activated by these cytokines, leading to an upregulation of their surface adhesion molecules and IE receptors, thereby contributing to their sequestration in CM. In addition, microparticles produced by IEs, leukocytes (not shown), platelets and activated endothelial cells during malaria infection are suspected to act as DAMPs and to amplify the DCs and macrophage stimulation and the consequent endothelial activation, which can cause endothelial damage, a key feature of CM pathogenesis

and RNA have also been demonstrated to activate PRRs, prompting a cascade of intracellular signalling through the phagolysosome of DCs and macrophages and leading to an increase in pro-inflammatory cytokine and type I interferon production [12]. The overproduction of pro-inflammatory cytokines has long been suspected to play a crucial role in the development of CM, especially via the upregulation of endothelial receptors for IEs and the alteration of the blood-brain barrier (BBB) due to the opening of the endothelial tight junctions [10, 19] (Fig. 1).

The host DAMPs, which are released from damaged cells as a result of malarial infection, may also contribute to the pathogenesis of CM by activating the PRRs and inflammasomes independently from and in addition to the PAMPs [20]. Malaria-associated DAMPs include uric acid, microparticles and haem. Uric acid and hypoxanthine are results of purine metabolism and accumulate in IEs during malaria infection. They are both released during schizogony, which has two inflammatory effects. First, when released in close proximity of endothelial cells by sequestered IEs, uric acid crystals induce severe endothelial damage [21], potentially increasing the response by the release of additional pro-inflammatory mediators. Second, once in circulation, hypoxanthine is converted into uric acid and urate crystals, which are recognised by macrophages and trigger a strong inflammatory response. Microparticles (MPs) are a heterogeneous population of plasma membrane extra-cellular vesicles that are generated and released when tissue and/or systemic homeostasis is disrupted [2]. These MPs have emerged as important biological effectors with demonstrated roles in cell-cell communication [22]. The production of MPs derived from platelets, endothelial cells, leukocytes and IEs is increased in both paediatric [23] and adult CM [24], inducing the release of cytokines by macrophages and the upregulation of adhesion molecules and IE receptors on endothelial cells [25, 26] through immunostimulatory pathways yet to be determined. A third DAMP is haem, which is produced by the oxidation of free haemoglobin once released in the circulation during malaria-induced hemolysis. The formation of reactive oxygen species is then catalysed by the haem moiety, resulting in oxidative stress, endothelial activation and microvascular damage through activation of PRRs in ECM [27] (Fig. 1).

3 Adaptive Immunity: T Cell Dependency of CM

Originally identified in a mouse model for CM, the requirement for T cells in the pathogenesis of the neurological syndrome has also been documented in the human disease, as reviewed in [7]. Similarities and differences between human and murine syndromes have been discussed [7]. Further analyses of the molecular mechanisms leading to T cell accumulation in brain microvessels include the identification of CCR5 as an important receptor, as the incidence of neurological signs is significantly reduced in CCR5 gene knockout (GKO) mice [28]. Additionally, the lymphotoxin beta receptor [29] and IP-10 [30] also play a crucial role in this intravascular arrest.

On the $CD8^+$ T cell, molecules such as perforin or granzyme B (GzmB) [31] appear to be important in promoting cerebral disease. GzmB-deficient mice are protected from CM and show lower parasite sequestration in the brain, as a consequence of enhanced antiparasitic $CD4^+$ T cell responses. The authors of the study outlined the importance of antigen-specific $CD8^+$ T cell, which could trigger CM upon adoptive transfer in CM-resistant (CM-R) mice. Upon infection, the numbers of PbA-specific $CD8^+$ T cells increase in CM-susceptible more than in CM-R mice. In wild-type mice, full activation of brain-recruited $CD8^+$ T cells also depends on a critical number of parasites in this tissue, which, in turn, is sustained by these tissue-recruited cells. Thus, an interdependent relationship between parasite burden and $CD8^+$ T cells dictates the onset of perforin/GzmB-mediated ECM. In PbA infection, there is a dramatic primary parasite-specific CTL response, reaching approximately

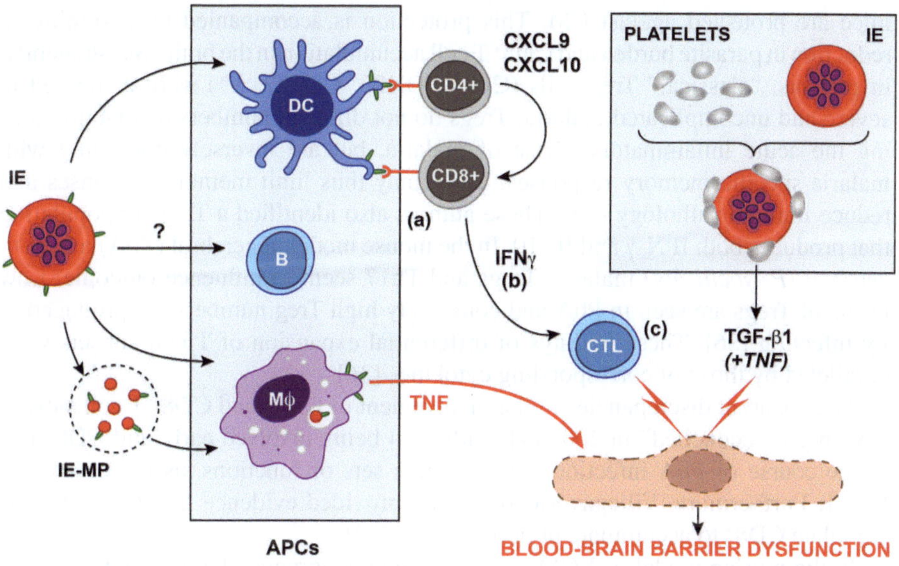

Fig. 2 Adaptive immune response mechanisms involved in the development of CM. After invasion by *P. falciparum* merozoites, infected erythrocytes (IEs) undergo plasma membrane modification and display parasite-expressed antigens, including *Plasmodium falciparum* erythrocyte membrane protein 1 (PfEMP-1). After IEs or their microparticles (IE-MPs) are recognised, they are phagocytosed by dendritic cells (DC) and macrophages (Mϕ), and parasite antigens are presented to CD4⁺ T cells by their major histocompatibility class (MHC) I. Concomitantly, stimulated macrophages secrete high levels of tumour necrosis factor (TNF), leading to the activation of endothelial cells locally. Once activated by antigen-presenting cells (APCs), CD4⁺ T cells recruit CD8⁺ T cells through the release of CXCL9 and CXCL10, resulting in (**a**) their activation by APCs via MHC II, (**b**) the secretion of gamma interferon (IFN-γ) and (**c**) the maturation of CD8⁺ T cells into cytotoxic T lymphocytes (CTLs). Lastly, platelets can be activated by contact with IEs, potentially leading to the formation of clumps but also to the release of TGFβ1 after degranulation, which acts in synergy with TNF to induce endothelial apoptosis and alter the blood-brain barrier

30 % of splenic CD81⁺ T cells, with many producing interferon gamma (IFN-γ) and TNF. These cells express GzmB and other markers of specific responders, are cytolytic, and react to a broad array of major histocompatibility complex (MHC) I-restricted epitopes, five of which have been identified so far. Vigorous CTL responses can therefore be induced against pathogens even when they largely reside in red blood cells, which lack MHC I processing machinery [32] (Fig. 2).

Among the newly elucidated cytokines that are instrumental in T cell-dependent pathology during CM, IL-33 and its receptor ST2 play a crucial role. Brain IL-33 is upregulated during CM, and ST2-deficient mice are resistant to PbA-induced neuropathology [33].

Aside from pathogenic T cells, regulatory subsets have been thought to counteract the development of pathology. Regulatory T (Treg) cells were first studied in CM by Amante et al. [34], who found paradoxically that these cells could contribute to pathology in the murine model. When depleted of Treg cells by anti-CD25 mAb, mice are protected against CM. This protection is accompanied by a significant reduction in parasite burden and $CD8^+$ T cell accumulation in the brain. Subsequently, in patients, "classical" Treg cells ($CD4^+$ $FOXP3^+$ $CD127^{-/low}$) were compared in severe and uncomplicated malaria. Tregs do not differ in numbers or function during the acute inflammatory phase of malaria, but are inversely correlated with malaria-specific memory responses. Tregs may thus limit memory responses and reduce immunopathology [35]. These authors also identified a Treg subpopulation that produces both IFN-γ and IL-10. In the mouse model of cerebral (PbA) and non-cerebral (*P. yoelii*, Py) malaria, Tregs and Th17 seem to influence outcome. Low levels of Tregs are seen in PbA and conversely high Treg numbers are produced in Py infection [36]. These findings of differential expansion of T cell subsets were paralleled by those of corresponding cytokines [36].

The apparent discrepancies in the involvement of $CD4^+$ and $CD8^+$ T cell subsets have been "reconciled" in 2003 [4], with CD4 being involved early and $CD8^+$ late in the course of PbA infection, with discrete sets of functions, as represented in Fig. 1. Furthermore, Villegas-Mendez et al. provided evidence that $CD4^+$ T cells stimulate $CD8^+$ to accumulate in brain vessels [37].

In the murine model of ECM at least, a time congruency between $CD8^+$ T cell activation and the rise of parasitaemia is needed for the neurological syndrome to develop [38]. Most interestingly, it was found recently that $CD8^+$ T cells accumulate in perivascular spaces but do not seem to trigger endothelial cell apoptosis [39]. It is in fact the majority of T cells that are compartmentalised to the perivascular side of the blood vessels during both PbA and Pb NK65 infections. These perivascular T cells form stable interactions with $CX3CR1^+$/GFP cells, i.e. subsets of monocytes, macrophages and DCs, and all microglia. Contrary to pre-existing hypotheses, these $CX3CR1^+$ cells are not required for CM development, and $CD8^+$ T cells do not cause significant endothelial apoptosis, at least not enough to cause the opening of the blood-brain barrier (BBB) seen in CM. Brain endothelial apoptosis is thus as rare in the PbA model as it is in the human disease [40].

The importance of cytokine overproduction [3, 41, 42] in CM has recently been corroborated by the demonstration that induction of pro-inflammatory cytokines by CpG oligonucleotides in CM-resistant BALB/c mice triggers CM. This reversal of susceptibility to CM is not seen in IFN-γ and IL-12 GKO mice, further highlighting the importance of these pathways [43].

4 Antigen-Presenting Cells (APCs): Monocytes, DC, DC Subsets

Immunosuppression induced by malarial infection had been foreseen in the early sixties by McGregor and Barr [44] and confirmed by numerous studies [45–47]. Seminal works by Urban et al., aiming at a better understanding of the obstacles in the development of protective immunity, have demonstrated that IEs can adhere to DCs in vitro and lead to a suppression of their functions [48]. Several subpopulations of migratory and lymphoid organ resident DCs have been described, with discrete roles for each in antigen presentation in vivo. In inflammatory conditions, the antigen presentation abilities of DCs can be severely impaired, but an additional population of monocyte-derived DCs then comes into play [49].

In the context of malaria, it has been shown that blood-stage infection leads to suppression of major histocompatibility (MHC) class I-restricted immunity to third-party (non-malarial) antigens as a consequence of systemic DC activation. In the *P. berghei* model, while *P. berghei*-expressed antigens are presented early in infection, presentation declines rapidly within 4 days, paralleling impairment in MHC class I- and II-restricted presentation of third-party antigens. Thus, *P. berghei* not only causes immunosuppression to subsequently encountered third-party antigens but also rapidly limits the capacity to generate effective parasite-specific immunity [50]. DCs do express C-type lectin receptors (CLRs), a family of pattern recognition receptors that recognise carbohydrate structures on pathogens and self-antigens. The DC immuno-receptor (DCIR) plays an important role in CM development: DCIR-/- mice are protected against the neurological syndrome and show markedly reduced brain inflammation and $CD8^+$ T cell sequestration, as well as decreased circulating TNF levels [51]. Equally important for CM development is the pro-inflammatory $Ly6C^{high}$ monocyte subset [52]. Depletion of this cell subset, using anti-CCR2 mAb, decreases IFN-γ levels and $IFN\text{-}\gamma^+CD8^+$ T effector cells in the brain. Interestingly, anti-CCR2 mAb injection does not prevent the generation of PbTg-specific T cell responses in the periphery. It is not plasmacytoid DCs but "conventional" DCs that seem to be the most critical APCs in CM [53]. This study also reemphasises the need for $CD4^+$ activation in CM prior to that of $CD8^+$ T cells.

Among other potential APCs, B cells have only been recently analysed in CM [54], and a modulatory role for regulatory B (Breg) cells has been demonstrated [55]. Adoptive transfer of IL-10-producing Breg cells to *P. berghei*-infected mice significantly reduces the brain accumulation of NK and $CD8^+$ T cells and cerebral haemorrhages. In contrast, adoptive transfer of $CD4^+$ $CD25^+$ Treg cells fails to prevent CM in infected mice. It is conceivable that the discrete roles of DC subsets described in the context of a viral infection are also at work in CM [56].

5 Antigen Processing, Co-stimulation and Cross Presentation

After antigens are picked up by APCs, they need to undergo a complex path of intracellular trafficking before they are loaded in MHC molecules, as detailed in Sollid and Villadangos [57]. Antigens must be trafficking via specific pathways before accessing MHC loading compartments. For MHC class I, cross presentation involves antigen trafficking to a specialised compartment. The features of this compartment and how it is accessed by different mechanisms of antigen capture and internalisation have been reviewed elsewhere [58].

Cross presentation is the process whereby exogenous antigens are presented via, or on, MHC class I molecules. It is essential for the induction of $CD8^+$ T cell responses and is carried out by specialised DC subsets [59]. While the mechanisms involved are incompletely understood, antigens can be transported by endocytic receptors, such as the mannose receptor (MR), into early endosomes in which the cross presentation machinery would be recruited. In these endosomal compartments, peptides would be trimmed by the aminopeptidase IRAP before loading onto MHC class I molecules. In vivo, cross presentation has been found to be impaired in monocyte-derived DC deficient in IRAP or MR, confirming the role of these two molecules in inflammatory DC [59].

Cross presentation might also have bearings on immunosuppression and even immune tolerance. Indeed, it has been shown that PbA infection in mice inhibits cross priming. Reduced cross priming is a consequence of downregulation of cross presentation by activated DCs due to systemic activation that do not otherwise globally inhibit T cell proliferation [60]. Furthermore, $CD8^+$ T cell tolerance can be mediated by the entry of exogenous antigen into the MHC class I-restricted cross presentation pathway. DCs appear to be the key cross presenting cells and are thought to carry specialised machinery dedicated to this purpose [61].

6 Endothelial Cells as APC

The classical immune response occurring within the microvessels involves IEs, DCs and T lymphocytes. Naturally, the close proximity of these cells to brain endothelial cells during sequestration may facilitate additional malaria antigen exchange sites, potentially leading to further T cell activation. This has been the subject of controversy, as summarised in [62] (Fig. 3). Endothelial cells are central in inflammation [63, 64], and there is compelling evidence for their capacity to act as semi-professional APCs—as originally shown by Male and colleagues [65]—in a variety of autoimmune diseases [66–68], even in settings involving sparse sequestration of lymphocytes in microvessels, as is the case in human CM, rheumatoid arthritis or multiple sclerosis. However, a recent histopathological study performed in Malawi showed that paediatric cases with autopsy-confirmed CM have significantly higher numbers of intravascular monocytes than children with non-malarial causes of coma, supporting the hypothesis that inflammation contributes to the pathogenesis of paediatric CM. This monocyte accumulation was significantly (>twofold) greater in HIV-positive patients [69], which indicates that immune dysregulation in HIV-positive children exacerbates the pathological features associated with CM.

Antigen-presenting functions have been described in ECM, where brain endothelial cells have the ability to capture and present antigens [70]. In addition, a conceptual link between APC function and CM pathogenesis is provided by IP-10/CXCL10, a chemokine involved both in antigen presentation [71] and in the development of neurologic syndrome in mice [72]. Brain endothelial cells can transfer antigens from IE onto their own surface in vitro [73], thereby potentially becoming a target for $CD8^+$ cytotoxic T lymphocytes (CTL), potentially leading to endothelial damage (Fig. 3) and a compromised BBB.

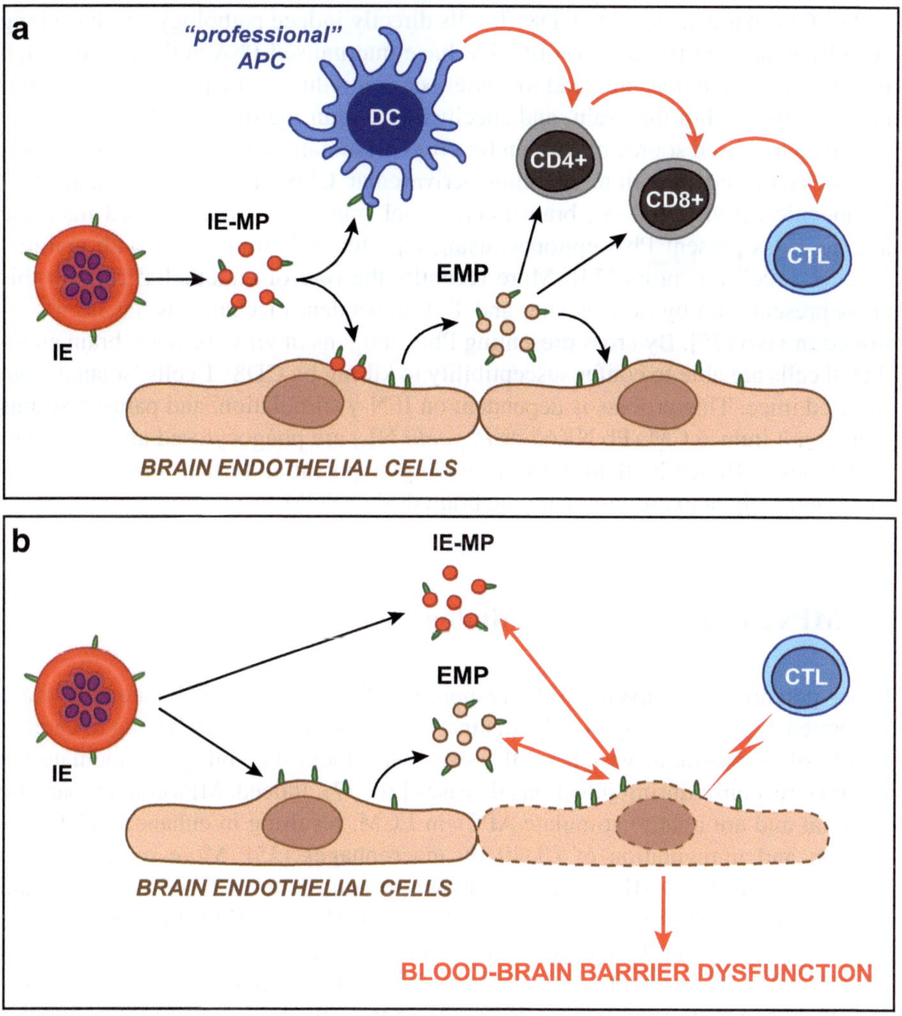

Fig. 3 The role of endothelial cells as antigen-presenting cells in the development of CM. *P. falciparum*-infected erythrocytes (IEs) produce parasite epitope-bearing microparticles (IE-MPs), which can amplify the stimulation of antigen-resenting cells (APCs), and the resulting immune cascade described in Fig. 2, which culminates in the activation of cytotoxic T lymphocytes (CTLs). IE-MPs can also bind and transfer their parasite antigens to the surface of endothelial cells. When stimulated by TNF, endothelial cells produce high numbers of microparticles (EMPs), which may carry the transferred parasite antigen and could (**a**) amplify the stimulation of other APCs and increase the immuno-stimulation of CD4$^+$ T cells, CD8$^+$ T cells and CTLs and (**b**) participate in the propagation of the parasite antigen to other endothelial cells (**a**). These are then presented on MHC I and MHC II molecules of TNF-stimulated endothelial cells, with the former marking them as targets for destruction by activated malaria specific CTLs. This contributes to the BBB damage and the pathogenesis of CM (**b**)

In ECM, parasite-specific $CD8^+$ T cells directly induce pathology and have long been hypothesised to kill brain EC that have internalised PbA antigens. Although PbA sequestration does not lead to vessel occlusion during the pathology, accumulation of IEs within the brain, and specifically within the perivascular space, may provide a localised source of antigen for cross presentation by endothelial or associated cells during infection, enabling perivascular $CD8^+$ T cells to mediate their pathogenic activity. Indeed, brain microvessel fragments from infected mice are able to cross present PbA epitopes, using reporter cells transduced with epitope-specific T cell receptors [74]. More recently, the role of endothelial cells in this cross presentation by proteasome- and TAP-dependent mechanisms has been confirmed in vivo [75]. By cross presenting PbA antigens in vitro, primary brain endothelial cells are able to confer susceptibility to killing by $CD8^+$ T cells isolated from infected mice. This process is dependent on IFN-γ stimulation, and parasite strains that do not induce CM (Pb NK65 or *P. yoelii* NL) are phagocytosed and cross presented less efficiently than PbA, providing a potential further mechanism for increased antigen expression with the brain during ECM.

7 MPs as Amplifiers of Pathology

Other potential participants in the response to Plasmodia are MPs, notably those generated by IEs. Although totally distinct from exosomes, which belong to another family of extracellular vesicles, MPs share with them the ability to modulate the immune response during infectious diseases [76, 77]. Indeed, MPs contain parasite material and are able to stimulate APCs in ECM, resulting in enhanced TNF production and upregulation of CD40 by macrophages [25]. More recently, brain endothelium-derived MPs have been shown to contribute to T cell activation and proliferation, in an in vitro human model of the CM lesion [78] (Fig. 3). Thus, the possibility of an endothelial presentation of malaria antigens to cognate T cells has established brain endothelial cells and potentially endothelium-derived MPs as critical players in malaria pathogenesis [2, 79]. Finally, the intricacy of several effector mechanisms of the pathogenetic immune responses in CM has been detailed elsewhere, with a focus on the role of MPs. These can assist the binding of infected erythrocytes to the cerebral vasculature as well as mediate and disseminate various inflammatory and immune processes [80–82].

8 Concluding Remarks

More than 120 years after the discovery of *P. falciparum*, the fundamental pathogenesis of fatal CM is still not well understood. Collaborative and multidisciplinary approaches using clinical samples from field sites in endemic areas, in vitro and ex vivo models as well as animal models of the disease are necessary to decipher its pathogenetic immune responses. Indeed, due to the lack of specific neuro- and vasculo-protective therapies, treatments for CM are currently still precariously limited to antimalarial drugs and emergency supportive care. The former are quickly dwindling, as the resistance of *P. falciparum* malaria against artemisinin combination treatments (ACTs) - the recommended first-line therapy for infected patients, is - on the rise in Southeast Asia. This is alarming because (1) resistance to the previous mainstays of antimalarial treatment—namely, chloroquine and sulfadoxine/pyrimethamine—has already spread across Southeast Asia into Africa, resulting in the deaths of millions of children, and (2) there are currently no alternative drugs to replace ACTs. A better understanding of the precise mechanisms underlying the development of CM is urgently needed to guide new adjunctive treatments directed towards its major immuno-pathogenetic processes.

References

1. Engwerda CR, Good MF (2005) Interactions between malaria parasites and the host immune system. Curr Opin Immunol 17(4):381–387
2. Combes V et al (2010) Microvesiculation and cell interactions at the brain-endothelial interface in cerebral malaria pathogenesis. Prog Neurobiol 91(2):140–151
3. Grau GE, Hunt NH (2014) Cytokines and some of their effector mechanisms in cerebral malaria pathogenesis. In: Kremsner PG, Hommel M, Krishna S (eds) Encyclopedia of malaria. Springer, New York, pp 1–11
4. Hunt NH, Grau GE (2003) Cytokines: accelerators and brakes in the pathogenesis of cerebral malaria. Trends Immunol 24(9):491–499
5. Idro R, Marsh K, John CC, Newton CR (2010) Cerebral malaria: mechanisms of brain injury and strategies for improved neurocognitive outcome. Pediatr Res 68(4):267–274
6. Wassmer SC et al (2015) Investigating the pathogenesis of severe malaria: a multidisciplinary and cross-geographical approach. Am J Trop Med Hyg 93(3 Suppl):42–56
7. Grau GE, Craig AG (2012) Cerebral malaria pathogenesis: revisiting parasite and host contributions. Future Microbiol 7:291–302
8. Combes V, De Souza JB, Renia L, Hunt NH, Grau GE (2005) Cerebral malaria: which parasite? Which model? Drug Discov Today Dis Models 2:141–148
9. Hearn J, Rayment N, Landon DN, Katz DR, de Souza JB (2000) Immunopathology of cerebral malaria: morphological evidence of parasite sequestration in murine brain microvasculature. Infect Immun 68(9):5364–5376
10. Coltel N, Combes V, Wassmer SC, Chimini G, Grau GE (2006) Cell vesiculation and immunopathology: implications in cerebral malaria. Microbes Infect 8(8):2305–2316
11. Schofield L, Grau GE (2005) Immunological processes in malaria pathogenesis. Nat Rev Immunol 5(9):722–735
12. Gazzinelli RT, Kalantari P, Fitzgerald KA, Golenbock DT (2014) Innate sensing of malaria parasites. Nat Rev Immunol 14(11):744–757
13. O'Neill LA, Golenbock D, Bowie AG (2013) The history of Toll-like receptors—redefining innate immunity. Nat Rev Immunol 13(6):453–460
14. Franchi L, Warner N, Viani K, Nunez G (2009) Function of Nod-like receptors in microbial recognition and host defense. Immunol Rev 227(1):106–128
15. Schofield L, Hackett F (1993) Signal transduction in host cells by a glycosylphosphatidylinositol toxin of malaria parasites. J Exp Med 177(1):145–153

16. Tachado SD et al (1996) Glycosylphosphatidylinositol toxin of *Plasmodium* induces nitric oxide synthase expression in macrophages and vascular endothelial cells by a protein tyrosine kinase-dependent and protein kinase C-dependent signaling pathway. J Immunol 156(5):1897–1907
17. Shio MT et al (2009) Malarial hemozoin activates the NLRP3 inflammasome through Lyn and Syk kinases. PLoS Pathog 5(8), e1000559
18. Dostert C et al (2009) Malarial hemozoin is a Nalp3 inflammasome activating danger signal. PLoS One 4(8), e6510
19. Wassmer SC, Combes V, Grau GE (2003) Pathophysiology of cerebral malaria: role of host cells in the modulation of cytoadhesion. Ann N Y Acad Sci 992:30–38
20. Matzinger P (1994) Tolerance, danger, and the extended family. Annu Rev Immunol 12:991–1045
21. Gallego-Delgado J, Ty M, Orengo JM, van de Hoef D, Rodriguez A (2014) A surprising role for uric acid: the inflammatory malaria response. Curr Rheumatol Rep 16(2):401
22. Jaiswal R, Grau GE, Bebawy M (2014) Cellular communication via microparticles: role in transfer of multidrug resistance in cancer. Future Oncol 10(4):655–669
23. Combes V et al (2004) Circulating endothelial microparticles in Malawian children with severe falciparum malaria complicated with coma. JAMA 291(21):2542–2544
24. Pankoui Mfonkeu JB et al (2010) Elevated cell-specific microparticles are a biological marker for cerebral dysfunctions in human severe malaria. PLoS One 5(10), e13415
25. Couper KN et al (2010) Parasite-derived plasma microparticles contribute significantly to malaria infection-induced inflammation through potent macrophage stimulation. PLoS Pathog 6(1), e1000744
26. Mantel PY, Marti M (2014) The role of extracellular vesicles in *Plasmodium* and other protozoan parasites. Cell Microbiol 16(3):344–354
27. Figueiredo RT et al (2007) Characterization of heme as activator of Toll-like receptor 4. J Biol Chem 282(28):20221–20229
28. Belnoue E et al (2003) CCR5 deficiency decreases susceptibility to experimental cerebral malaria. Blood 101(11):4253–4259
29. Togbe D et al (2008) Both functional LTbeta receptor and TNF receptor 2 are required for the development of experimental cerebral malaria. PLoS One 3(7), e2608
30. Nie CQ et al (2009) IP-10-mediated T cell homing promotes cerebral inflammation over splenic immunity to malaria infection. PLoS Pathog 5(4), e1000369
31. Haque A et al (2011) Granzyme B expression by $CD8^+$ T cells is required for the development of experimental cerebral malaria. J Immunol 186(11):6148–6156
32. Lau LS et al (2011) Blood-stage *Plasmodium berghei* infection generates a potent, specific $CD8^+$ T-cell response despite residence largely in cells lacking MHC I processing machinery. J Infect Dis 204(12):1989–1996
33. Palomo J et al (2015) Critical role of IL-33 receptor ST2 in experimental cerebral malaria development. Eur J Immunol 45(5):1354–1365
34. Amante FH et al (2007) A role for natural regulatory T cells in the pathogenesis of experimental cerebral malaria. Am J Pathol 171(2):548–559
35. Walther M et al (2009) Distinct roles for FOXP3 and FOXP3 CD4 T cells in regulating cellular immunity to uncomplicated and severe *Plasmodium falciparum* malaria. PLoS Pathog 5(4), e1000364
36. Keswani T, Bhattacharyya A (2014) Differential role of T regulatory and Th17 in Swiss mice infected with *Plasmodium berghei* ANKA and *Plasmodium yoelii*. Exp Parasitol 141:82–92
37. Villegas-Mendez A et al (2012) IFN-gamma-producing $CD4^+$ T cells promote experimental cerebral malaria by modulating $CD8^+$ T cell accumulation within the brain. J Immunol 189(2):968–979
38. McQuillan JA et al (2011) Coincident parasite and CD8 T cell sequestration is required for development of experimental cerebral malaria. Int J Parasitol 41(2):155–163
39. Shaw TN et al (2015) Perivascular arrest of $CD8^+$ T cells is a signature of experimental cerebral malaria. PLoS Pathog 11(11), e1005210

40. Newton CR, Taylor TE, Whitten RO (1998) Pathophysiology of fatal falciparum malaria in African children. Am J Trop Med Hyg 58(5):673–683
41. Grau GE et al (1987) Tumor necrosis factor (cachectin) as an essential mediator in murine cerebral malaria. Science 237(4819):1210–1212
42. Artavanis-Tsakonas K, Tongren JE, Riley EM (2003) The war between the malaria parasite and the immune system: immunity, immunoregulation and immunopathology. Clin Exp Immunol 133(2):145–152
43. Schmidt KE et al (2011) Induction of pro-inflammatory mediators in *Plasmodium berghei* infected BALB/c mice breaks blood-brain-barrier and leads to cerebral malaria in an IL-12 dependent manner. Microbes Infect 13(10):828–836
44. Barr M, Mc GI (1962) Diphtheria antitoxin levels in the serum of Gambian Africans. Trans R Soc Trop Med Hyg 56:368–370
45. Greenwood BM, Bradley-Moore AM, Bryceson AD, Palit A (1972) Immunosuppression in children with malaria. Lancet 1(7743):169–172
46. Chizzolini C, Grau GE, Geinoz A, Schrijvers D (1990) Lymphocyte-T interferon-gamma production induced by *Plasmodium falciparum* antigen is high in recently infected non-immune and low in immune subjects. Clin Exp Immunol 79:95–99
47. Ho M et al (1986) Antigen-specific immunosuppression in human malaria due to *Plasmodium falciparum*. J Infect Dis 153(4):763–771
48. Urban BC et al (1999) *Plasmodium falciparum*-infected erythrocytes modulate the maturation of dendritic cells. Nature 400(6739):73–77
49. Segura E, Villadangos JA (2009) Antigen presentation by dendritic cells in vivo. Curr Opin Immunol 21(1):105–110
50. Lundie RJ et al (2010) Blood-stage *Plasmodium berghei* infection leads to short-lived parasite-associated antigen presentation by dendritic cells. Eur J Immunol 40(6):1674–1681
51. Maglinao M, Klopfleisch R, Seeberger PH, Lepenies B (2013) The C-type lectin receptor DCIR is crucial for the development of experimental cerebral malaria. J Immunol 191(5):2551–2559
52. Schumak B et al (2015) Specific depletion of Ly6C^{hi} inflammatory monocytes prevents immunopathology in experimental cerebral malaria. PLoS One 10(4), e0124080
53. deWalick S et al (2007) Cutting edge: conventional dendritic cells are the critical APC required for the induction of experimental cerebral malaria. J Immunol 178(10):6033–6037
54. Sullivan RT et al (2016) B cell sub-types following acute malaria and associations with clinical immunity. Malar J 15(1):139
55. Liu Y et al (2013) Role of IL-10-producing regulatory B cells in control of cerebral malaria in *Plasmodium berghei* infected mice. Eur J Immunol 43(11):2907–2918
56. Mintern JD, Villadangos JA (2015) Antigen-presenting cells look within during influenza infection. Nat Med 21(10):1123–1125
57. Sollid LM, Villadangos JA (2013) Antigen processing. Curr Opin Immunol 25(1):71–73
58. Mintern JD, Macri C, Villadangos JA (2015) Modulation of antigen presentation by intracellular trafficking. Curr Opin Immunol 34:16–21
59. Segura E, Albiston AL, Wicks IP, Chai SY, Villadangos JA (2009) Different cross-presentation pathways in steady-state and inflammatory dendritic cells. Proc Natl Acad Sci U S A 106(48):20377–20381
60. Wilson NS et al (2006) Systemic activation of dendritic cells by Toll-like receptor ligands or malaria infection impairs cross-presentation and antiviral immunity. Nat Immunol 7(2):165–172
61. Villadangos JA, Heath WR, Carbone FR (2007) Outside looking in: the inner workings of the cross-presentation pathway within dendritic cells. Trends Immunol 28(2):45–47
62. Wheway J, Obeid S, Couraud PO, Combes V, Grau GE (2013) The brain microvascular endothelium supports T cell proliferation and has potential for alloantigen presentation. PLoS One 8(1), e52586
63. Lichtman AH (2007) Endothelial antigen presentation. In: Aird WC (ed) Endothelial biomedicine. Cambridge University Press, New York, pp 1098–1107

64. Manes TD, Pober JS (2011) Identification of endothelial cell junctional proteins and lymphocyte receptors involved in transendothelial migration of human effector memory CD4+ T cells. J Immunol 186(3):1763–1768
65. Male DK, Pryce G, Hughes CC (1987) Antigen presentation in brain: MHC induction on brain endothelium and astrocytes compared. Immunology 60(3):453–459
66. Becher B, Prat A, Antel JP (2000) Brain-immune connection: immuno-regulatory properties of CNS-resident cells. Glia 29(4):293–304
67. Engelhardt B (2008) The blood-central nervous system barriers actively control immune cell entry into the central nervous system. Curr Pharm Des 14(16):1555–1565
68. Engelhardt B (2008) Immune cell entry into the central nervous system: involvement of adhesion molecules and chemokines. J Neurol Sci 274(1-2):23–26
69. Hochman SE et al (2015) Fatal pediatric cerebral malaria is associated with intravascular monocytes and platelets that are increased with HIV coinfection. MBio 6(5), e01390-01315
70. Razakandrainibe R, Pelleau S, Grau GE, Jambou R (2012) Antigen presentation by endothelial cells: what role in the pathophysiology of malaria? Trends Parasitol 28(4):151–160
71. Campanella GS et al (2006) Oligomerization of CXCL10 is necessary for endothelial cell presentation and in vivo activity. J Immunol 177(10):6991–6998
72. Campanella GS et al (2008) Chemokine receptor CXCR3 and its ligands CXCL9 and CXCL10 are required for the development of murine cerebral malaria. Proc Natl Acad Sci U S A 105(12):4814–4819
73. Jambou R et al (2010) *Plasmodium falciparum* adhesion on human brain microvascular endothelial cells involves transmigration-like cup formation and induces opening of intercellular junctions. PLoS Pathog 6(7), e1001021
74. Howland SW et al (2013) Brain microvessel cross-presentation is a hallmark of experimental cerebral malaria. EMBO Mol Med 5(7):916–931
75. Howland SW, Poh CM, Renia L (2015) Activated brain endothelial cells cross-present malaria antigen. PLoS Pathog 11(6), e1004963
76. Ling ZL, Combes V, Grau GE, King NJ (2011) Microparticles as immune regulators in infectious disease—an opinion. Front Immunol 2:67
77. Walters SB et al (2013) Microparticles from mycobacteria-infected macrophages promote inflammation and cellular migration. J Immunol 190(2):669–677
78. Wheway J, Latham SL, Combes V, Grau GE (2014) Endothelial microparticles interact with and support the proliferation of T cells. J Immunol 193(7):3378–3387
79. Cockburn IA, Zavala F (2016) Dendritic cell function and antigen presentation in malaria. Curr Opin Immunol 40:1–6
80. Wassmer SC, Combes V, Grau GE (2011) Platelets and microparticles in cerebral malaria: the unusual suspects. Drug Discov Today Dis Mech 8:e15–e23
81. Wassmer SC, Grau GE (2016) Platelets as pathogenetic effectors and killer cells in cerebral malaria. Expert Rev Hematol 9(6):515–517
82. El-Assaad F, Combes V, Grau GE (2014) Experimental models of microvascular immunopathology: the example of cerebral malaria. J Neuroinfect Dis 5(1):134

A Role for Autoimmunity in the Immune Response Against Malaria

Juan Rivera-Correa and Ana Rodriguez

Contents

1 Introduction 81
2 Pathologies Driven by Autoimmunity in Complicated Malaria 83
  2.1 Inflammation and Innate Immunity-Induced Pathology 83
  2.2 Autoantibody-Mediated Pathology 84
  2.3 T-Cell-Mediated Pathology 86
3 Protective Autoimmunity During Malaria 86
  3.1 Recognition of *Plasmodium* Parasite by Natural Antibodies 86
  3.2 Role of Self-Reactive Lymphocytes 87
4 Genetic Insights Between Malaria and Autoimmunity 88
  4.1 Fc Receptors 89
  4.2 Inhibitory Receptors 90
  4.3 Other Immune Genetic Variants 91
5 Implications 91
References 92

1 Introduction

The immune system is a highly complex collection of both cellular and molecular components whose purpose is to defend against foreign or danger signals in its host [1]. These foreign and danger signals usually include infections or cancer. The immune system is highly adapted to respond quickly to control the threat (innate immunity), develop a more specific targeted response to eradicate it (adaptive immunity), and create a long-lasting protection against it (memory response). Due to this, this system has evolved various ways to distinguish "self from nonself"

J. Rivera-Correa • A. Rodriguez (✉)
Division of Parasitology, Department of Microbiology, New York University School of Medicine, New York, NY 10010, USA
e-mail: jrc621@nyumc.org

M.M. Mota, A. Rodriguez (eds.), *Malaria*, DOI 10.1007/978-3-319-45210-4_5

or "danger vs. non danger" in order to attack foreign threats while evolving tolerance to the host. Autoimmunity is a consequence of the breakdown of this tolerance to the host molecules or epitopes. This breakdown leads to a disseminated attack on various organs and tissues leading to diseases with high mortality and morbidity, as seen mostly in the developed world. The development of autoimmune disease is highly complex and multifactorial, involving both genetic and environmental factors. Autoimmune diseases are the third leading cause of morbidity and mortality in the developed world [2]. These associations with the developed world already suggest a possible relation with infectious agents that have driven human evolution, such as the *Plasmodium* parasites that cause human malaria.

Autoimmunity during infection, including during malaria, has been an extensively reported phenomenon. Polyclonal activation of B-cells and autoantibody production has been reported during murine malaria since the 1970s [3]. Additionally, autoantibodies against all kind of host molecules have been reported extensively in malaria patients infected with any of the human *Plasmodium* species [4, 5]. The development of autoimmunity, particularly production of autoantibodies during malaria, has been correlated with disease severity [6]. The mechanisms leading to autoimmunity during infection are poorly understood, but some likely candidates have been hypothesized to be involved. Among these hypothesized mechanisms are molecular mimicry, epitope spreading, bystander activation, persistent infection, and polyclonal activation [2]. During malaria, evidence has been reported that would support each of these as a likely mechanism leading to autoimmunity during infection. In fact, *Plasmodium* and other eukaryotic parasites have been deemed master manipulators of the immune system. Mechanisms such as molecular mimicry can be supported by the fact that the reported inflammatory *Plasmodium* molecules posses great similarity to host molecules, such as nucleic acids. Additionally, the fact that *Plasmodium* parasites required an intracellular life cycle within the host cells already suggests that many host molecules will be presented along with parasite antigens, facilitating other mechanisms such as epitope spreading and bystander activation. Moreover, the highly inflammatory response to *Plasmodium* along with its lack of sterile immunity supports autoreactive mechanisms such as persistent infection and polyclonal activation. Furthermore, there have been numerous reports showing great inverse correlations between malaria and development of autoimmune diseases, such as systemic lupus erythematosus (SLE) and rheumatoid arthritis (RA). Genetic mutations that correlate with the development of autoimmunity have also been reported to confer resistance to malarial infection [7, 8]. With studies showing how rodent malaria parasites prevented the development of lupus in mice and arthritis in rats [9], mechanistic studies linking malaria and autoimmunity are needed.

Lastly, some groups have long hypothesized that autoimmunity during malaria can have a protective effect [10, 11]. These protective effects are deemed to the ability to recognize host antigens that are present in the infected red blood cells and could help facilitate parasite clearance. In the first section of this chapter, we summarize the evidence reporting autoimmunity as a major promoter of the pathology seen during complicated malaria. Conversely, in the following section, we first explore the protective role that autoimmunity could play during malarial infection. We follow up by discussing various mechanistic insights that have been hypothesized to drive autoimmunity during malaria. Then, we discuss the striking genetic and evolutionary links that have been done with malarial infection and different autoimmune diseases. Lastly, we overview the general concept and role that autoimmunity may play during infection.

2 Pathologies Driven by Autoimmunity in Complicated Malaria

2.1 Inflammation and Innate Immunity-Induced Pathology

The inflammatory cytokine "storm" correlating with the peaks of high fevers has been a hallmark of clinical malaria. The massive upregulation of all proinflammatory cytokines seen in malaria patients can lead to an overreactive immune system promoting autoimmunity and multiple organ damage. Inflammatory cytokines during malaria play a significant role in pathology leading to the associated malarial complications such as cerebral malaria and severe anemia. Autoimmune disorders, such SLE and RA, have also been promoted and aggravated by specific inflammatory cytokines. Perhaps the most obvious inflammatory cytokine known to be an important mediator to disease in both malaria and autoimmunity is tumor necrosis factor alpha (TNF-α) [12]. For example, this cytokine has been attributed to be a promoter of pathology on joint inflammation during RA, while it has also been reported to be a major factor contributing to the development of cerebral malaria both in mice models and patients. In fact, anti-TNF-α monoclonal antibodies have been a successful therapeutic for many autoimmune disorders such as Crohn's disease and RA [13]. Unfortunately, this same therapeutic target was not found to be protective during cerebral malaria in patients, showing the great complexity involved in this syndrome [12]. Other cytokines, such as IL-6 and IL-10, have been correlated with mediating severe malarial anemia by inducing bone marrow suppression [14]. Type I interferons are potent proinflammatory cytokines mainly induced by nucleic acid sensing. These cytokines have also been correlated with disease in both malaria and autoimmune disorders. *Plasmodium* parasites have been known to induce upregulation of type I interferon during multiple stages of their life cycle [15]. Collectively, type I interferons have also been known to be a hallmark of disease during SLE and RA mediating many of the pathologies associated with the disorders [16]. Particularly, SLE is characterized by excessive inflammatory response and autoantibodies against nuclear antigens such as nucleic acids. These inflammatory correlations between malaria and autoimmune disorders suggest a common mechanism leading to this excessive immune response, particularly against self-antigens such as nucleic acids. The massive inflammatory response during both autoimmune disorders and malaria leads to increased oxidative stress due to release of reactive oxygen species by immune cells. This uncontrolled oxidative stress can also lead to oxidatively modified autoantigens, which can become targets for the immune system [17]. Lastly, all this uncontrolled inflammation can lead to nonspecific responses that can serve as an advantageous mechanism of immune evasion to the parasite. One example is the high titers of nonspecific IgM in the serum of malaria patients, which can mask infected erythrocytes and protect them from clearance [18].

Another key molecular component of the immune system is the complement system. The complement cascade is a set of molecules from the immune system involved in mounting a quick and low specificity response against the threat. This system works by recognizing specific molecular patterns found on pathogen cell surfaces and mediating their destruction either by lysis or opsonization. The complement system has been attributed an important role in maintaining self-tolerance [19]. Host cells are not targeted by this system because they posses complement inhibitory and regulatory proteins, such as CD59 and CD55. Both malaria and autoimmunity have been characterized by the lost of these complement regulatory proteins on many host cells. For example, the loss of both CD59 and CD55 on erythrocytes has been associated with severe anemia in malaria patients [20]. This association with the loss of complement regulatory proteins is also related to accumulation of immune complexes, which are opsonized by complement. CD55 has also been described to be an essential receptor for red blood cell invasion by merozoites, suggesting a possible mechanism for its downregulation [21]. Additionally, lymphocytes possess specific complement receptors, such as CR2/CD21 in B-cells, which control their threshold of activation and antibody production [22]. Alterations in surface CR2/CD21 on patients' B-cells have been reported in RA and SLE and even on patients with severe malaria [23, 24]. Conversely, engagement of CR2/CD21 on B-cells has been hypothesized to be an essential signal for the expansion of anti-self DNA antibody-producing cells during SLE [25]. All of this evidence supports a role for inappropriate complement activation during autoimmune disease and malaria. These similarities in inflammatory cytokines and the complement system just reinforce the strong relationships between how autoimmunity plays a role in malaria.

2.2 Autoantibody-Mediated Pathology

Autoantibody production and polyclonal activation have been observed in experimental malaria mice models and patients since the 1970s [3, 26]. The immune response against malaria has also been characterized by hyper-IgG and IgM globulinemia. These antibodies are hypothesized to be induced by nonspecific activation of B-cells, while only a small proportion of these antibodies has anti-malaria antigen activity [27]. A high percentage of these antibodies has been identified to react against self-antigens such as nucleic acids, membrane components, and nuclear proteins. Particularly, a lot of these autoantibodies can recognize very similarly uninfected erythrocytes during malaria as they recognized infected erythrocyte antigens [28–30]. Although understudied, these antibodies have been hypothesized to be involved in various malarial complications such as glomerulonephritis and severe anemia. Two of these antibody specificities, anti-DNA and anti-phosphatidylserine (anti-PS), have been directly shown to contribute to these associated malarial syndromes. These autoantibodies have also been a hallmark in autoimmune disorders, particularly in SLE, reinforcing again the shared immune mechanism between them.

Antinuclear antibodies (ANAs) are autoantibodies that target nuclear antigens such DNA, RNA, histones, and nuclear proteins. These antibodies are the primordial mediator of pathology during SLE, which can lead to renal complications. These antibodies have been found to mediate a similar renal pathology in experimental malaria mice models. Wozencraft et al. demonstrated that mice infection with any of the three different rodent *Plasmodium* species (*P. vinckei*, *P. yoelii*, and *P. berghei*) resulted in increased single-stranded DNA-binding antibody titers and resulted in kidney damage and dysfunction [31]. This study showed that anti-DNA monoclonal antibodies could bind glomeruli within the kidneys extracted from infected mice, after the initial damage had occurred. The renal pathology induced by these anti-DNA antibodies has been attributed mainly to the fact that they can form large immune complexes. If these immune complexes are not removed from circulation, by receptors such as CR1/CD35 and CR2/CD21, they could accumulate in the kidney and lead to widespread inflammation. There have been numerous reports describing how malarial infection leads to downregulation of these immune complex receptors (CR1/CR2) in both mice models and patients [23, 32]. These downregulations can then lead to immune complex accumulation in the kidneys, hence explaining the renal pathology observed during malaria. In agreement, Fernandez-Arias et al. reported great accumulation of immune complexes during *P. yoelii* infection in mice along with widespread downregulation of immune complex receptor CR1/CD35, supporting the role of immune complexes in renal damage during malaria [32]. Immune complexes have also been correlated to contribute to severe anemia [33] and cerebral malaria [34, 35]. DNA-containing immune complexes have also been implicated to be a source of high inflammation during malaria [36, 37].

Another autoantibody specificity that has been shown to play a role in malaria pathology is antiphospholipid antibodies. Antiphospholipid antibodies are commonly seen in many autoimmune diseases, such as SLE. These antibodies have been attributed to be involved in thrombosis, thrombocytopenia, and anemia [11, 26, 38]. Particularly during malaria, antiphospholipid antibodies that target the host membrane phospholipid phosphatidylserine (PS) have been shown to directly promote malarial anemia. In a recent study, Fernandez-Arias et al. reported how anti-PS antibodies recognized PS on uninfected erythrocytes promoting their clearance by circulating macrophages [29]. Apart from anti-PS antibodies, autoantibodies against all kinds of phospholipids have been reported in malaria patients and infected mice [39, 40]. In contrast to SLE and autoimmune diseases, these antiphospholipid antibodies seem to be more specific and cofactor independent (β2GP1 dependent), which is similar to autoantibodies seen in other infectious diseases [4, 41, 42].

2.3 T-Cell-Mediated Pathology

The role of autoreactive T-cells during malaria is poorly understood and understudied. These could be due to the fact that T-cell immunity is mostly correlated with protection in malaria vaccine studies [43]. In autoimmune disorders, T-cells have been described to mediate pathology by direct cytotoxicity and by epitope spreading of subdominant (cryptic) self-antigens leading to expansion of autoantibody-producing B-cells [44, 45]. Additionally, activated T-cells are potent inflammatory cytokine producers, such as TNF-α and IFN-γ. These T-cell-secreted cytokines have been known to play a vital role in parasite killing but can also contribute to tissue pathology as mentioned above [46]. A recent report correlated activation of $CD8^+$ T-cells with anemia development in *P. berghei ANKA*-infected rats, although the mechanism remains elusive [47]. In the autoimmune disorder multiple sclerosis, myelin-specific T-cells have been implicated an essential role in mediating the associated pathology [48]. Similarly, $CD8^+$ T-cells have also been shown to be pathological agents during experimental cerebral malaria model [49, 50] although whether they are self-reactive and their role in human cerebral malaria remains controversial. Overall, more mechanistic studies are needed in order to understand the presence and role of autoreactive T-cells in malaria pathology.

3 Protective Autoimmunity During Malaria

There is no doubt that one of the main reasons our immune system exists is to battle infectious diseases. Even though a potent and sensitive immune system has been regarded as negative in the developed world due to the development of autoimmune disorders, it can be highly beneficial in a setting where complex infectious diseases are present. The various studies reporting the inverse correlation between malaria and autoimmune disorders suggest a role for autoimmunity in resistance against malaria. The surge of autoimmunity during malaria could be influenced by the proximity or hapten-like presentation of self-antigens along with antigenic parasite molecules. In this section we discuss the various evidences reporting how both natural and induced recognition of host self-antigens can mediate an antiparasitic immune response.

3.1 *Recognition of* Plasmodium *Parasite by Natural Antibodies*

The human immune system keeps low titers of self-reactive IgM antibodies, called natural antibodies. These antibodies are mainly secreted by innate-like B1 cells and have been suggested to have homeostatic role in the clearance of apoptotic cells with anti-inflammatory properties [51, 52]. Some of the self-specificities described by these antibodies include membrane phospholipids like phosphatidylcholine, erythrocyte membrane proteins like Band 3, and sugar moieties, among others. Absence of these natural antibodies in circulation has been reported to contribute to autoimmunity development, mostly likely through mounting an immune response to self-antigens in apoptotic cells [52]. Since these antibodies could recognize damaged erythrocyte membrane antigens that would be present in *Plasmodium*-infected erythrocytes, various groups have suggested a role for these naturally occurring antibodies in mediating parasite clearance at various stages of its life cycle.

Plasmodium parasites and their human host share a lot of common phospholipid epitopes that could cross-react. Mice deficient on CD5+ B1a cells have been reported to experience a more severe murine malarial infection, which correlated with decreased titers of antiphospholipid antibodies [11]. In fact, there have been various studies reporting how these antiphospholipid antibodies can recognize infected erythrocytes, enhance parasite clearance [53], and control inflammation [54] in mice models. However, most of these studies have been purely correlative and have not shown direct mechanisms involving antiphospholipid antibodies and parasite clearance. Additionally, some antiphospholipid antibodies, such as anti-PS, antibodies, have been directly shown to be pathogenic rather than beneficial in a mouse model of malarial anemia [29]. Furthermore, as discussed above, antiphospholipid antibodies have been reported extensively in malaria patients, and no correlation with protection has been observed; instead, a correlation with pathology has been suggested [29, 40]. More studies of the individual antiphospholipid antibodies are needed to understand this relationship.

A more successful natural antibody that has been observed to be antiparasitic is anti-glycan antibodies such α-gal IgM-specific antibodies. In a recent report, Yilmaz et al. reported how anti-α-gal antibodies target *Plasmodium* sporozoites for complement-mediated cytotoxicity in the skin and how immunization with the antigen could reduce liver-stage parasite burden. These α-gal natural antibodies have a homeostatic role in microbiota control and do not recognize similar host glycan moieties. Additionally, these α-gal antibodies have been suggested a role in controlling malaria transmission stages [55]. Unfortunately, these antibodies described are mostly of the IgM isotype whose role in blood-stage parasite clearance is unclear [18]. Similarly, natural antibodies against sugar moieties have been known to play a role during Chagas disease caused by protozoan parasite *Trypanosoma cruzi*. The role of these antibodies has been controversial since the same antibodies that recognized the parasite were also attributed to be mediators of the cardiac pathology seen during Chagas disease [56]. Naturally occurring antibodies seem to provide another evidence of convergent evolution between our immune system and protozoan parasite resistance.

3.2 *Role of Self-Reactive Lymphocytes*

Lymphocytes have an essential role in mediating parasite clearance as proven in both mouse and human malaria [57]. T-cells secrete potent cytokines, such as TNF-α and IFN-γ, while B-cells produce anti-parasite antibodies that have been attributed to be essential for parasite clearance. The production of these potent inflammatory cytokines has also been implicated in the development of autoimmune disorder, supporting the inverse correlation between these two. Additionally, T-cells and B-cells would provide effective anti-parasite memory, which would prevent future pathological effects. Even though a hyperactive T-cell and B-cell response would be viewed as autoimmunity in the developed world, it could have its benefits in the setting of complex pathogens such as *Plasmodium* parasites.

Like autoimmune disorders, *Plasmodium* infection is characterized by polyclonal B-cell activation and increased autoantibody production. Although the pathogenic role of these autoantibodies is evident, their role in parasite clearance is less clear. Anti-DNA antibodies compose a great part of the repertoire of antibodies identified in malaria patients [28]. Although these high titers of anti-DNA antibodies mediate pathologies as discussed before, they have also been reported to recognize parasite DNA [36]. Some groups have even reported this anti-DNA response to be critical in the protective immune response in murine models of malaria. This was evidenced in the study of Manoor et al., where they found over 50 % increase in mortality on a nonlethal *P. yoelii* infection after depletion of single-stranded DNA (ssDNA)-binding autoreactive B-cells. Alternatively, adopted transfer of these cells to infected mice provided inhibition of parasitemia [58]. This group also reported that these anti-ssDNA IgG antibodies were cross-reactive with *P. yoelii* antigens. This evidence suggests a role for autoantibodies in mediating parasite clearance. As mentioned before, anti-DNA antibodies play a crucial role in the pathology of SLE, hence reinforcing the relationship between the development of autoimmunity and malaria resistance. Rheumatoid factor (RF) is an antibody that targets the Fc portion of other IgG antibodies, being present in high titers in autoimmune diseases such as RA. RF has also been reported in the serum of malaria patients, probably as a consequence of polyclonal B-cell activation. This autoantibody has also been implicated to have a role in parasite clearance, as shown by *P. falciparum* schizont inhibition in vitro [59]. A lot of these autoantibodies have been shown to be T-cell dependent, supporting the role for both self-reactive T and B lymphocytes [44]. Lastly, basigin is a novel autoantigen that has been recently attributed to mediate parasite inhibition. Basigin was identified as an essential receptor for *P. falciparum* invasion of erythrocytes. A recent study reported how monoclonal antibodies blocking this receptor inhibited blood stage of *P. falciparum* in a humanized mice model [60]. Other host surface proteins that have been considered as target for enhancing anti-malarial immunity are the liver-stage receptor CD68 and inhibitory molecules such as PD-1 and Lag-3 [61]. The mechanisms by which targeting of these inhibitory molecules would benefit anti-malaria immunity is discussed in the next section of this chapter.

4 Genetic Insights Between Malaria and Autoimmunity

Plasmodium parasites have been top pathogens that have influenced human evolution and genetics. Autoimmune diseases have been considered "modern diseases" for their high prevalence in developed countries where complex infectious diseases, such as malaria, are no longer a public health problem. Genetic factors play a big role in the development of autoimmune disorders as concluded from twin studies [2]. The hygiene hypothesis is a hypothesis proposed by scientist and clinicians which states that the lack of exposure to infectious diseases during early age, especially parasites, can increase this susceptibility to hypersensitivity due to an inappropriate development of the immune system. This hypothesis has been mostly proposed to apply to a Th2-driven anti-inflammatory response by parasitic helminthes infections in relation to the development of allergies. Some groups have proposed that the hygiene hypothesis could also apply to explain malaria and autoimmune disease, such as SLE and RA. The rationale with malaria would be the opposite as for the helminthes, where a potent inflammatory immune system has benefited a host in malaria-endemic areas, while it has led to misguided immune system promoting autoimmune disorders in the absence of malaria [50]. Various genetic polymorphisms and co-disease models have supported this hypothesis.

Various polymorphisms and genetic variants of different immunological agents have been described to promote autoimmunity development. Interestingly, some of the same variants have been attributed to provide resistance to malarial infection. Some of the most reported genetic variants include antibody Fc receptors, inhibitory receptors, and inflammatory cytokine genes.

4.1 Fc Receptors

Fc receptors are antibody receptors expressed in various immune cells like macrophages and B lymphocytes. These receptors are isotype specific and bind the constant Fc region of antibodies to promote phagocytosis of opsonized pathogens or immune complexes. Most Fc receptors are regarded as inflammatory since their activation would lead to a signal cascade leading to secretion of proinflammatory cytokines. Genetic variants for some of these inflammatory receptors have been rendered important for anti-malaria immunity. IgG receptor FcγRIIa homozygotes displayed higher IgG2 levels that were protective against high parasitemia and onset of malaria symptoms [62].

Out of all the Fc receptors, there is only one inhibitory receptor called FcγRIIb (CD32b). These inhibitory receptors have an immunoreceptor tyrosine-based inhibitory motif (ITIM) within their cytoplasmic domain. The main function of FcγRIIb is to inhibit activating signals to modulate inflammatory and antibody responses and contribute to immune tolerance, especially on B lymphocytes. Cross-linking of FcγRIIb and the B-cell receptor (BCR) can induce apoptosis, being hypothesized to occur during negative selection to eliminate autoreactive B-cells. The frequency of some of the homozygous FcγRIIb variant that are associated with reduced inhibitory activity is subject to considerable ethnic variation and is lower in Caucasians (1 %) than Africans (8–11 %) or Southeast Asians (5–7 %) [7]. *FCGR2B* is one of the genes thought to influence susceptibility to several autoimmune diseases in humans, especially SLE and RA. These genetic haplotypes have been observed in

SLE and RA patients and correlated with decreased protein expression on patient memory B-cells. Both SLE and RA are primordially autoantibody-mediated diseases, hence attributing an important role for FcγRIIb mutations to the break of self-tolerance in these diseases. Potential mechanisms by which FcγRIIb could be directly mediating pathology during SLE and RA include lack of clearance of immune complexes and increased autoantibody production by the lack of negative selection against autoreactive B-cells during development. Even a modest increase in the expression of FcγRIIb on B-cells can ameliorate spontaneous SLE in mice [63]. These mechanistic associations attribute an important role to the reduced FcγRIIb expression in the development of autoimmune disorders. There has been a consistent relation of FcγRIIb mutations in malaria-endemic areas. The incidence of SLE is at least two- to fourfold higher in populations of African or Asian descent than in Caucasians. This has led to the hypothesis that decreased FcγRIIb function could provide a survival advantage against malaria. This mechanism could be mediated by reduction of FcγRIIb activity in both macrophages and B-cells [46, 64]. The hypothesis would be that reduced FcγRIIb activity would lead to a more potent immune system that could clear the parasite better. This enhanced inflammatory activity includes increased phagocytosis, malaria-specific antibody titers, and TNF production, hence correlating with protection against severe malaria as found in Kenyan children [65]. Additionally, it has been described that FcγRIIb deficiency, a genetic susceptibility to SLE, can protect against experimental cerebral malaria in mice [66]. All of these inverse correlations between SLE development and resistance to malaria have been attributed to an enhanced immune response against parasitized erythrocytes.

4.2 Inhibitory Receptors

Inhibitory receptors have an essential role in regulating autoreactivity. Some of the most studied inhibitory receptors include PD-1, Lag-3, and CTLA-4. Even though these inhibitory receptors can be expressed on innate immune cells, they have been mostly studied for their essential role in T and B lymphocytes [67].

Polymorphisms of these inhibitory receptors on T- and B-cells have been linked to susceptibility to several autoimmune diseases. Additionally, these receptors have been observed on pathogen-specific lymphocytes during HIV and malarial infection. Specifically expression of these receptors on B-cells has been studied and observed to be largely expanded in malaria patients in endemic areas being titled atypical memory B-cells [68]. Expression of these inhibitory receptors on lymphocytes renders them nonresponsive, hence being given the title of "exhausted" and being correlated with chronic exposure to the pathogen [69]. These associations provide us with yet another genetic link between autoimmunity and malarial infection. These inhibitory receptors have an immunoreceptor tyrosine-based inhibitory motif (ITIM) within their cytoplasmic domain and provide inhibitory signals to the cell, similarly as FcγRIIb.

The hypothesis linking inhibitory receptors on lymphocytes and malarial infections involves a similar protective mechanism to the one proposed to FcγRIIb: a more potent immune system. PD-1 and Lag-3 have been observed on *Plasmodium*-specific memory B-cells, suggesting that anti-malaria immunity is being restricted by normal inhibitory mechanisms on immune cells [70]. This observation led to the targeting of PD-1 and Lag-3 to investigate their role in anti-parasite immunity. Butler et al. reported that targeting of these two inhibitory molecules led to increased protective antibody titers and rapid clearance of rodent blood-stage malaria parasites [71]. Similar therapeutic targeting approaches have been regarded as the breakthrough treatment in cancer immunotherapy against many different cancers [72]. It seems that even though these inhibitory receptors play an essential role in preventing autoreactive lymphocyte expansion, they are mistakenly inhibiting beneficial anti-pathogen/cancer immunity. Conversely, it could be suggesting that autoimmunity is needed for clearance of complex pathogens and cancer, at least to some degree.

4.3 Other Immune Genetic Variants

Other genetic genes of different immunological genes have been attributed to influence malarial infection and autoimmunity. Some of these immunological genes include antigen presentation genes, inflammatory cytokine genes, and complement receptor genes. For antigen presentation, polymorphisms of class I HLA and class II HLA are involved in resistance to *Plasmodium falciparum* malaria [73]. Even though some HLA variants have been used as markers for the development of some autoimmune disorders, no studies have reported the presence of these specific variants during malaria. Conversely polymorphisms of inflammatory cytokine genes, such as TNF-α, are shared between both malaria and autoimmune disorders such as RA. Excessive production of TNF-α has been a key pathological agent during RA and in the development of cerebral malaria. Another immunological gene involved in both autoimmunity and malaria is complement receptor 1 (CR1/CD35). CR1 has also being identified as receptor used by *Plasmodium falciparum* merozoites for erythrocyte invasion [21]. The pathological factor for CR1 deficiency during autoimmune disorders and malaria is mainly due to decreased immune complex clearance. As mentioned before, immune complex accumulation can lead to organ damage and even increased risk of cerebral malaria [32, 34].

5 Implications

Autoimmunity during and after infection has been extensively reported although the mechanisms leading to it are poorly understood. *Plasmodium* parasites, like other globally relevant pathogens, are complex infectious agents that trigger a strong immune response. Additionally, *Plasmodium* parasites have co-inhabited and shaped human evolution. Furthermore, antigens being targeted during *Plasmodium* and other complex infections shared many similar epitopes to host antigens, such as nucleic acids. The human immune response against malaria parasites has been regarded as complex and noneffective. This dysfunction could be explained partly by the pathology mediated by the development of autoimmunity during malaria. Conversely, this dysfunction could be useful as the reported beneficial role of autoimmunity in aiding the clearance malaria parasites. A strong immune system proves to be an evolutionary advantage against many complex pathogens. Conversely, a potent immune system can lead to the development of autoimmune disorders in the absence of complex infectious agents. Whether autoimmunity during malarial infection, or any infection, is beneficial or pathogenic is not a trivial question to answer. Regardless, much evolutionary and mechanistic evidence strongly supports a role for autoimmunity during malarial infection.

References

1. Pradeu T, Cooper EL (2012) The danger theory: 20 years later. Front Immunol 3:287. doi:10.3389/fimmu.2012.00287
2. Kivity S, Agmon-Levin N, Blank M, Shoenfeld Y (2009) Infections and autoimmunity—friends or foes? Trends Immunol 30(8):409–414. doi:10.1016/j.it.2009.05.005
3. Rosenberg YJ (1978) Autoimmune and polyclonal B cell responses during murine malaria. Nature 274(5667):170–172
4. Consigny PH, Cauquelin B, Agnamey P, Comby E, Brasseur P, Ballet JJ, Roussilhon C (2002) High prevalence of co-factor independent anticardiolipin antibodies in malaria exposed individuals. Clin Exp Immunol 127(1):158–164
5. Liew J, Amir A, Chen Y, Fong MY, Razali R, Lau YL (2015) Autoantibody profile of patients infected with knowlesi malaria. Clin Chim Acta 448:33–38. doi:10.1016/j.cca.2015.06.006
6. Zandman-Goddard G, Shoenfeld Y (2009) Parasitic infection and autoimmunity. Lupus 18(13):1144–1148. doi:10.1177/0961203309345735
7. Smith KG, Clatworthy MR (2010) FcγRIIB in autoimmunity and infection: evolutionary and therapeutic implications. Nat Rev Immunol 10(5):328–343. doi:10.1038/nri2762
8. Adebajo AO (1997) Low frequency of autoimmune disease in tropical Africa. Lancet 349(9048):361–362
9. Butcher G (2008) Autoimmunity and malaria. Trends Parasitol 24(7):291–292. doi:10.1016/j.pt.2008.03.010
10. Jarra W (1983) Protective immunity to malaria and anti-erythrocyte autoimmunity. Ciba Found Symp 94:137–158
11. Daniel-Ribeiro CT, Zanini G (2000) Autoimmunity and malaria: what are they doing together? Acta Trop 76(3):205–221
12. Gimenez F, Barraud de Lagerie S, Fernandez C, Pino P, Mazier D (2003) Tumor necrosis factor alpha in the pathogenesis of cerebral malaria. Cell Mol Life Sci 60(8):1623–1635. doi:10.1007/s00018-003-2347-x
13. Chatzantoni K, Mouzaki A (2006) Anti-TNF-alpha antibody therapies in autoimmune diseases. Curr Top Med Chem 6(16):1707–1714
14. Perkins DJ, Were T, Davenport GC, Kempaiah P, Hittner JB, Ong'echa JM (2011) Severe malarial anemia: innate immunity and pathogenesis. Int J Biol Sci 7(9):1427–1442
15. Gazzinelli RT, Kalantari P, Fitzgerald KA, Golenbock DT (2014) Innate sensing of malaria parasites. Nat Rev Immunol 14(11):744–757. doi:10.1038/nri3742

16. Niewold TB (2014) Type I interferon in human autoimmunity. Front Immunol 5:306. doi:10.3389/fimmu.2014.00306
17. Kurien BT, Scofield RH (2008) Autoimmunity and oxidatively modified autoantigens. Autoimmun Rev 7(7):567–573. doi:10.1016/j.autrev.2008.04.019
18. Pleass RJ, Moore SC, Stevenson L, Hviid L (2016) Immunoglobulin M: restrainer of inflammation and mediator of immune evasion by *Plasmodium falciparum* malaria. Trends Parasitol 32(2):108–119. doi:10.1016/j.pt.2015.09.007
19. Prodeus AP, Goerg S, Shen LM, Pozdnyakova OO, Chu L, Alicot EM, Goodnow CC, Carroll MC (1998) A critical role for complement in maintenance of self-tolerance. Immunity 9(5):721–731
20. Stoute JA, Odindo AO, Owuor BO, Mibei EK, Opollo MO, Waitumbi JN (2003) Loss of red blood cell-complement regulatory proteins and increased levels of circulating immune complexes are associated with severe malarial anemia. J Infect Dis 187(3):522–525. doi:10.1086/367712
21. Egan ES, Jiang RH, Moechtar MA, Barteneva NS, Weekes MP, Nobre LV, Gygi SP, Paulo JA, Frantzreb C, Tani Y, Takahashi J, Watanabe S, Goldberg J, Paul AS, Brugnara C, Root DE, Wiegand RC, Doench JG, Duraisingh MT (2015) Malaria. A forward genetic screen identifies erythrocyte CD55 as essential for *Plasmodium falciparum* invasion. Science 348(6235):711–714. doi:10.1126/science.aaa3526
22. Carroll MC (1998) CD21/CD35 in B cell activation. Semin Immunol 10(4):279–286. doi:10.1006/smim.1998.0120
23. Korir JC, Magambo JK, Mwatha JK, Waitumbi JN (2012) B-cell activity in children with malaria. Malar J 11:66. doi:10.1186/1475-2875-11-66
24. Kremlitzka M, Polgar A, Fulop L, Kiss E, Poor G, Erdei A (2013) Complement receptor type 1 (CR1, CD35) is a potent inhibitor of B-cell functions in rheumatoid arthritis patients. Int Immunol 25(1):25–33. doi:10.1093/intimm/dxs090
25. Leadbetter EA, Rifkin IR, Hohlbaum AM, Beaudette BC, Shlomchik MJ, Marshak-Rothstein A (2002) Chromatin-IgG complexes activate B cells by dual engagement of IgM and Toll-like receptors. Nature 416(6881):603–607. doi:10.1038/416603a
26. Rosenberg EB, Strickland GT, Yang SL, Whalen GE (1973) IgM antibodies to red cells and autoimmune anemia in patients with malaria. Am J Trop Med Hyg 22(2):146–152
27. Abu-Shakra M, Shoenfeld Y (1991) Parasitic infection and autoimmunity. Autoimmunity 9(4):337–344
28. Daniel-Ribeiro C, Druilhe P, Monjour L, Homberg JC, Gentilini M (1983) Specificity of auto-antibodies in malaria and the role of polyclonal activation. Trans R Soc Trop Med Hyg 77(2):185–188
29. Fernandez-Arias C, Rivera-Correa J, Gallego-Delgado J, Rudlaff R, Fernandez C, Roussel C, Gotz A, Gonzalez S, Mohanty A, Mohanty S, Wassmer S, Buffet P, Ndour PA, Rodriguez A (2016) Anti-self phosphatidylserine antibodies recognize uninfected erythrocytes promoting malarial anemia. Cell Host Microbe 19(2):194–203. doi:10.1016/j.chom.2016.01.009
30. Lefrancois G, Bouvet E, le Bras J, Vroklans M, Simonneau M, Vachon F (1982) Anti-erythrocyte autoimmunisation during chronic Falciparum malaria. Lancet 1(8266):280–281
31. Wozencraft AO, Lloyd CM, Staines NA, Griffiths VJ (1990) Role of DNA-binding antibodies in kidney pathology associated with murine malaria infections. Infect Immun 58(7):2156–2164
32. Fernandez-Arias C, Lopez JP, Hernandez-Perez JN, Bautista-Ojeda MD, Branch O, Rodriguez A (2013) Malaria inhibits surface expression of complement receptor 1 in monocytes/macrophages, causing decreased immune complex internalization. J Immunol 190(7):3363–3372. doi:10.4049/jimmunol.1103812
33. Owuor BO, Odhiambo CO, Otieno WO, Adhiambo C, Makawiti DW, Stoute JA (2008) Reduced immune complex binding capacity and increased complement susceptibility of red cells from children with severe malaria-associated anemia. Mol Med 14(3–4):89–97. doi:10.2119/2007-00093.Owuor
34. de Oliveira RB, Wang JP, Ram S, Gazzinelli RT, Finberg RW, Golenbock DT (2014) Increased survival in B-cell-deficient mice during experimental cerebral malaria suggests a role for circulating immune complexes. MBio 5(2), e00949-00914. doi:10.1128/mBio.00949-14
35. Eisenhut M (2009) Causes of reduced immune complex clearance in cerebral malaria. Parasite Immunol 31(2):59. doi:10.1111/j.1365-3024.2008.01074.x, author reply 60

36. Hirako IC, Gallego-Marin C, Ataide MA, Andrade WA, Gravina H, Rocha BC, de Oliveira RB, Pereira DB, Vinetz J, Diamond B, Ram S, Golenbock DT, Gazzinelli RT (2015) DNA-containing immunocomplexes promote inflammasome assembly and release of pyrogenic cytokines by CD14+ CD16+ CD64 high CD32 low inflammatory monocytes from malaria patients. MBio 6(6):e01605–e01615. doi:10.1128/mBio.01605-15
37. Wu X, Gowda NM, Kumar S, Gowda DC (2010) Protein-DNA complex is the exclusive malaria parasite component that activates dendritic cells and triggers innate immune responses. J Immunol 184(8):4338–4348. doi:10.4049/jimmunol.0903824
38. Lacerda MV, Mourao MP, Coelho HC, Santos JB (2011) Thrombocytopenia in malaria: who cares? Mem Inst Oswaldo Cruz 106(Suppl 1):52–63
39. Facer CA, Agiostratidou G (1994) High levels of anti-phospholipid antibodies in uncomplicated and severe *Plasmodium falciparum* and in *P. vivax* malaria. Clin Exp Immunol 95(2): 304–309
40. Owens S, Chamley LW, Ordi J, Brabin BJ, Johnson PM (2005) The association of anti-phospholipid antibodies with parity in placental malaria. Clin Exp Immunol 142(3):512–518. doi:10.1111/j.1365-2249.2005.02936.x
41. Berlin T, Zandman-Goddard G, Blank M, Matthias T, Pfeiffer S, Weis I, Toubi E, Singh S, Asherson R, Fraser A, Gilburd B, Sapir T, Levy Y, Lukac J, Rozman B, Kveder T, Shoenfeld Y (2007) Autoantibodies in nonautoimmune individuals during infections. Ann N Y Acad Sci 1108:584–593
42. Sene D, Piette JC, Cacoub P (2008) Antiphospholipid antibodies, antiphospholipid syndrome and infections. Autoimmun Rev 7(4):272–277. doi:10.1016/j.autrev.2007.10.001
43. Casares S, Richie TL (2009) Immune evasion by malaria parasites: a challenge for vaccine development. Curr Opin Immunol 21(3):321–330. doi:10.1016/j.coi.2009.05.015
44. Poels LG, van Niekerk CC, van der Sterren-Reti V, Jerusalem C (1980) *Plasmodium berghei*: T cell-dependent autoimmunity. Exp Parasitol 49(1):97–105
45. Lehmann PV, Targoni OS, Forsthuber TG (1998) Shifting T-cell activation thresholds in autoimmunity and determinant spreading. Immunol Rev 164:53–61
46. Butcher GA (1991) Does malaria select for predisposition to autoimmune disease? J R Soc Med 84(8):451–453
47. Safeukui I, Gomez ND, Adelani AA, Burte F, Afolabi NK, Akondy R, Velazquez P, Holder A, Tewari R, Buffet P, Brown BJ, Shokunbi WA, Olaleye D, Sodeinde O, Kazura J, Ahmed R, Mohandas N, Fernandez-Reyes D, Haldar K (2015) Malaria induces anemia through CD8+ T cell-dependent parasite clearance and erythrocyte removal in the spleen. MBio 6(1), e02493-14. doi:10.1128/mBio.02493-14
48. Fletcher JM, Lalor SJ, Sweeney CM, Tubridy N, Mills KH (2010) T cells in multiple sclerosis and experimental autoimmune encephalomyelitis. Clin Exp Immunol 162(1):1–11. doi:10.1111/j.1365-2249.2010.04143.x
49. Howland SW, Claser C, Poh CM, Gun SY, Renia L (2015) Pathogenic CD8+ T cells in experimental cerebral malaria. Semin Immunopathol 37(3):221–231. doi:10.1007/s00281-015-0476-6
50. Sotgiu S, Angius A, Embry A, Rosati G, Musumeci S (2008) Hygiene hypothesis: innate immunity, malaria and multiple sclerosis. Med Hypotheses 70(4):819–825. doi:10.1016/j.mehy.2006.10.069
51. Elkon KB, Silverman GJ (2012) Naturally occurring autoantibodies to apoptotic cells. Adv Exp Med Biol 750:14–26. doi:10.1007/978-1-4614-3461-0_2
52. Nagata S, Hanayama R, Kawane K (2010) Autoimmunity and the clearance of dead cells. Cell 140(5):619–630. doi:10.1016/j.cell.2010.02.014
53. Bordmann G, Rudin W, Favre N (1998) Immunization of mice with phosphatidylcholine drastically reduces the parasitaemia of subsequent *Plasmodium chabaudi* chabaudi blood-stage infections. Immunology 94(1):35–40
54. Bate CA, Kwiatkowski D (1994) A monoclonal antibody that recognizes phosphatidylinositol inhibits induction of tumor necrosis factor alpha by different strains of *Plasmodium falciparum*. Infect Immun 62(12):5261–5266
55. Soares MP, Yilmaz B (2016) Microbiota control of malaria transmission. Trends Parasitol 32(2):120–130. doi:10.1016/j.pt.2015.11.004

56. Galili U (2013) Anti-Gal: an abundant human natural antibody of multiple pathogeneses and clinical benefits. Immunology 140(1):1–11. doi:10.1111/imm.12110
57. Stevenson MM, Riley EM (2004) Innate immunity to malaria. Nat Rev Immunol 4(3): 169–180. doi:10.1038/nri1311
58. Mannoor K, Li C, Inafuku M, Taniguchi T, Abo T, Sato Y, Watanabe H (2013) Induction of ssDNA-binding autoantibody secreting B cell immunity during murine malaria infection is a critical part of the protective immune responses. Immunobiology 218(1):10–20. doi:10.1016/j.imbio.2012.01.018
59. Green TJ, Packer BJ (1984) A role for rheumatoid factor enhancement of *Plasmodium falciparum* schizont inhibition in vitro. Infect Immun 46(3):668–672
60. Zenonos ZA, Dummler SK, Muller-Sienerth N, Chen J, Preiser PR, Rayner JC, Wright GJ (2015) Basigin is a druggable target for host-oriented antimalarial interventions. J Exp Med 212(8):1145–1151. doi:10.1084/jem.20150032
61. Langhorne J, Duffy PE (2016) Expanding the antimalarial toolkit: targeting host-parasite interactions. J Exp Med 213(2):143–153. doi:10.1084/jem.20151677
62. Grant AV, Roussilhon C, Paul R, Sakuntabhai A (2015) The genetic control of immunity to *Plasmodium* infection. BMC Immunol 16:14. doi:10.1186/s12865-015-0078-z
63. Brownlie RJ, Lawlor KE, Niederer HA, Cutler AJ, Xiang Z, Clatworthy MR, Floto RA, Greaves DR, Lyons PA, Smith KG (2008) Distinct cell-specific control of autoimmunity and infection by FcγRIIb. J Exp Med 205(4):883–895. doi:10.1084/jem.20072565
64. Butcher GA (1996) Malaria and macrophage function in Africans: a possible link with autoimmune disease? Med Hypotheses 47(2):97–100
65. Willcocks LC, Carr EJ, Niederer HA, Rayner TF, Williams TN, Yang W, Scott JA, Urban BC, Peshu N, Vyse TJ, Lau YL, Lyons PA, Smith KG (2010) A defunctioning polymorphism in FCGR2B is associated with protection against malaria but susceptibility to systemic lupus erythematosus. Proc Natl Acad Sci U S A 107(17):7881–7885. doi:10.1073/pnas.0915133107
66. Clatworthy MR, Willcocks L, Urban B, Langhorne J, Williams TN, Peshu N, Watkins NA, Floto RA, Smith KG (2007) Systemic lupus erythematosus-associated defects in the inhibitory receptor FcγRIIb reduce susceptibility to malaria. Proc Natl Acad Sci U S A 104(17):7169–7174. doi:10.1073/pnas.0608889104
67. Odorizzi PM, Wherry EJ (2012) Inhibitory receptors on lymphocytes: insights from infections. J Immunol 188(7):2957–2965. doi:10.4049/jimmunol.1100038
68. Weiss GE, Crompton PD, Li S, Walsh LA, Moir S, Traore B, Kayentao K, Ongoiba A, Doumbo OK, Pierce SK (2009) Atypical memory B cells are greatly expanded in individuals living in a malaria-endemic area. J Immunol 183(3):2176–2182. doi:10.4049/jimmunol.0901297
69. Portugal S, Tipton CM, Sohn H, Kone Y, Wang J, Li S, Skinner J, Virtaneva K, Sturdevant DE, Porcella SF, Doumbo OK, Doumbo S, Kayentao K, Ongoiba A, Traore B, Sanz I, Pierce SK, Crompton PD (2015) Malaria-associated atypical memory B cells exhibit markedly reduced B cell receptor signaling and effector function. Elife 4, e07218. doi:10.7554/eLife.07218
70. Muellenbeck MF, Ueberheide B, Amulic B, Epp A, Fenyo D, Busse CE, Esen M, Theisen M, Mordmuller B, Wardemann H (2013) Atypical and classical memory B cells produce *Plasmodium falciparum* neutralizing antibodies. J Exp Med 210(2):389–399. doi:10.1084/jem.20121970
71. Butler NS, Moebius J, Pewe LL, Traore B, Doumbo OK, Tygrett LT, Waldschmidt TJ, Crompton PD, Harty JT (2012) Therapeutic blockade of PD-L1 and LAG-3 rapidly clears established blood-stage *Plasmodium* infection. Nat Immunol 13(2):188–195. doi:10.1038/ni.2180
72. Sharpe AH, Wherry EJ, Ahmed R, Freeman GJ (2007) The function of programmed cell death 1 and its ligands in regulating autoimmunity and infection. Nat Immunol 8(3):239–245. doi:10.1038/ni1443
73. Bonilla-Abadia F, Tobon GJ, Canas CA (2012) Possible influence of resistance to malaria in clinical presentation of rheumatoid arthritis: biological significance of natural selection. Arthritis 2012:670579. doi:10.1155/2012/670579

Part II
Immune Response to Malaria Vaccines: Liver Stage Vaccines

Whole-Sporozoite Malaria Vaccines

António M. Mendes, Anja Scholzen, Ann-Kristin Mueller, Shahid M. Khan, Robert W. Sauerwein, and Miguel Prudêncio

Contents

1 Introduction 100
2 Radiation-Attenuated Sporozoites (RAS) 103
 2.1 Immune Correlates in RAS Immunization 103
 2.2 Recent Progress in RAS Immunization 108
3 Genetically Attenuated Parasites (GAPs) 111
 3.1 Creation of GAPs 111
 3.2 Immunity Induced After GAP Immunization 113
4 Chemoprophylaxis and Sporozoite (CPS) Immunization 116
 4.1 Parasite Life Cycle Target for CPS-Induced Protection 118
 4.2 Humoral Immunity After CPS Immunization 119
 4.3 Cellular Immunity After CPS Immunization 119
5 Other Models of Sporozoite-Based Vaccination 120
 5.1 Chemically Attenuated Sporozoites 121
 5.2 Rodent *Plasmodium*-Based Immunization Against Human Malaria 121
6 Future Directions and Concluding Remarks 122
References 124

António M. Mendes and Anja Scholzen contributed equally with all other contributors.

A.M. Mendes • M. Prudêncio (✉)
Instituto de Medicina Molecular, Faculdade de Medicina, Universidade de Lisboa, Avenida Professor Egas Moniz, 1649-028 Lisbon, Portugal
e-mail: mprudencio@medicina.ulisboa.pt

A. Scholzen • R.W. Sauerwein
Department of Medical Microbiology, Radboud University Medical Center, P.O. Box 9101, 6500 HB Nijmegen, The Netherlands

A.-K. Mueller
Centre for Infectious Diseases, Parasitology Unit, Heidelberg University Hospital, Heidelberg, Germany

German Centre for Infection Research, D 69120 Heidelberg, Germany

S.M. Khan
Leiden Malaria Research Group, Department of Parasitology, Leiden University Medical Center, 2333 ZA Leiden, The Netherlands

M.M. Mota, A. Rodriguez (eds.), *Malaria*, DOI 10.1007/978-3-319-45210-4_6

1 Introduction

More than two centuries have passed since Edward Jenner's breakthrough postulates on whole-organism vaccination and more than one since Pasteur's formulation of the idea of immunization through microorganism attenuation [1]. Nowadays, health-care systems around the world rely on numerous successful vaccines to prevent morbidity and mortality in a cost-effective manner [2]. However, despite significant advances in molecular biology, approximately half of all currently approved vaccines continue to rely on the use of live attenuated microorganisms to elicit immunity against the diseases caused by their non-attenuated counterparts [1].

Malaria is one of the most important infectious diseases for which an effective vaccine is still lacking [3]. The gold standard strategies for malaria immunization rely on the administration of live *Plasmodium* sporozoites, the malaria parasite form transmitted to man by mosquitoes. Sporozoite-based vaccination strategies aim at preventing the parasite's life cycle progression from hepatic stages to the symptomatic blood stages of infection while eliciting potent preerythrocytic immune responses. Such whole-sporozoite malaria vaccination strategies are unique in their potential to induce sterile protection against a new infection and have led to the development of various vaccine candidates, currently ongoing preclinical and clinical development. This chapter will explore in detail our current knowledge of the protective immunity elicited by *Plasmodium* sporozoite-based malaria vaccination.

Although it was not until the 1960s that protective immunity against human malaria was first demonstrated [4, 5], the long list of classical studies exploring the use of sporozoites for immunization against malaria spans over a century, with the first studies using heat-inactivated avian parasites dating back to 1910 [6]. However, it was the discovery of the preerythrocytic stages of *Plasmodium* [7], followed by the establishment of a mouse model of malaria [8], that enabled the laboratory production of all stages of the parasite's life cycle [9], which eventually led to the landmark demonstration that live sporozoites attenuated by X-irradiation (RAS) could be used to elicit sterile protection against a new infection [10, 11]. This discovery was soon expanded to humans with the demonstration that volunteers could be protected against homologous and heterologous strains of *P. falciparum* parasites [12–14] (Fig. 1).

The excitement generated by these successes in both animal models and humans ensured that a large number of studies would continue into the following decades, aiming at optimizing the potential of sporozoite-based immunization, as well as at characterizing the immune responses elicited by these strategies [36, 60–64]. Progress also included exploring alternative methods that did not rely on the use of radiation, such as the administration of sporozoites under the cover of antimalarial drugs [37, 38]. Such strategies are based on sporozoite administration with the concomitant administration of a drug that does not interfere with the parasite's ability to complete liver-stage development but prevents blood-stage replication, enabling the induction of a strong immune response in the liver while avoiding the onset of pathology.

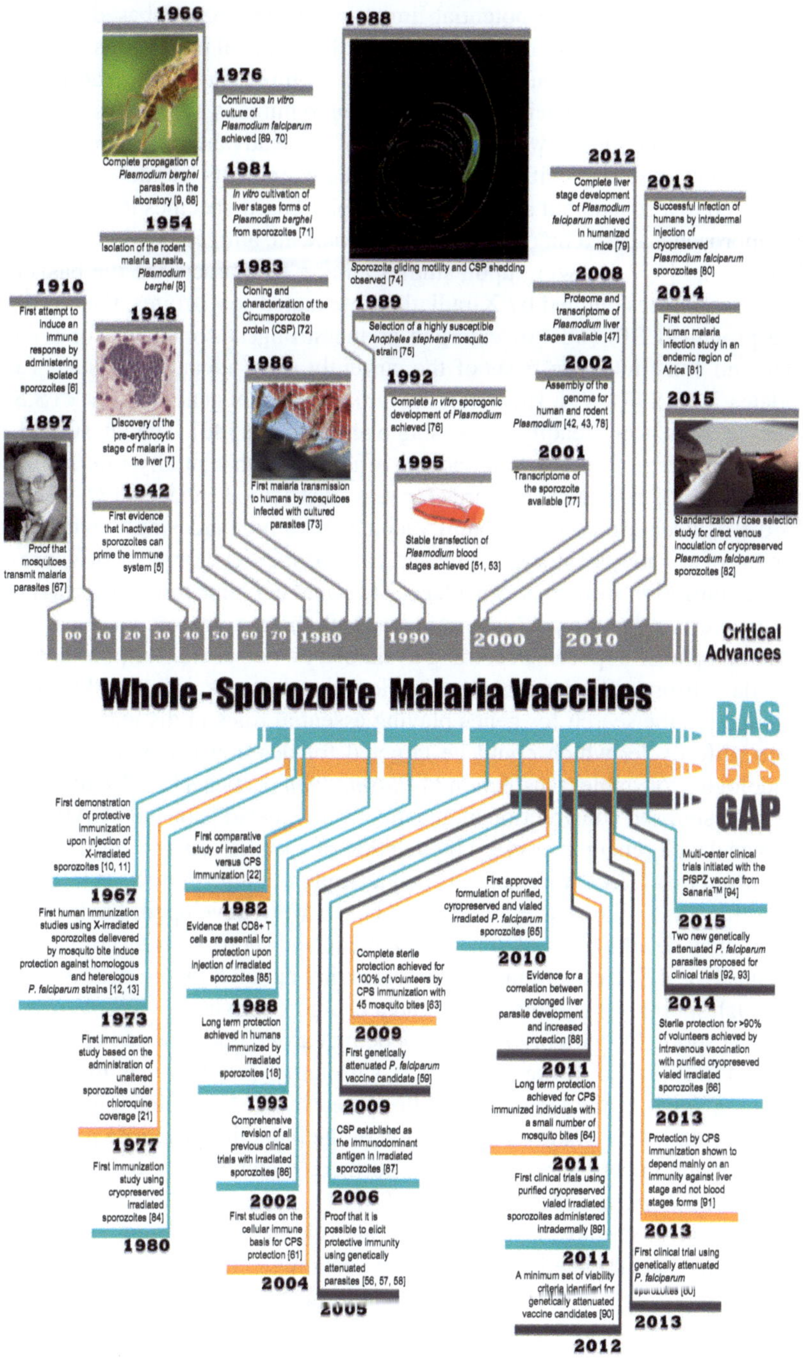

Fig. 1 Timeline of critical events in whole-sporozoite malaria vaccine development. *Top* [5–9, 15–35], *bottom* [10, 13, 36–59]

Nonetheless, some of the potential limitations of sporozoite-based vaccination strategies were already evident in the 1970s [65]. Technical procedures to manufacture and store the large amounts of sporozoites required for immunization, as well as to provide safe and efficacious administration to humans, were always a concern and justified the skepticism with which some of these advances were received [66]. These difficulties, along with extraordinary developments in molecular biology methods, led to a substantial shift from sporozoite-based vaccines to subunit vaccination approaches, based on only one or a few parasite antigens with high immunogenic potential [67]. Drawing upon studies aiming to characterize the basis of the protective responses elicited by X-radiation-attenuated sporozoites, the circumsporozoite protein (CSP) [68–70] emerged as the strongest contender for a subunit vaccine and constitutes the basis of the currently most advanced of such vaccine candidates, RTS,S [71–79]. However, the initial optimism generated by RTS,S over 20 years ago has been steadily decreasing over the years [80]. The latest field studies in endemic regions show that vaccine efficacy is substantially inferior to what are the commonly accepted standards for mass distributed vaccines [81–83].

As the reduced efficacy of subunit vaccines became increasingly evident at the beginning of the new century, a renewed call for the development of sporozoite-based immunization strategies took place. At around the same time, malaria research was also entering into the post-genomic era, with the genome sequences of various *Plasmodium* parasite species becoming available, as well as transcriptomic and proteomic data from different parasite developmental stages [15–17, 84–87]. This knowledge fed the search for genes playing essential roles in distinct points of the parasite's life cycle, which could be targeted for deletion using well-established methodologies for stable transfection of *Plasmodium* parasites [18, 19, 88–92]. This led to the design and construction of genetically attenuated parasites (GAPs), whose liver-stage development is arrested by deletion of specific gene(s). Initial studies in mice showed that GAPs were able to elicit a strong immune protection [39, 40, 93]. Shortly afterwards, the first *P. falciparum* GAPs were developed, paving the way for the clinical development of genetically attenuated sporozoites as human vaccine candidates [41, 42]. Concomitantly, strategies that entailed the induction of immunity through sporozoite administration under chemoprophylaxis (CPS) were brought back to the spotlight, with pivotal studies being carried out in mice [43, 94] and in humans [44, 45]. Also in the last decade, substantial progress was made towards overcoming some of the technical hurdles faced by RAS vaccination [46], which eventually culminated in the demonstration of the induction of sterile protection by the intravenous injection of aseptically purified, metabolically active, radiation-attenuated *P. falciparum* sporozoites [47] (Fig. 1).

Recent clinical studies played an important role in consolidating and extending the knowledge accumulated throughout the years regarding the immune responses elicited by sporozoite-based immunization approaches. We now possess a significant understanding of the protective mechanisms at play during whole-sporozoite vaccination. Undoubtedly, our ever-increasing knowledge of these mechanisms will play an instrumental role in guiding future efforts toward the development of a truly effective malaria vaccine.

2 Radiation-Attenuated Sporozoites (RAS)

Radiation-attenuated sporozoites (RAS) have been considered the "gold standard" of whole-sporozoite vaccination [95]. The concept of RAS vaccination was originally described in the late 1960s, when sterile protection from *Plasmodium* challenge was achieved in mice immunized by the mosquito bite administration of *P. berghei* sporozoites attenuated through the X-irradiation of the mosquito vector [10]. These initial studies with rodents paved the way for early studies in humans that established that immunization of volunteers through the bites of irradiated mosquitoes carrying *P. falciparum* or *P. vivax* sporozoites afforded protection against a subsequent *P. falciparum* or *P. vivax* infection [12–14, 96–98]. Between 1989 and 1999, an additional 11 volunteers were immunized by the bites of irradiated *P. falciparum*-infected mosquitoes at the Naval Medical Research Center. Of note, volunteers in these studies averaged nine immunizations with a mean of over 1000 immunizing mosquito bites per volunteer over 9–10 months before the first challenge [51]. Challenges were performed by the bites of mosquitoes infected from cultured *P. falciparum* gametocytes [26, 99], which has since become the method of choice for controlled human malaria infections (CHMIs). A total of 26 challenges were performed in these studies, and protection was observed in 24 of them, with the reported persistence of protective immunity of at least 42 weeks [51].

Despite the protective immunity elicited by these immunization protocols, for a long time, large-scale vaccination with irradiated sporozoites was considered unfeasible, due to the large numbers of parasites required and the need to deliver them alive by infected mosquitoes. As we will see, the twenty-first century brought along significant developments in this regard, to the extent that many researchers no longer consider RAS vaccination impractical. However, recent advances notwithstanding, earlier studies not only established the potential of attenuated sporozoites for malaria vaccination but also began to shed light on the immune responses that govern sterilizing immunity against *Plasmodium* infection.

2.1 Immune Correlates in RAS Immunization

2.1.1 Antibody and T-Cell Responses in Mice and Monkeys

Antibodies have been shown to be effective at limiting the number of parasites that successfully reach the liver [100]. CSP is the most abundant protein on the surface of *Plasmodium* sporozoites and plays a pivotal role in their characteristic gliding motility [101] (Fig. 1). Antibodies against the repeat region of CSP function by blocking both sporozoite motility and invasion of host cells [102]. Passive protection of mice and monkeys by monoclonal or polyclonal antibodies against the central repeat of *P. berghei*, *P. yoelii*, or *P. vivax* CSP has been amply demonstrated (reviewed in [103]). The efficacy of the protective humoral responses targeted to the extracellular, infective sporozoite depends on the concentration and specificity of the anti-sporozoite antibody response [104, 105]. However, besides humoral responses, cell-mediated immune responses of the RAS-immunized host also play a crucial role in the generation of immunity against sporozoite challenge.

$CD8^+$ T cells have been shown to be important for eliminating parasites that successfully invade and replicate within hepatocytes, making the liver stage the primary target for the vaccine-inducible T-cell responses and the presumed target of the RAS vaccination model [100]. It has been suggested that antigens present in the skin following sporozoite injection are presented in the skin-draining lymph nodes, where they prime specific $CD8^+$ T cells which then migrate to the liver [106], where $CD8^+$ T-cell-mediated elimination of *Plasmodium* hepatic stages occurs [107]. The transporter associated with antigen processing (TAP)-associated processing of exoerythrocytic antigens was also shown to be critical for the presentation of liver-stage antigens by infected hepatocytes [108], and, very recently, it was proposed to play a crucial role in $CD8^+$ T-cell-mediated, *P. berghei* RAS-induced sterile protection [109].

The role of T cells in the protection conferred by RAS immunization was originally established by results showing that whereas immunization of T-cell-deficient mice did not result in the generation of protective immunity, B-cell-deficient mice could still be protected following immunization with irradiated sporozoites [110]. Later, passive and adoptive transfer studies in mice further demonstrated that irradiated sporozoites induce potent cell-mediated immunity in the absence of antibodies [111, 112]. Selective depletion of T-cell subsets in RAS-immunized mice by treatment with monoclonal antibodies against $CD4^+$ or $CD8^+$ T cells subsequently showed that, whereas in vivo depletion of $CD4^+$ T cells did not reduce immunity, depletion of $CD8^+$ T cells completely reversed protection [50, 113]. $CD8^+$ T cells were also shown to play an essential role in sterile immunity of *rhesus* monkeys following attenuated sporozoite vaccination [114]. The exact effector mechanisms utilized by the protective memory $CD8^+$ T cells to eliminate liver-stage parasites are yet to be fully elucidated. Studies in mice immunized with *P. berghei* RAS have suggested that IFNγ produced in response to parasite-specific stimulation of $CD8^+$ T cells is a critical effector molecule for protection [113, 115, 116]. However, whether protective mechanisms are indeed mediated by IFNγ produced by $CD8^+$ T cells or by cytolytic perforin and granzyme through direct contact in the absence of IFNγ is not yet absolutely clear (reviewed in [100, 117, 118]). $CD3^+$ γδ T cells have also been implicated in RAS-elicited protective immunity against *P. yoelii* in the absence of αβ T cells [119]. Besides, a role for interleukin (IL)-12, nitric oxide (NO), and NK cells for RAS-induced protective immunity initiated by $CD8^+$ T cells has also been proposed [120, 121].

The pivotal role of $CD8^+$ cytolytic T-cell-mediated protection following RAS vaccination of mice is now fully established, although the quantity or functionality of the protective $CD8^+$ T-cell response can differ based on the rodent model [95]. In fact, although most studies suggest that effective RAS immunization in mice appears to depend on $CD8^+$ T cells, in some strains of mice, protection mediated by $CD8^+$ T cells is not absolute, in which case $CD4^+$ T cells are also crucial [103]. Depletion of $CD8^+$ T cells in some strains of mice does not affect protective immunity against

P. yoelii [122]. Moreover, *P. yoelii* and *P. berghei* RAS-induced sterile immunity has been observed in CD8$^+$ T-cell-deficient mice, where protection appears to be mediated by antibodies and CD4$^+$ T-cell-derived IFNγ [123].

Sporozoites and intrahepatic parasite stages contain over 1000 potential antigens [31]. This has led to alternative suggestions that the effectiveness of RAS immunization might result from broad immune responses against multiple antigen targets [124] or, instead, from a few immunodominant antigens that mediate the protection [52]. Several studies have pointed to CSP as a crucial determinant of T-cell responses following RAS immunization. The first evidence for a role for CSP in CD8$^+$ T-cell-mediated immunity elicited by irradiated sporozoites came from passive transfer and in vitro studies that identified epitopes in the carboxyl terminus of the CSP of *P. berghei* [125] and *P. yoelii* [126], which are recognized by T cells from immunized mice. An epitope of *P. falciparum* CSP was later identified in studies with mice immunized with sporozoites or with recombinant vaccinia virus expressing *P. falciparum* CSP [127]. More recently, it was shown that in the absence of T-cell-dependent immune responses to CSP, protection induced by immunization with two doses of irradiated *P. yoelii* sporozoites was greatly reduced [52]. Another study has shown that protective immunity induced by *P. yoelii* RAS in transgenic mice expressing K^d molecules under the MHC-I promoter is mediated by CSP-specific, Kd-restricted CD8$^+$ T cells [128], further supporting the notion that CSP is indeed an immunodominant protective antigen in mice. However, it has also been shown that, after RAS hyperimmunization, complete CD8$^+$ T-cell-mediated protection can occur in transgenic mice that are T-cell tolerant to CSP and cannot produce antibodies [52]. In an effort to identify these non-CSP-protective T-cell antigens, the synthetic peptides corresponding to 34 *P. yoelii* sporozoite antigens that were predicted to contain strong CD8$^+$ T-cell epitopes were screened for the presence of peptide-specific CD8$^+$ T cells secreting IFNγ in splenocytes of the same hyperimmunized transgenic mice. This study revealed that the numbers of IFNγ-secreting splenocytes specific for the non-CSP antigen-derived peptides were 20–100 times lower than those specific for the CSP-specific peptide. Besides, when mice were immunized with recombinant adenoviruses expressing selected non-CSP antigens, the animals were not protected against challenge with *P. yoelii* sporozoites, despite the large numbers of CD8$^+$-specific T cells generated [129]. While the immunodominance of CSP has been largely accepted, its role in immunity has been questioned by studies employing the expression of heterologous CSP proteins by *P. berghei* and *P. yoelii* sporozoites [130, 131]. Interestingly, adoptive transfer of CD4$^+$ CTLs from mice immunized with *P. berghei* RAS that recognized an unidentified non-CSP sporozoite and blood-stage antigen conferred protection to naïve mice [132]. Nevertheless, immunization of mice with a peptide representing a CD4$^+$ T-cell epitope in the N-terminus of *P. berghei* [133] or *P. yoelii* [134] CSP also conferred protection. It has also been argued that protective subdominant antigens may be expressed both by the sporozoite and by liver-stage parasites to allow recognition by CD8$^+$ T cells primed in the lymph nodes by sporozoites, an expression that may be critical to induce protective CD8$^+$ T cells [100]. In any event, the overwhelming evidence accumulated over the last few decades strongly suggests that CSP plays a pivotal role in the protection conferred by RAS immunization.

2.1.2 Early Studies of Antibody and T-Cell Responses in Humans

Ever since their identification, anti-CSP antibodies have been considered candidates for mediating protective immunity against malaria [67]. RAS immunization of human volunteers has been shown to elicit the production of antibodies to both the repeat and the flanking regions of CSP [61, 63], with antibody levels paralleling the serum inhibitory activity of sporozoite invasion of hepatoma cells in vitro [63]. Antibodies against the immunodominant B-cell epitope of *P. falciparum* CSP, identified as a repetitive $(NANP)_3$ sequence [69, 135, 136], inhibit sporozoite infectivity in vitro [70, 137] and in vivo [138]. However, the efficacy of a $(NANP)_3$ peptide-based vaccine was limited by the absence of *Plasmodium* T-cell epitopes [139, 140], in agreement with the notion that, in naturally exposed individuals, anti-CSP antibody levels seem to correlate with exposure but not necessarily with protection (reviewed in [141]). Antibodies against *P. falciparum* sporozoite surface protein 2 (SSP2) have also been identified in RAS-immunized volunteers protected against malaria [142].

CSP-specific cellular immune responses were described in RAS-immunized volunteers as determined by the proliferation of peripheral blood mononuclear cells (PBMCs) upon in vitro stimulation with recombinant *P. falciparum* CSP [61, 143]. An epitope mapping to the 5′ repeat region of *P. falciparum* CSP was identified in T-cell lines and clones obtained from a sporozoite-immunized human volunteer [144]. Another epitope (peptide 326–345) of the *P. falciparum* CSP was later shown to be recognized by human cytolytic class II-restricted $CD4^+$ T cells [145]. This epitope contains both a polymorphic [146] and a conserved [69] region of *P. falciparum* CSP, consistent with strain cross-reactivity of RAS-induced protection. A subsequent analysis of the genetic restriction of a series of T-cell clones derived from three RAS-immunized volunteers showed that peptide 326–345 can be presented by multiple MHC class II HLA-DR alleles [147]. Most of the clones analyzed in this study recognized a series of variant peptides representing the amino acid substitutions found in the polymorphic region of different *P. falciparum* strains, suggesting that polymorphism might not constitute a serious obstacle for recognition of this region of CSP by $CD4^+$ T cells [147].

Despite the wide array of direct evidence regarding the contribution of *Plasmodium*-specific $CD8^+$ T cells in protection in mouse models of RAS immunization, the inability to conduct $CD8^+$ T-cell depletion studies in humans makes direct evidence of $CD8^+$ T-cell involvement in immunity harder to obtain. However, as we will see below, liver-stage-specific cytokine-producing $CD8^+$ T-cell responses are induced by RAS immunization in humans and may indeed contribute to protection.

2.1.3 RAS Immunization-Based Discovery of Preerythrocytic *P. falciparum* Antigens

Following the discovery that particular HLA class I and class II alleles were associated with resistance to severe malaria in Gambian children [148], an HLA-based approach termed reverse immunogenetics has been employed to identify epitopes from preerythrocytic-stage antigens of *P. falciparum*. This approach enabled the identification of CTL epitopes for two common HLA-B alleles in the liver-stage antigen 1 (LSA-1) protein of *P. falciparum* [149, 150] as well as epitopes for several class I antigens that are found at high frequencies in Caucasians and/or Africans, including CSP, SSP2, and sporozoite threonine- and asparagine-rich protein (STARP) [149, 151].

Antigen discovery studies in naturally infected populations have been significantly complemented and extended by analyses performed in the context of RAS immunization. Proliferative T-cell responses to *P. falciparum* SSP2 have been reported in protected RAS-immunized volunteers suggesting that this antigen is a target of protective immunity [142]. HLA-B8-restricted responses against two epitopes of SSP2, one of which is conserved and the other variant among *P. falciparum* isolates, have also been reported in two *P. falciparum* RAS-immunized individuals [152]. Later, a panel of 27 open reading frames (ORFs) previously identified by a proteomic analysis [31], representing antigens potentially expressed in the sporozoite and intrahepatic stage of *P. falciparum* life cycle, was interrogated, leading to the identification of 16 antigenic proteins recognized by *P. falciparum* RAS-immunized volunteers [153]. Peptides derived from four previously well-characterized *P. falciparum* preerythrocytic-stage antigens [CSP, SSP2, LSA-1, and exported protein 1 (EXP-1)] were analyzed in parallel. Noteworthy, the reactivity against several of the newly identified antigens, most notably antigen 2 (later designated CelTOS—cell-traversal protein for ookinetes and sporozoites [154]), exceeded those observed against the well-characterized antigens [153]. In a subsequent study, protein microarrays representing 23 % of the entire *P. falciparum* proteome were probed with plasma from individuals either showing sterile protection or not protected against infectious *P. falciparum* challenge, following experimental *P. falciparum* RAS immunization [155]. Overall, a markedly different pattern in antibody recognition was observed between the protected and non-protected groups of individuals, in agreement with previously obtained data [156]. A panel of 19 preerythrocytic-stage antigens, 16 of which were novel, was identified as strongly associated with RAS-induced protective immunity, which may form a potential signature associated with sporozoite-induced protection [155]. More recently, 27 out of 151 recombinant *P. falciparum* preerythrocytic antigens selected bioinformatically were recognized by plasma from RAS-immunized volunteers. Twenty-one of these antigens induced detectable antibody responses in mice and rabbits. Moreover, PBMCs from RAS-immunized subjects elicited positive ex vivo or cultured ELISpot responses against peptides from 20 of 22 of these antigens [157]. This study also showed that peptides spanning the full length of *P. falciparum* CelTOS recalled significantly higher positive responses from protected than non-protected subjects [157].

Collectively, these results suggested that immune responses to *Plasmodium* are complex and multispecific. These data further suggest that serodominance does not necessarily correlate with sporozoite-induced immunity and that some of the novel antigens identified by recently employed strategies may represent good candidates for vaccine development [153, 155].

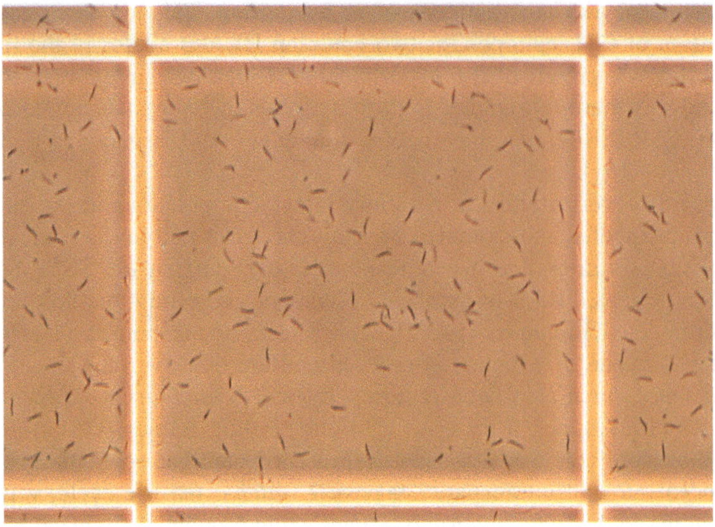

Fig. 2 Purified PfSPZ. The purification process significantly reduces the amount of salivary gland and mosquito material contaminating the PfSPZ (200× magnification). Photo kindly provided by Sanaria™ Inc.

2.2 *Recent Progress in RAS Immunization*

The twenty-first century witnessed a renewed interest in RAS immunization, which, to a significant extent, was due to the efforts of the company Sanaria™. This company has developed a radiation-attenuated, metabolically active, non-replicating *P. falciparum* sporozoite vaccine, the PfSPZ vaccine (Fig. 2) [46, 66]. The vialed PfSPZ vaccine is aseptic purified and cryopreserved in liquid nitrogen vapor phase (LNVP) [158], by an undisclosed method. Non-attenuated PfSPZ, cryopreserved by the same method, seems to be substantially less infective than their freshly dissected counterparts [159]. Nevertheless, they have been successfully employed in various CHMI studies where they have been administered by intradermal (id; [33, 34, 160]), intramuscular (im; [160–162]), and intravenous (iv; [35, 162]) routes, paving the way to PfSPZ vaccine immunization studies in humans.

2.2.1 The PfSPZ Vaccine Immunization and the Search for Immune Correlates of Protection

The first attempt at vaccination with the PfSPZ vaccine to humans was reported in 2011, when the vaccine was administered to 80 volunteers by id or subcutaneous (sc) injection, prior to challenge with infectious *P. falciparum* sporozoites [54]. Although the vaccine administered by these routes proved safe, it was only poorly immunogenic and protective, with only two individuals protected out of 44 immunized volunteers challenged by the bites of five *P. falciparum*-infected mosquitoes. Immunized volunteers produced generally low levels of T-cell responses in response to a stimulus with PfSPZ, as measured by IFNγ production, which increased with vaccine dose and number of boosts for the sc but not for the id group of volunteers [54]. Furthermore, PBMCs from immunized volunteers showed a low frequency of PfSPZ-specific $CD4^+$ T cells producing any combination of the IFNγ, tumor necrosis factor-α (TNF-α), and interleukin-2 (IL-2) cytokines and no $CD8^+$ T-cell responses whatsoever [54]. Also of note, responses to whole sporozoites were more pronounced than to any of the individual *P. falciparum* proteins CSP, SSP2, LSA-1, or CelTOS. The titers of antibodies against whole *P. falciparum* sporozoites and *P. falciparum* CSP were found to increase with vaccine dose and number of doses, but immune sera revealed at best a modest capacity to inhibit *P. falciparum* sporozoite invasion in vitro [54]. These results prompted additional studies in nonhuman primate (NHP) and rabbit models to assess the impact of the route of immunization on protection. The results obtained strongly indicated that immunogenicity and protective efficacy could be greatly improved by iv administration of the PfSPZ vaccine. The suboptimal immunogenicity and protection elicited by vaccine administration by other routes may be explained by the reduced liver load that results from the latter, as was observed in mouse studies employing *P. berghei* [163, 164] and *P. yoelii* [164] sporozoites.

Collectively, the data obtained in this study argue in favor of iv vaccine administration to elicit sterile protection by RAS immunization. Indeed, this is the subject of a groundbreaking study in 2013, where various doses of the PfSPZ vaccine were administered iv to 40 volunteers, prior to challenge with fully infectious *P. falciparum* sporozoites [47]. The results of this study showed that the vaccine was protective, with six out of six and three out of nine volunteers immunized with five and four doses of 135,000 PfSPZ vaccine, respectively, fully protected against malaria. Humoral responses in protected and unprotected subjects were assessed 2 weeks after the last immunization by measuring antibody titers against CSP and PfSPZ, as well as by in vitro assays of inhibition of PfSPZ invasion (ISI). A dose-dependent increase in anti-CSP and anti-PfSPZ antibody titers, as well as in ISI, was observed. However, despite a clear trend for higher antibody titers and ISI in protected than in unprotected individuals, neither of these parameters could directly predict protection. Multiparameter flow cytometry was also employed to assess the frequency of PfSPZ-specific IFNγ, IL-2, TNF-α, or perforin-producing $CD3^+CD4^+$, $CD3^+CD8^+$, $CD3^+$ γδ T cells and NK cells from PBMCs 2 weeks after the final immunization. Although no absolute correlates of cell-mediated protection could be derived from this analysis, important information about the immune responses elicited by RAS immunization could be obtained: (1) a dose-dependent increase in frequency of PfSPZ-specific $CD3^+CD4^+$ T cells and $CD3^+CD8^+$ T cells producing any combination of IFNγ, IL-2, or TNF-α was observed; (2) there was no significant difference between protected and unprotected individuals for PfSPZ-specific $CD3^+CD4^+$ IFNγ-producing T cells, whereas protected subjects showed a trend toward higher and more consistent PfSPZ-specific $CD3^{+}CD8^{+}$ IFNγ-producing T-cell responses; (3) no differences were observed between protected and unprotected subjects in terms of the quality of the PfSPZ-specific $CD3^{+}CD4^{+}$ T-cell responses, while a somewhat higher percentage of PfSPZ-specific $CD3^{+}CD8^{+}$ T cells that produced IFNγ only was observed in protected than in non-protected individuals; and (4) the overall frequency of $CD3^{+}$ γδ T cells increased in subjects who received the highest dose of vaccine. Finally, ELISpot analyses showed that IFNγ responses to PfSPZ were highest in the group that received the highest vaccine load, but IFNγ responses to CSP, SSP2, LSA-1, and CelTOS were low or undetectable in all subjects that received 135,000 PfSPZ vaccine [47].

More recently, another study assessed long-term protection of human volunteers following PfSPZ vaccination. In this report, 7 out of 9 and 6 out of 11 volunteers immunized with four doses of 270,000 iv-administered PfSPZ were protected following CHMI at 3 and 21 weeks after immunization, respectively. Five of the individuals protected at 21 weeks were re-challenged at 59 weeks after immunization and none developed parasitemia [165]. This study further showed that im injection of PfSPZ was substantially less efficient in inducing protection than iv administration of the vaccine, as only 3 out of 8 subjects vaccinated im with 2.2×10^6 PfSPZ were protected 3 weeks after vaccination, and all three developed parasitemia upon repeat CHMI at 25 weeks [165]. On average, anti-CSP and anti-PfSPZ antibody levels measured 2 weeks after the last immunization were significantly higher in protected than in non-protected individuals who underwent CHMI 3 and 21–25 weeks after the final immunization. Interestingly, the percentage of IFNg-, IL-2- and/or TNFα-producing *P. falciparum*-specific $CD4^{+}$ and $CD8^{+}$ T cells in the blood did not correlate with outcome at the 3-week or the 21- to 25-week CHMI. However, the absolute frequency of unstimulated $V\delta2^{+}$ T cells as a percentage of total lymphocytes correlated with outcome at the 21- to 25-week CHMI, while the frequency of the $V\delta2^{+}$ T cell subset measured prior to the first immunization also correlated with outcome of CHMI at 3 and 21–25 weeks [165]. Nevertheless, it is important to note that neither the antibody nor the cellular correlates found in this study constitute absolute predictors of protection, as no clear threshold of antibody levels or $V\delta2^{+}$ T cell frequency exists, above which all subjects are protected and below which none are.

Despite the encouraging results obtained with the PfSPZ vaccine, several challenges remain. These include the high numbers of parasites required for immunization, the requirement for iv delivery, the relatively high number of doses required for protection, the possibility that the vaccine might be strain specific, and the duration of protection after immunization [166, 167]. However, efforts to tackle these and other issues are currently being made by Sanaria™ [168] and others. With five stage 1 clinical trials already completed, and an additional seven stage 2 trials in the USA, Europe, and Africa planned to address a set of well-defined objectives [59], significant progress in the clinical development of the PfSPZ vaccine can safely be expected in the near future.

3 Genetically Attenuated Parasites (GAPs)

3.1 Creation of GAPs

As discussed above, human test subjects immunized with *P. falciparum* RAS can be effectively protected from a subsequent challenge of fully infectious *P. falciparum* wild-type sporozoites. In 2005, employing rodent models of malaria, it was reported that similar sporozoite attenuation can be achieved by targeted gene deletion, by removing genes essential for liver-stage development, thereby creating so-called genetically attenuated parasites (GAPs) [40, 93]. Importantly, mice immunized with rodent *Plasmodium* GAPs can induce sterile immunity that is comparable to RAS immunization [169]. An advantage of GAPs over RAS immunization is that GAPs constitute a homogeneous population of parasites with a defined attenuation phenotype. This removes issues related to the delivery of correct doses of irradiation in order to ensure sufficient attenuation without killing the parasites or leaving them competent to produce a blood infection. The conceptual basis of vaccines consisting of GAP, just like RAS, is that after inoculation sporozoites invade but only partially develop in the liver. In the years following the first description of GAPs, a number of gene deletion mutants have been described in the rodent malaria models, *P. berghei* and *P. yoelii*, which are completely or partially attenuated, and manifest an arrest phenotype at different points during liver-stage development which provokes different levels of protective immunity (Fig. 3) [171].

The generation of GAPs, which can serve as a malaria vaccine, requires the creation of genetically engineered sporozoites that can invade liver cells but are unable to complete hepatic development. Furthermore, these parasites must provoke a strong protective immunity against a subsequent human malaria infection. These two features are critical to the development of a malaria vaccine consisting of attenuated parasites: first and foremost it must be safe (i.e., complete attenuation in the liver) and next it needs to be potent (generates strong protective immunity). *Plasmodium* genes that may govern exclusively sporozoite and/or liver-stage-specific functions were first identified by characterizing mRNA transcripts that are only expressed (or highly upregulated) in salivary gland sporozoites [30, 172]. Deletion of some of these gene candidates from the genomes of rodent malaria parasites resulted in the creation of some of the first GAPs [39, 93]. Moreover, as with irradiated sporozoites, immunization with sporozoites lacking expression of these proteins generated sterile protective immunity against malaria in mice. Independent studies, also in rodent models, investigating proteins of the *Plasmodium* 6-Cys protein family revealed that one member of this family, P52, was vital for parasite development in the liver and immunization of mice with sporozoites lacking P52 could also induce protective immunity [40]. Mutants lacking the 6-Cys protein P52 either by itself or in combination with the deletion of the gene encoding the closely related protein, P36, were among the first GAP to be created in *P. falciparum* [41, 55, 173]. Recently, a newly identified member of the 6-Cys protein family, B9, has

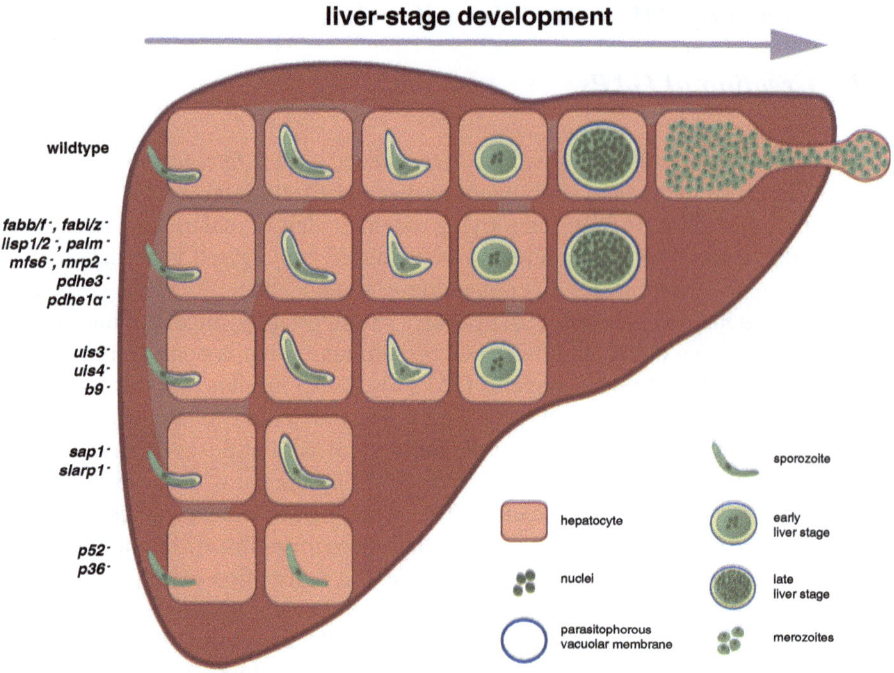

Fig. 3 Liver-stage developmental arrest of GAPs in rodent malaria models. Adapted from [170] and kindly provided by Britta Nyboer

also been shown to be critical to parasite development in the liver, and mutants lacking this protein have been shown to elicit strong protective immunity in rodent models [58, 174]. After the initial identification of these rodent GAPs, a number of other gene deletion mutants have been identified that are completely or partially attenuated and shown to induce protective immunity [171, 175] (Fig. 3). However, of all the GAP candidates in rodent models that could be advanced as a potential *P. falciparum* GAP vaccine, only mutants lacking the gene *slarp* (alternatively known as *sap1*), which encodes a protein involved in the regulation of transcripts in sporozoites, have been shown to fully arrest during liver-stage development, even at very high sporozoite doses (up to 5×10^6 sporozoites inoculated intravenously) [176–178]. Recently, GAPs generated in both *P. berghei* and *P. falciparum* lacking the gene *mrp2* that arrest mid-late during liver-stage development are only the second mutant that appears to be fully arrested in the liver cell even at very high sporozoite doses [179]. All other GAPs have been shown to be capable of leading to breakthrough blood infections when the dose of sporozoites is increased [171]. Consequently, the GAPs that are most advanced for human use and currently ready for clinical evaluation consist of mutants where *slarp/sap1* has been removed in addition to the deletion of one or more of the 6-Cys genes from the *P. falciparum* genome. Specifically, the *P. falciparum* GAPs "*p52(−)/p36(−)/sap1(−)*" and "*Δb9Δslarp*" have both been examined in blood-stage culture, in mosquitoes, in cultured human hepatocytes, and in mice engrafted with human liver tissue and have been shown to only exhibit a growth defect after liver cell invasion [57, 58]. They completely abort intrahepatic development, demonstrating that they are likely to be safe for use in humans; currently these GAPs await clinical testing to evaluate their protective efficacy in humans. Importantly, these *P. falciparum* GAPs are expected to arrest early in hepatic development, soon after invasion of hepatocytes by sporozoites.

It has been reported that a late-arresting rodent GAP was a superior immunogen to irradiated sporozoites and early-arresting GAPs [53]. GAPs that progress into late liver-stage development will express both a greater quantity and a greater diversity of antigens, compared to early-arresting GAPs and RAS. The hypothesis is that parasites that arrest late into liver-stage development will not only expose the immune system to a greater magnitude of antigens (a mature liver stage contains up to 40,000 times more protein than an invading sporozoite) but also to a greater diversity of antigens, as they will express antigens expressed in irradiated sporozoites as well as antigens expressed later in the liver and in blood stages (Fig. 3).

3.2 Immunity Induced After GAP Immunization

Depending on the type and/or strength of attenuation, parasites arrest at different time points during liver-stage development or shortly thereafter. Heat-killed or over-irradiated sporozoites fail to invade hepatocytes and hence do not confer protection [180]. This emphasizes the importance of the preerythrocytic stage and the requirement for metabolically active, attenuated parasites that progress at least to early hepatic development before they arrest [181]. Sterile protective immunity in whole-sporozoite experimental vaccinations highly depends on the parasite species, mouse strains, and the immunization regimens. As such, sterile protection is more easily achieved in the *P. yoelii*/Balb/c experimental model than in the *P. berghei*/C57/Bl6 model [121, 182].

Protective immunity has been reported to rely on $CD8^+$ T cells and IFNγ as the key mediators of protection in all different GAP models [169, 183, 184]. Depletion of $CD4^+$ T cells did not abrogate protection, although adoptive transfer of $CD4^+$ T cells from, e.g., *uis3(−)*-GAP-immunized mice protected 50 % of naïve animals from wild-type infection, indicating a role also for this T-cell subset in GAP-induced immunity. Humoral responses to CSP were measured in the *P. berghei* GAP model but appeared to be dispensable since B-cell-deficient mice were capable of sterile protection [183].

Similarly to RAS, GAP immunization induces a significant increase in intrahepatic $CD8^+$ T cells displaying a T effector memory phenotype (Tem) that is clearly associated with long-term protection [185, 186]. Concerning direct effector mechanisms, Trimnell et al. hypothesized that contact-dependent cytotoxicity is mediated by $CD8^+$ T cells since sterile protection was abolished in perforin-deficient mice. Moreover, $CD8^+$ T cells induced apoptosis in infected hepatocytes in vitro [169, 186].

One dose of *P. yoelii uis4(−)* sporozoites was sufficient to induce protection against challenge infection in a Balb/c mouse background [184] that is mediated by the significant upregulation of specific effector CD8⁺ T-cell activation markers such as CD11c. It was suggested that the upregulated CD11c expression phenotype on effector CD8⁺ T cells induced by *P. yoelii* GAP vaccination is not only responsible for their potent inflammatory function but also marks their highly proliferative but short-lived, antigen-specific effector activity, which will ultimately lead to controlling both infectious sporozoite hepatocyte invasion and intrahepatic differentiation [187].

A second generation of GAP leading to a late arrest in liver-stage development was introduced more recently. Immunization with *Pyfabb/f(−)* parasites that are depleted of a gene encoding an essential enzyme of the apicoplast-localized, type II fatty acid biosynthesis (FAS II) pathway induced long-lasting protection in rodent models [53, 188], despite later evidence of breakthrough infections by *Pbfabb/f(−)* parasites [55]. The results of the underlying study further suggested that a larger number of effector memory CD8⁺ T cells with a broader antigenic specificity were elicited by immunization with *Pyfabb/f(−)* GAPs as compared to early-arresting GAP or even RAS. These characteristics of *Pyfabb/f(−)*-induced immune responses correlated with enhanced protection, and thus it was postulated that late-arresting GAP confers superior protective immunity than early-arresting attenuated parasites. Besides, it was shown that this superior protection is stage transcending, i.e., mice immunized with *Pyfabb/f(-)* are not only sterile protected against sporozoite-induced challenge infection but also enjoy protective immunity after intravenous challenge with homologous *P. yoelii* blood-stage parasites [53].

As such late-arresting live attenuated parasites are promising for next-generation vaccine design, it is now imperative to gain a more detailed overview about the underlying immunological functions triggered during experimental vaccination, before such attenuated parasites can be optimized for human clinical trials. Protective immunity induced by the late-arresting experimental whole-organism model parasite *Pyfabb/f(−)* was comprehensively studied over the last few years. It was recently found that not only CD8⁺ T cells but also CD4⁺ T cells contribute to protective responses and that the co-stimulatory molecule CD40 is key in mediating robust protection. CD40 signaling was demonstrated to control intrahepatic DC licensing during *Pyfabb/f(−)* immunization and seems to be instrumental for establishing robust CD8⁺ effector and memory T-cell responses [189]. Very recently, the immunity mechanisms underlying stage-transcending protection exclusively induced by late-arresting *Pyfabb/f(−)* GAP [53] were reported to involve both the cellular and humoral arm of the immune system. Hence, it is proposed that during experimental vaccination with late-arresting GAPs, the immune system gets equipped to establish immunity against both the clinically silent, intrahepatic and pathological, blood-stage phase. As for the humoral response, it is thought that antigenic targets are shared between the hepatic and blood-stage phase and protective antibodies rely on F_c-mediated functions such as F_c receptor binding and complement fixation [190]. Indeed, a study by Keitany et al. showed for the first time that functional antibodies are induced in *Pyfabb/f(−)* GAP-immunized mice and inhibit liver cell invasion as well as the capacity to decrease intrahepatic parasite burden [191]. It is a matter of course that such GAPs not only inform about the underlying immunological mechanisms involved in protection against parasites but will also be ideal to further isolate novel antigens and/or correlates of (transcending) sterile protection. The latter will ideally assist in the development of novel subunit-anti-infective vaccination strategies. Interestingly, a study headed by Chen et al. reported the identification of *Py*Tmp21 as a promising protective antigen candidate that shows the capacity to reduce intrahepatic parasite burden and contribute to sterile protection during *Pyfabb/f(−)* GAP experimental immunization [192, 193].

Experimental immunization of rodents with a knockout parasite line for the *Plasmodium*-specific apicoplast protein important for liver merozoite formation (PALM) elicits potent and long-lived protective immunity against sporozoite-induced malaria by only two immunization doses. Indeed *palm(−)* knockout parasites are very similar to the *Plasmodium* late-arresting *fabb/f(−)* strain, as PALM seems to be important for the successful transition from liver to blood-stage parasites, i.e., display a growth arrest at a very late time point in intrahepatic development [194]. Indeed, a thorough study of the underlying immunity mechanisms of *palm(−)*-vaccinated rodents revealed persistence of some intrahepatic antigen-specific IFNγ-secreting $CD8^+$ memory T cells in aging immunized mice [195, 196].

The involvement of innate immunity in GAP-mediated immune responses still remains to be investigated. GAP immunization of *RAG1 (−/−)* mice that lack adaptive immune cells (which are traditionally considered to mediate memory responses to vaccinations) resulted in a delayed disease outbreak after challenge with viable sporozoites, suggesting that the innate immune system in these mice is sufficient to confer partial protection after vaccination, e.g., through NK memory cells [183]. However, the cellular events and molecular pathways underlying the process of memory generation in NK cells remain largely elusive.

Regarding antigenic specificity, only CSP-specific, IFNγ-secreting $CD8^+$ T cells, as well as CSP-specific antibodies, were reported to be elicited by GAP immunizations. Indeed, Kumar et al. measured no significant differences in these CSP-specific responses in Balb/c mice that were either immunized with *Py*RAS or *Pyuis3(−)* and *Pyuis4(−)* genetically attenuated parasites. The authors therefore postulated conserved and similar mechanisms of protection irrespective of the method of attenuation [183, 197].

Recently, the results from a first clinical trial demonstrated safety of *Pf*GAP vaccination in humans using *Pfp52(−)/p36(−)* double knockout parasites. Initial immunological profiling showed CSP-specific antibody titers after 200-bite exposure of volunteers and moderate memory responses of $CD8^+$ and $CD4^+$ T cells to CSP and non-CSP antigens such as LSA-1 or AMA-1. Of importance, a breakthrough infection was observed in one of the *Pf*GAP-immunized volunteers suggesting that development of more severely attenuated *Pf*GAP, possibly with multiple gene deletions, should be pursued in future developments [42].

It has been demonstrated that immunization of mice with late liver-stage-arresting GAP elicits broader and better $CD8^+$ T-cell responses when compared to irradiated (early-arresting) sporozoites, producing superior long-lasting sterile protection against a malaria infection [53]. These parasites are believed to present a greater diversity and amount of parasite antigen to the host immune system. However, *P. falciparum* parasites lacking FabB/F expression fail to produce sporozoites [198]. Thus, discrepancies in attenuation phenotypes and potency between GAPs of different *Plasmodium* species indicate that the importance of the same gene for liver-stage development may differ between rodent models and *P. falciparum*. Consequently, the identification of *Plasmodium* genes that are critical to mid-/late liver-stage development to create late-arresting *P. falciparum* GAPs is actively being sought, and a number of gene expression studies on rodent and human sporozoite and/or intrahepatic liver stages are currently being mined to identify these genes.

4 Chemoprophylaxis and Sporozoite (CPS) Immunization

While sterile protection has been most elaborately investigated using RAS, induction of protective preerythrocytic immunity is most potent and efficient when sporozoite and liver-stage development remain fully intact, while asexual-stage multiplication is abrogated at the earliest stages [59, 199, 200]. Attempts with targeted deletions of genes encoding late-stage liver antigens are promising, but, as outlined above, safety has thus far not been appropriately ensured in humans because of the occurrence of breakthrough infections with asexual-stage parasites [42, 175, 199]. Successes, however, have been reported with the use of antimalarial drugs in combination with wild-type parasites: chemoprophylaxis and sporozoites (CPS) immunization (or infection-treatment-vaccination (IVT)) can safely induce fully protective immune responses as was first demonstrated in rodents [37, 38, 43, 201]. The first drug used in these *P. berghei* studies to kill parasites at early blood-stage level was chloroquine, which disrupts heme detoxification and does not affect preerythrocytic stages [202, 203]. Other antimalarials have since been successfully used in rodents, including artesunate, azithromycin, clindamycin, mefloquine, piperaquine, primaquine, and pyrimethamine with variable effects on parasite liver-stage development [204–208]. Similar results have been obtained in the CHMI model where malaria-naïve adult volunteers receiving mosquito bites from a total of 36–45 *P. falciparum*-infected mosquito under chloroquine prophylaxis (Fig. 4a) show complete protection against a homologous challenge 3–5 months after the last immunization and (partial) protection up to 2.5 years later [44, 45, 56]. Chloroquine and mefloquine are equipotent as prophylactic drugs [209], and other partner drugs are under investigation in ongoing trials [59]. As in murine models [43, 210, 211], induction of sterile CPS-induced protection is dose dependent (Fig. 4b) [209]. Both partial and full protection against a heterologous *P. falciparum* strain after CPS immunization have been demonstrated in a rechallenge trial [212] and are under further investigation (clinicaltrials.gov NCT02098590).

The potency of the CPS-chloroquine regimen is unprecedented compared to radiation-attenuated sporozoite (RAS) immunization and to protection obtained

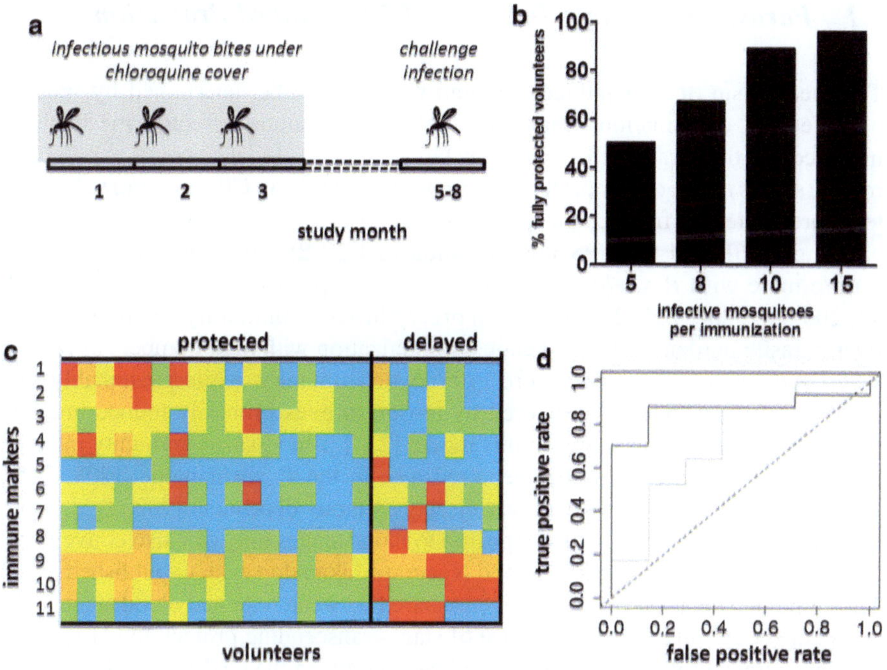

Fig. 4 CPS immunization regime, protection, and cellular immune signature in human volunteers. (**a**) Malaria-naïve adult volunteers are subjected monthly to bites of *P. falciparum*-infected mosquitoes while taking chemoprophylaxis. Protection is assessed by challenge infection via infected mosquitoes 3–5 months after the last immunization. (**b**) Sterile protection defined as the absence of parasitemia by microscopy until 21 days after challenge infection is dose dependent as assessed for $n=58$ volunteers enrolled in four clinical trials using either chloroquine or mefloquine prophylaxis [44, 56, 209]. (**c**) *Rows* show eleven biomarkers that can distinguish $n=17$ fully protected and $n=7$ partially protected/delayed volunteers in a dose escalation CPS trial [209], identified by penalized logistic regression. *Colors* indicate the degree of responses, with strongest responses in *red*. (**d**) Accuracy of prediction of protection from mosquito bite challenge assessed with the area under the receiver operator curve based on leave-one-out cross validation (LOOCV), using one parameter alone (parasite-specific degranulating CD107a$^+$ CD4$^+$ T cells, *light gray line*, AUC 0.73) or in combination with ten additional markers (AUC 0.87, *dark gray line*) (unpublished data)

after natural infections [59, 213]. While the dogma that protective malaria immunity is difficult to acquire is challenging, possible explanations including the broader antigenic repertoire, higher antigen load, and potential immunomodulatory effects of chloroquine remain speculative [200]. The CPS model, however, opens avenues for a better understanding of immune mechanisms of protective immunity, identification of immune correlates of protection, and novel target antigens for inclusion in subunit vaccines. Moreover, clinical development of a vaccine based on the CPS regime is currently explored with cryopreserved sporozoites as PfSPZ-CVac (clinicaltrials.gov NCT02511054 and NCT02115516 and [59, 214]).

4.1 Parasite Life Cycle Target for CPS-Induced Protection

The mechanism of CPS-induced immunity appears to be determined by specific parasite/host combinations regarding both the immune effector mechanisms involved and the parasite life cycle stage targeted. Most evidence points to preerythrocytic stages as targets for protective immunity: (1) human CPS-immunized volunteers are protected from challenge by mosquito bite, but not after a blood-stage challenge [56], and (2) CPS immunization of C57/Bl6 mice with *P. berghei* or Balb/c mice with *P. yoelii* with 10,000 or more sporozoites intravenously [37, 43, 203, 207, 208, 215, 216] results in preerythrocytic immunity and reduction of liver parasite burden [43]. Intravenous immunization with high numbers of *P. chabaudi* sporozoites also induces preerythrocytic immunity, while presumably low numbers of sporozoites as delivered by mosquito bites primarily induce immune responses against blood stages in this model [211]. Blood-stage immunity induced by CPS immunization has been reported also in the *P. yoelii* model [208, 215], where control of parasite growth was clearly antibody dependent [208, 215]. More strikingly, there is evidence that exposure to blood stages only can also convey preerythrocytic immunity ([201, 211] and Nganou-Makamdop et al. unpublished data). The combined data suggest that antigens shared between liver and blood stages [17] create the possibility for the existence of stage-transcending protection [217].

Since clinical follow-up of prolonged parasitemia in the CHMI model is limited for obvious safety reasons, CPS studies in humans primarily highlight induction of liver-stage immunity [56]. There are nevertheless hints for the presence not only of immune recognition but also of blood-stage immunity: (1) although humoral responses directed against blood-stage antigens are minimal ([44, 218] and Behet et al. unpublished data) and show no growth inhibition activity in vitro [56], IFNγ responses to blood-stage parasites are enhanced both in vivo [56] and in vitro [44, 45, 209, 219], and (2) immunized volunteers show a somewhat reduced peak parasitemia after blood-stage challenge [56]. These data feed the possibility that at least some functional blood-stage immunity might be present which only becomes apparent after a number of asexual multiplication cycles required for boosting. This hypothesis is in line with a correlation between prepatent period, as determined by thick smear, and the interval between a positive qPCR and positive thick smear as a proxy for parasite growth rate (Bijker et al. unpublished data), in partially protected volunteers (24). Since prepatency itself was not dependent on parasite density at the time of positive qPCR, these data suggest that parasite growth becomes slower when parasitemia is longer lasting. Thus, the CPS model efficiently induces sterile protection that is, in principle, accomplished at the preerythrocytic level. In addition, a blood-stage component may be present, which may contribute in case of partial protection and might become more evident in individuals possessing some degree of anti-disease immunity that allows longer follow-up. Albeit insufficient by itself, the short period of low-grade parasitemia as obtained under chloroquine prophylaxis in humans might be an asset for induction of at least some contributing blood-stage immunity. Indeed, low parasitemia has been shown before to efficiently induce blood-stage protection in the CHMI model [220].

4.2 Humoral Immunity After CPS Immunization

Parasite-specific antibodies induced by CPS immunization may interfere at several levels with preerythrocytic parasite development where sporozoite integrity, motility (gliding), hepatocyte invasion, and/or intrahepatic development may be compromised. In the *P. berghei* murine model, the functional contribution of antibodies to CPS-induced preerythrocytic protection is unclear: in CPS-immunized C57/Bl6 mice, antibodies induced against sporozoites and liver stages inhibit hepatocyte infection in vitro [208], but are unable to confer protection against sporozoite challenge in vivo [43, 208]. In human volunteers, CPS immunization induces both a robust plasma antibody and long-lasting memory B-cell response [218]. This humoral response is largely directed against preerythrocytic parasite antigens with CSP being the major target identified thus far [44, 209, 218, 221]. Plasma IgG from CPS-immunized volunteers inhibits sporozoite traversal in vitro, as well as liver-stage infection in human liver-chimeric mice following challenge by *P. falciparum*-infected mosquito bites [222]. However, anti-CSP titers per se appear to be a correlate of exposure rather than protection in the human CPS model [218]. In fact, anti-CSP titers are the lowest in individuals that become already protected during the immunization period [218]. Since CSP is not only expressed in sporozoites but also in liver stages [32, 223, 224], one possible explanation might be that at least a proportion of the parasites is eliminated by CPS-induced immune responses early during liver-stage development. It remains to be investigated to what level human anti-CSP antibodies will be sufficient to prevent sporozoite infectivity. There is evidence that targets other than CSP might be involved to accomplish sterile protection [52, 130]. The use of protein microarrays probing the antibody compartment for proteome-wide antigen reactivity [156, 225] has already revealed novel protection-associated antigen targets in RAS-immunized individuals [155], and similar investigations are currently ongoing in CPS-immunized volunteers.

4.3 Cellular Immunity After CPS Immunization

As in other whole-sporozoite vaccination approaches [95], cellular responses induced after CPS immunization are considered to be responsible for the key effector mechanisms driving elimination of infected hepatocytes. In the C57/Bl6 *P. berghei* CPS model, there is a sustained $CD8^+$ T-cell IFNγ response [205, 216] correlating with protective efficacy [216], and immunity can be transferred by total splenocytes [203] and $CD4^+$ and $CD8^+$ T cells [43]. Despite a strong $CD8^+$ T-cell response, protection of *P. yoelii* CPS-immunized C57/Bl6 mice, in contrast, was independent of $CD8^+$ T cells, suggesting a role for $CD4^+$ T cells or antibodies instead. CPS immunization in humans induces long-lasting cellular immune responses [44, 45, 209, 219], which are still detectable even 2.5 years after the initial immunization [45]. In line with a role for both Th1 and cytotoxic responses, CPS-immunized volunteers show increased expression of granzyme B and the Th1 transcription factor T-bet in activated and proliferating T cells during immunization [214]. However, a clear immune correlate of protection has not yet been identified, as neither polyfunctional effector memory T cells that coproduce IFNγ and interleukin-2 [44, 45] nor total IFNγ-producing CD4⁺, CD8⁺, or γδ T cells that can differentiate between fully and partially protected volunteers [209]. Parasite-specific degranulation by CD4⁺ T cells and granzyme B production by CD8⁺ T cells, in contrast, are significantly higher in fully protected individuals [209]. Nevertheless, these cytotoxic responses also do not allow for a distinct differentiation between the two groups. Given the fact that individuals differ in their "immunological fingerprint" and protection likely relies on the interaction of multiple immune effector pathways, a combination of multiple immune markers in the form of an immune signature may be of more predictive of protection than individual responses (Bijker and Teirlinck et al. unpublished data, Fig. 4c, d). Next to adaptive responses, this may also include innate lymphocytes such as NK cells but particularly γδ T cells, which are expanded following CHMI, CPS, and high-dose RAS [47, 219, 226] and show memory-like responses following CPS immunization [209, 219].

Based on observations from natural immunity in the field, the current dogma is that acquisition of protective immunity against malaria per se is a lengthy and difficult process involving many exposures and is rapidly lost in the absence of exposure. The efficient induction and persistence of immunity following CPS immunization, however, clearly refutes this statement and indicates that this may only apply to protection from disease, but not infection. A plausible explanation can be found in the composition of immune responses targeting the different parts of the life cycle involving distinct parasite immune regulation and evasion strategies [200]. CPS immunization induces protection from sporozoite challenge, in line with predominantly preerythrocytic targeted antibodies that reduce sporozoite infectivity and long-lasting cellular cytokine and cytotoxic responses. None of these responses, however, are a clear-cut correlate of protection, and further research is necessary to identify which (combination) of immune responses predicts protection. Importantly, while this immunization regimen has been primarily tested against homologous parasites, heterologous challenge studies are underway and indicate at least some protection. Future studies will need to focus on the identification of target antigens of the induced immune responses and their functionality also against heterologous parasites. Another focus should be to elucidate the potential contribution of blood-stage immunity in this model, particularly in preexposed individuals. Thereby, CPS immunization may not only aid future subunit vaccine development but—once satisfactory—also be considered for clinical development as a vaccine to be marketed for special groups including travelers or the military.

5 Other Models of Sporozoite-Based Vaccination

RAS, GAP, and CPS are, by far, the most thoroughly investigated approaches for whole-sporozoite vaccination against malaria. However, alternative strategies for eliciting protective immune responses against human-infective *Plasmodium* parasites have also been proposed and will be briefly addressed here.

5.1 Chemically Attenuated Sporozoites

Chemical attenuation of sporozoites (CAS) has been investigated as an alternative strategy for the production of a liver-stage vaccine against malaria. Similarly to other whole-sporozoite immunization approaches, the concept of CAS relies on the immune responses elicited during hepatic infection by chemically treated sporozoites, which are unable to progress into a patent blood-stage infection and cause disease. The strategy has been evaluated by the use of centamycin [227], a DNA-binding agent that is effective against blood-stage *Plasmodium* parasites and blocks sexual differentiation of the parasites in mosquitoes [228]. Centamycin-treated *P. berghei* sporozoites were shown to display a significantly reduced hepatocyte infection rate and impaired preerythrocytic development and to be unable to generate blood-stage infections in mice [229]. Immunization of mice with *P. berghei* [229] and *P. yoelii* [229] CAS was shown to produce sterile immunity against challenge with fully infectious sporozoites. Vaccination with *P. yoelii* or *P. berghei* CAS induced sporozoite-specific antibodies and CSP-specific IFNγ-producing $CD8^+$ T-cell responses at levels similar to those generated by RAS immunization [229]. More recently, it was shown that chemical attenuation of *P. berghei* parasites with isopentaquine during their liver-stage development alters disease outcome and protects mice from experimental cerebral malaria [230]. It has been argued that the CAS vaccine presents certain advantages over the RAS approach, most notably the fact that the chemical attenuation process can be strictly controlled, leading to a vaccine that is reproducibly attenuated and does not present the risks potentially associated with improper parasite irradiation [229]. However, further investigations are clearly necessary before the true potential of CAS vaccination can be fully ascertained.

5.2 Rodent Plasmodium-Based Immunization Against Human Malaria

A yet unpublished novel approach for whole-sporozoite vaccination against malaria has recently been proposed, based on the use of genetically modified rodent *Plasmodium* parasites that were genetically engineered to express and present antigens of their human-infective counterparts. The concept relies on the notion that such genetically modified rodent parasites may elicit cross-species immune responses arising from similarities between the antigenic compositions of the two species of parasites (interestingly, immunization with *P. falciparum* CelTOS has previously been shown to confer protection against *P. berghei* [231]), along with antigen-targeted responses resulting from the introduction of specific human *Plasmodium* immunogens on the rodent parasite platform. The proof of concept of this idea has been established through the use of *P. berghei*, a rodent parasite species that is widely recognized as nonpathogenic to humans. *P. berghei* is readily amenable to genetic modification [232], and strategies to generate transgenic parasites expressing human-infective *Plasmodium* proteins have been developed [233]. A method for transgene expression and gene complementation [234] was employed to generate selectable marker-free *P. berghei* parasites that express *P. falciparum* CSP under the control of the *P. berghei* upregulated in sporozoites 4 (UIS4) promoter [*Pb*(*Pf*CS@UIS4)]. *P. berghei* was shown to effectively infect human hepatocytes of human liver-chimeric mice, a requisite for any whole-sporozoite vaccine against malaria. Immunization of mice with *Pb*(*Pf*CS@UIS4) was shown to elicit the production of antibodies against whole *P. falciparum* sporozoites as well as against *P. falciparum* CSP. Passive transfer of the immune serum of these mice into liver-humanized mice followed by challenge by *P. falciparum*-infected mosquito bites led to a significant blockage of hepatic infection by this human-infective parasite. Following completion of its preclinical validation, the *Pb*(*Pf*CS@UIS4) vaccine candidate is expected to enter Phase I/IIa clinical trials. If successful, the use of "naturally attenuated" rodent parasites for immunization against human malaria could gain further momentum, and next-generation vaccine candidates can be envisaged to protect not only against multiple species of human malaria but also against various stages of the parasite's life cycle.

6 Future Directions and Concluding Remarks

The application of a whole-sporozoite vaccination approach has raised various types of concerns, ranging from safety to deployment in the field. Safety-wise, whole-sporozoite immunization requires ensuring that sporozoites cannot complete their development process in the liver or that merozoites are eliminated as soon as they reach the blood while retaining immunogenicity [60, 235]. On the other hand, the *P. falciparum* sporozoites required for immunization must be obtained from infected mosquitoes, which must be reared under appropriate containment conditions to prevent accidental release. Sporozoites are then obtained from the dissection of mosquito salivary glands and must subsequently be purified and adequately cryopreserved for long-term storage [46]. Finally, application to the field requires knowledge of total dose required for protection and timing of booster immunizations [95], as well as a feasible vaccine administration method that ensures the development of protective immune responses.

Many important aspects to be considered for the design of a next-generation preerythrocytic vaccine may equally account for the development of a blood-stage vaccine. The ultimate question to be answered is what kind of immune response must be induced to confer high-level and long-lived protection and how to accomplish this. This task is both supported and exacerbated by the complex and not always unequivocal data from basic research, preclinical, and clinical studies. In general, it will be vital to improve the knowledge about protective immune responses, i.e., to properly understand the difference between vaccine-induced protection and naturally acquired immunity, to exploit the data on *P. falciparum* RAS-mediated protection in humans or the large past clinical trials of RTS,S in order to determine which responses are the true mediators of protection.

A substantial amount of data advocates the need to induce antibody response against the sporozoite to prevent liver infection or at least to reduce the number of sporozoites infecting hepatocytes. The latter mechanism is assumed to contribute to a delay in prepatency in RTS,S-vaccinated individuals which consequently limits severe disease. Likewise, it seems unrealistic that complete protection can be mediated solely by humoral responses that were even shown to be dispensable in animal models. In fact, numerous studies have pointed out the essential role of T-cell responses against liver-stage parasites and have explicitly demonstrated the critical function of intrahepatic $CD8^+$ T cells in protective immunity. This has important implications for the quality and/or quantity of the $CD8^+$ T-cell response but also for the liver as the site of T-cell priming and effector function.

It seems clear that research into the immune responses induced by whole-sporozoite immunization approaches has given first insights into the immune mechanisms involved, but an actual correlate of sterile protective immunity has yet to be revealed. Such a correlate is unlikely to be a single common readout, but instead a signature of multiple immune effector pathways acting in synergy. This will likely include both phenotypic and functional readouts of humoral and cellular immune responses as well as a combination of various antigen targets. Complementing ongoing efforts using the protein microarray for genome-wide screening of antimalarial antibody responses, T cells which target antigen can also be identified by large-scale screen approaches, such as the Atlas™ assay using protein plasmid and expression libraries [225]. Application of this screening technology to samples from RAS- as well as CPS-immunized individuals is currently under way [225] and should be extended to GAP trials in the future. Such comparative analysis will be highly informative to dissect the differences and overlaps in immune signatures between the three main whole-sporozoite immunization approaches to (1) clarify why some approaches are more efficient in inducing protection than others and (2) home in on a minimal signature of antigen targets associated with protection. Target antigen identification will be useful not only for subunit vaccine design but also for generation of next-generation whole-sporozoite immunization regimens using parasites transgenic for variants of key antigens to induce efficient heterologous protection.

It can safely be said that further investigations of the immunological mechanism(s) whereby whole-sporozoite inoculation elicits protective immunity will greatly facilitate whole-sporozoite vaccine development [167]. Such knowledge, along with the expanded use of controlled human malaria infection studies [236, 237] and the envisioned progress in tackling the technical and logistical hurdles that still persist [59], can be expected to lead toward the ultimate goal of obtaining an effective vaccine with a pivotal role in the eventual global eradication of malaria.

References

1. Plotkin S (2014) History of vaccination. Proc Natl Acad Sci U S A 111(34):12283–12287
2. Ozawa S, Clark S, Portnoy A, Grewal S, Brenzel L, Walker DG (2016) Return on investment from childhood immunization in low- and middle-income countries, 2011–20. Health Aff 35(2):199–207
3. World Health Organization (2015) World malaria report 2015. World Health Organization, Geneva
4. McGregor IA (1964) The passive transfer of human malarial immunity. Am J Trop Med Hyg 13(Suppl):237–239
5. Russell PF, Mohan BN (1942) The immunization of fowls against mosquito-borne *Plasmodium gallinaceum* by injections of serum and of inactivated homologous sporozoites. J Exp Med 76(5):477–495
6. Sergent E, Sergent E (1910) Sur l'immunite dans le paludisme des oiseaux. Conservation in vitro des sporozoites de *Plasmodium relictum*. Immunite relative obtenue par inoculation de ces sporozoites. C R Acad Sci 151:407–409
7. Shortt HE, Garnham PC et al (1948) The pre-erythrocytic stage of human malaria, *Plasmodium vivax*. Br Med J 1(4550):547
8. Vincke IH (1954) Natural history of *Plasmodium berghei*. Indian J Malariol 8(4):245–256
9. Yoeli M, Upmanis RS, Vanderberg J, Most H (1966) Life cycle and patterns of development of *Plasmodium berghei* in normal and experimental hosts. Mil Med 131(9 Suppl):900–914
10. Nussenzweig RS, Vanderberg J, Most H, Orton C (1967) Protective immunity produced by the injection of x-irradiated sporozoites of *Plasmodium berghei*. Nature 216(5111):160–162
11. Nussenzweig R, Vanderberg J, Most H (1969) Protective immunity produced by the injection of x-irradiated sporozoites of *Plasmodium berghei*. IV. Dose response, specificity and humoral immunity. Mil Med 134(10):1176–1182
12. Clyde DF, McCarthy VC, Miller RM, Hornick RB (1973) Specificity of protection of man immunized against sporozoite-induced falciparum malaria. Am J Med Sci 266(6):398–403
13. Rieckmann KH, Carson PE, Beaudoin RL, Cassells JS, Sell KW (1974) Letter: sporozoite induced immunity in man against an Ethiopian strain of *Plasmodium falciparum*. Trans R Soc Trop Med Hyg 68(3):258–259
14. Rieckmann KH, Beaudoin RL, Cassells JS, Sell KW (1979) Use of attenuated sporozoites in the immunization of human volunteers against falciparum malaria. Bull World Health Organ 57(Suppl 1):261–265
15. Carlton JM, Angiuoli SV, Suh BB, Kooij TW, Pertea M, Silva JC, Ermolaeva MD, Allen JE, Selengut JD, Koo HL et al (2002) Genome sequence and comparative analysis of the model rodent malaria parasite *Plasmodium yoelii yoelii*. Nature 419(6906):512–519
16. Gardner MJ, Hall N, Fung E, White O, Berriman M, Hyman RW, Carlton JM, Pain A, Nelson KE, Bowman S et al (2002) Genome sequence of the human malaria parasite *Plasmodium falciparum*. Nature 419(6906):498–511
17. Tarun AS, Peng X, Dumpit RF, Ogata Y, Silva-Rivera H, Camargo N, Daly TM, Bergman LW, Kappe SH (2008) A combined transcriptome and proteome survey of malaria parasite liver stages. Proc Natl Acad Sci U S A 105(1):305–310
18. Wu Y, Sifri CD, Lei HH, Su XZ, Wellems TE (1995) Transfection of *Plasmodium falciparum* within human red blood cells. Proc Natl Acad Sci U S A 92(4):973–977
19. van Dijk MR, Waters AP, Janse CJ (1995) Stable transfection of malaria parasite blood stages. Science 268(5215):1358–1362
20. Ross R (1897) On some peculiar pigmented cells found in two mosquitos fed on malarial blood. Br Med J 2(1929):1786–1788
21. Vanderberg JP, Yoeli M (1966) Effects of temperature on sporogonic development of *Plasmodium berghei*. J Parasitol 52(3):559–564
22. Haynes JD, Diggs CL, Hines FA, Desjardins RE (1976) Culture of human malaria parasites *Plasmodium falciparum*. Nature 263(5580):767–769

23. Trager W, Jensen JB (1976) Human malaria parasites in continuous culture. Science 193(4254):673–675
24. Hollingdale MR, Leef JL, McCullough M, Beaudoin RL (1981) In vitro cultivation of the exoerythrocytic stage of *Plasmodium berghei* from sporozoites. Science 213(4511):1021–1022
25. Ozaki LS, Svec P, Nussenzweig RS, Nussenzweig V, Godson GN (1983) Structure of the *plasmodium knowlesi* gene coding for the circumsporozoite protein. Cell 34(3):815–822
26. Chulay JD, Schneider I, Cosgriff TM, Hoffman SL, Ballou WR, Quakyi IA, Carter R, Trosper JH, Hockmeyer WT (1986) Malaria transmitted to humans by mosquitoes infected from cultured *Plasmodium falciparum*. Am J Trop Med Hyg 35(1):66–68
27. Stewart MJ, Vanderberg JP (1988) Malaria sporozoites leave behind trails of circumsporozoite protein during gliding motility. J Protozool 35(3):389–393
28. Feldmann AM, Ponnudurai T (1989) Selection of *Anopheles stephensi* for refractoriness and susceptibility to *Plasmodium falciparum*. Med Vet Entomol 3(1):41–52
29. Warburg A, Miller LH (1992) Sporogonic development of a malaria parasite in vitro. Science 255(5043):448–450
30. Kappe SH, Gardner MJ, Brown SM, Ross J, Matuschewski K, Ribeiro JM, Adams JH, Quackenbush J, Cho J, Carucci DJ et al (2001) Exploring the transcriptome of the malaria sporozoite stage. Proc Natl Acad Sci U S A 98(17):9895–9900
31. Florens L, Washburn MP, Raine JD, Anthony RM, Grainger M, Haynes JD, Moch JK, Muster N, Sacci JB, Tabb DL et al (2002) A proteomic view of the *Plasmodium falciparum* life cycle. Nature 419(6906):520–526
32. Vaughan AM, Mikolajczak SA, Wilson EM, Grompe M, Kaushansky A, Camargo N, Bial J, Ploss A, Kappe SH (2012) Complete *Plasmodium falciparum* liver-stage development in liver-chimeric mice. J Clin Invest 122(10):3618–3628
33. Roestenberg M, Bijker EM, Sim BK, Billingsley PF, James ER, Bastiaens GJ, Teirlinck AC, Scholzen A, Teelen K, Arens T et al (2013) Controlled human malaria infections by intradermal injection of cryopreserved *Plasmodium falciparum* sporozoites. Am J Trop Med Hyg 88(1):5–13
34. Shekalaghe S, Rutaihwa M, Billingsley PF, Chemba M, Daubenberger CA, James ER, Mpina M, Ali Juma O, Schindler T, Huber E et al (2014) Controlled human malaria infection of Tanzanians by intradermal injection of aseptic, purified, cryopreserved *Plasmodium falciparum* sporozoites. Am J Trop Med Hyg 91(3):471–480
35. Mordmuller B, Supan C, Sim KL, Gomez-Perez GP, Ospina Salazar CL, Held J, Bolte S, Esen M, Tschan S, Joanny F et al (2015) Direct venous inoculation of *Plasmodium falciparum* sporozoites for controlled human malaria infection: a dose-finding trial in two centres. Malar J 14:117
36. Edelman R, Hoffman SL, Davis JR, Beier M, Sztein MB, Losonsky G, Herrington DA, Eddy HA, Hollingdale MR, Gordon DM et al (1993) Long-term persistence of sterile immunity in a volunteer immunized with X-irradiated *Plasmodium falciparum* sporozoites. J Infect Dis 168(4):1066–1070
37. Beaudoin RL, Strome CP, Mitchell F, Tubergen TA (1977) *Plasmodium berghei*: immunization of mice against the ANKA strain using the unaltered sporozoite as an antigen. Exp Parasitol 42(1):1–5
38. Orjih AU, Cochrane AH, Nussenzweig RS (1982) Comparative studies on the immunogenicity of infective and attenuated sporozoites of *Plasmodium berghei*. Trans R Soc Trop Med Hyg 76(1):57–61
39. Mueller AK, Labaied M, Kappe SH, Matuschewski K (2005) Genetically modified *Plasmodium* parasites as a protective experimental malaria vaccine. Nature 433(7022):164–167
40. van Dijk MR, Douradinha B, Franke-Fayard B, Heussler V, van Dooren MW, van Schaijk B, van Gemert GJ, Sauerwein RW, Mota MM, Waters AP et al (2005) Genetically attenuated, P36p-deficient malarial sporozoites induce protective immunity and apoptosis of infected liver cells. Proc Natl Acad Sci U S A 102(34):12194–12199

41. VanBuskirk KM, O'Neill MT, De La Vega P, Maier AG, Krzych U, Williams J, Dowler MG, Sacci JB Jr, Kangwanrangsan N, Tsuboi T et al (2009) Preerythrocytic, live-attenuated *Plasmodium falciparum* vaccine candidates by design. Proc Natl Acad Sci U S A 106(31):13004–13009
42. Spring M, Murphy J, Nielsen R, Dowler M, Bennett JW, Zarling S, Williams J, de la Vega P, Ware L, Komisar J et al (2013) First-in-human evaluation of genetically attenuated *Plasmodium falciparum* sporozoites administered by bite of Anopheles mosquitoes to adult volunteers. Vaccine 31(43):4975–4983
43. Belnoue E, Costa FT, Frankenberg T, Vigario AM, Voza T, Leroy N, Rodrigues MM, Landau I, Snounou G, Renia L (2004) Protective T cell immunity against malaria liver stage after vaccination with live sporozoites under chloroquine treatment. J Immunol 172(4):2487–2495
44. Roestenberg M, McCall M, Hopman J, Wiersma J, Luty AJ, van Gemert GJ, van de Vegte-Bolmer M, van Schaijk B, Teelen K, Arens T et al (2009) Protection against a malaria challenge by sporozoite inoculation. N Engl J Med 361(5):468–477
45. Roestenberg M, Teirlinck AC, McCall MB, Teelen K, Makamdop KN, Wiersma J, Arens T, Beckers P, van Gemert G, van de Vegte-Bolmer M et al (2011) Long-term protection against malaria after experimental sporozoite inoculation: an open-label follow-up study. Lancet 377(9779):1770–1776
46. Hoffman SL, Billingsley PF, James E, Richman A, Loyevsky M, Li T, Chakravarty S, Gunasekera A, Chattopadhyay R, Li M et al (2010) Development of a metabolically active, non-replicating sporozoite vaccine to prevent *Plasmodium falciparum* malaria. Hum Vaccin 6(1):97–106
47. Seder RA, Chang LJ, Enama ME, Zephir KL, Sarwar UN, Gordon IJ, Holman LA, James ER, Billingsley PF, Gunasekera A et al (2013) Protection against malaria by intravenous immunization with a nonreplicating sporozoite vaccine. Science 341(6152):1359–1365
48. Clyde DF, Most H, McCarthy VC, Vanderberg JP (1973) Immunization of man against sporozite-induced falciparum malaria. Am J Med Sci 266(3):169–177
49. Orjih AU, Nussenzweig RS (1980) Immunization against rodent malaria with cryopreserved irradiated sporozoites of *Plasmodium berghei*. Am J Trop Med Hyg 29(3):343–347
50. Weiss WR, Sedegah M, Beaudoin RL, Miller LH, Good MF (1988) $CD8^+$ T cells (cytotoxic/suppressors) are required for protection in mice immunized with malaria sporozoites. Proc Natl Acad Sci U S A 85(2):573–576
51. Hoffman SL, Goh LM, Luke TC, Schneider I, Le TP, Doolan DL, Sacci J, de la Vega P, Dowler M, Paul C et al (2002) Protection of humans against malaria by immunization with radiation-attenuated *Plasmodium falciparum* sporozoites. J Infect Dis 185(8):1155–1164
52. Kumar KA, Sano G, Boscardin S, Nussenzweig RS, Nussenzweig MC, Zavala F, Nussenzweig V (2006) The circumsporozoite protein is an immunodominant protective antigen in irradiated sporozoites. Nature 444(7121):937–940
53. Butler NS, Schmidt NW, Vaughan AM, Aly AS, Kappe SH, Harty JT (2011) Superior antimalarial immunity after vaccination with late liver stage-arresting genetically attenuated parasites. Cell Host Microbe 9(6):451–462
54. Epstein JE, Tewari K, Lyke KE, Sim BK, Billingsley PF, Laurens MB, Gunasekera A, Chakravarty S, James ER, Sedegah M et al (2011) Live attenuated malaria vaccine designed to protect through hepatic $CD8^+$ T cell immunity. Science 334(6055):475–480
55. Annoura T, Ploemen IH, van Schaijk BC, Sajid M, Vos MW, van Gemert GJ, Chevalley-Maurel S, Franke-Fayard BM, Hermsen CC, Gego A et al (2012) Assessing the adequacy of attenuation of genetically modified malaria parasite vaccine candidates. Vaccine 30(16):2662–2670
56. Bijker EM, Bastiaens GJ, Teirlinck AC, van Gemert GJ, Graumans W, van de Vegte-Bolmer M, Siebelink-Stoter R, Arens T, Teelen K, Nahrendorf W et al (2013) Protection against malaria after immunization by chloroquine prophylaxis and sporozoites is mediated by preerythrocytic immunity. Proc Natl Acad Sci U S A 110(19):7862–7867

57. Mikolajczak SA, Lakshmanan V, Fishbaugher M, Camargo N, Harupa A, Kaushansky A, Douglass AN, Baldwin M, Healer J, O'Neill M et al (2014) A next-generation genetically attenuated *Plasmodium falciparum* parasite created by triple gene deletion. Mol Ther 22(9):1707–1715
58. van Schaijk BC, Ploemen IH, Annoura T, Vos MW, Foquet L, van Gemert GJ, Chevalley-Maurel S, van de Vegte-Bolmer M, Sajid M, Franetich JF et al (2014) A genetically attenuated malaria vaccine candidate based on *P. falciparum* b9/slarp gene-deficient sporozoites. Elife 3, e03582
59. Richie TL, Billingsley PF, Sim BK, James ER, Chakravarty S, Epstein JE, Lyke KE, Mordmuller B, Alonso P, Duffy PE et al (2015) Progress with *Plasmodium falciparum* sporozoite (PfSPZ)-based malaria vaccines. Vaccine 33(52):7452–7461
60. Mellouk S, Lunel F, Sedegah M, Beaudoin RL, Druilhe P (1990) Protection against malaria induced by irradiated sporozoites. Lancet 335(8691):721
61. Herrington D, Davis J, Nardin E, Beier M, Cortese J, Eddy H, Losonsky G, Hollingdale M, Sztein M, Levine M et al (1991) Successful immunization of humans with irradiated malaria sporozoites: humoral and cellular responses of the protected individuals. Am J Trop Med Hyg 45(5):539–547
62. Malik A, Egan JE, Houghten RA, Sadoff JC, Hoffman SL (1991) Human cytotoxic T lymphocytes against the *Plasmodium falciparum* circumsporozoite protein. Proc Natl Acad Sci U S A 88(8):3300–3304
63. Egan JE, Hoffman SL, Haynes JD, Sadoff JC, Schneider I, Grau GE, Hollingdale MR, Ballou WR, Gordon DM (1993) Humoral immune responses in volunteers immunized with irradiated *Plasmodium falciparum* sporozoites. Am J Trop Med Hyg 49(2):166–173
64. Silvie O, Semblat JP, Franetich JF, Hannoun L, Eling W, Mazier D (2002) Effects of irradiation on *Plasmodium falciparum* sporozoite hepatic development: implications for the design of pre-erythrocytic malaria vaccines. Parasite Immunol 24(4):221–223
65. Vanderberg J, Nussenzweig R, Most H (1970) Protective immunity produced by the injection of x-irradiated sporozoites of *Plasmodium berghei*. J Parasitol 56(SectionII):350–351
66. Luke TC, Hoffman SL (2003) Rationale and plans for developing a non-replicating, metabolically active, radiation-attenuated *Plasmodium falciparum* sporozoite vaccine. J Exp Biol 206(Pt 21):3803–3808
67. Nussenzweig V, Nussenzweig RS (1989) Rationale for the development of an engineered sporozoite malaria vaccine. Adv Immunol 45:283–334
68. Yoshida N, Nussenzweig RS, Potocnjak P, Nussenzweig V, Aikawa M (1980) Hybridoma produces protective antibodies directed against the sporozoite stage of malaria parasite. Science 207(4426):71–73
69. Dame JB, Williams JL, McCutchan TF, Weber JL, Wirtz RA, Hockmeyer WT, Maloy WL, Haynes JD, Schneider I, Roberts D et al (1984) Structure of the gene encoding the immunodominant surface antigen on the sporozoite of the human malaria parasite *Plasmodium falciparum*. Science 225(4662):593–599
70. Enea V, Ellis J, Zavala F, Arnot DE, Asavanich A, Masuda A, Quakyi I, Nussenzweig RS (1984) DNA cloning of *Plasmodium falciparum* circumsporozoite gene: amino acid sequence of repetitive epitope. Science 225(4662):628–630
71. Gordon DM, McGovern TW, Krzych U, Cohen JC, Schneider I, LaChance R, Heppner DG, Yuan G, Hollingdale M, Slaoui M et al (1995) Safety, immunogenicity, and efficacy of a recombinantly produced *Plasmodium falciparum* circumsporozoite protein-hepatitis B surface antigen subunit vaccine. J Infect Dis 171(6):1576–1585
72. Stoute JA, Slaoui M, Heppner DG, Momin P, Kester KE, Desmons P, Wellde BT, Garcon N, Krzych U, Marchand M (1997) A preliminary evaluation of a recombinant circumsporozoite protein vaccine against *Plasmodium falciparum* malaria. RTS,S Malaria Vaccine Evaluation Group. N Engl J Med 336(2):86–91
73. Bojang KA, Milligan PJ, Pinder M, Vigneron L, Alloueche A, Kester KE, Ballou WR, Conway DJ, Reece WH, Gothard P et al (2001) Efficacy of RTS,S/AS02 malaria vaccine

against *Plasmodium falciparum* infection in semi-immune adult men in The Gambia: a randomised trial. Lancet 358(9297):1927–1934
74. Alonso PL, Sacarlal J, Aponte JJ, Leach A, Macete E, Milman J, Mandomando I, Spiessens B, Guinovart C, Espasa M et al (2004) Efficacy of the RTS,S/AS02A vaccine against *Plasmodium falciparum* infection and disease in young African children: randomised controlled trial. Lancet 364(9443):1411–1420
75. Bojang KA, Olodude F, Pinder M, Ofori-Anyinam O, Vigneron L, Fitzpatrick S, Njie F, Kassanga A, Leach A, Milman J et al (2005) Safety and immunogenicity of RTS,S/AS02A candidate malaria vaccine in Gambian children. Vaccine 23(32):4148–4157
76. Aponte JJ, Aide P, Renom M, Mandomando I, Bassat Q, Sacarlal J, Manaca MN, Lafuente S, Barbosa A, Leach A et al (2007) Safety of the RTS,S/AS02D candidate malaria vaccine in infants living in a highly endemic area of Mozambique: a double blind randomised controlled phase I/IIb trial. Lancet 370(9598):1543–1551
77. Agnandji ST, Lell B, Soulanoudjingar SS, Fernandes JF, Abossolo BP, Conzelmann C, Methogo BG, Doucka Y, Flamen A, Mordmuller B et al (2011) First results of phase 3 trial of RTS,S/AS01 malaria vaccine in African children. N Engl J Med 365(20):1863–1875
78. Rts SCTP, Agnandji ST, Lell B, Fernandes JF, Abossolo BP, Methogo BG, Kabwende AL, Adegnika AA, Mordmuller B, Issifou S et al (2012) A phase 3 trial of RTS,S/AS01 malaria vaccine in African infants. N Engl J Med 367(24):2284–2295
79. Cohen J, Nussenzweig V, Nussenzweig R, Vekemans J, Leach A (2010) From the circumsporozoite protein to the RTS,S/AS candidate vaccine. Hum Vaccin 6(1):90–96
80. Greenwood B, Doumbo OK (2016) Implementation of the malaria candidate vaccine RTS,S/AS01. Lancet 387(10016):318–319
81. Minsoko PA, Lell B, Fernandes JF, Abossolo BP, Kabwende AL, Adegnika AA, Mordmuller B, Issifou S, Kremsner PG, Loembe MM et al (2014) Efficacy and safety of the RTS,S/AS01 malaria vaccine during 18 months after vaccination: a phase 3 randomized, controlled trial in children and young infants at 11 African sites. PLoS Med 11(7), e1001685
82. Tinto H, D'Alessandro U, Sorgho H, Valea I, Tahita MC, Kabore W, Kiemde F, Lompo P, Ouedraogo S, Derra K et al (2015) Efficacy and safety of RTS,S/AS01 malaria vaccine with or without a booster dose in infants and children in Africa: final results of a phase 3, individually randomised, controlled trial. Lancet 386(9988):31–45
83. Olotu A, Fegan G, Wambua J, Nyangweso G, Awuondo KO, Leach A, Lievens M, Leboulleux D, Njuguna P, Peshu N et al (2013) Four-year efficacy of RTS,S/AS01E and its interaction with malaria exposure. New Engl J Med 368(12):1111–1120
84. Le Roch KG, Zhou Y, Blair PL, Grainger M, Moch JK, Haynes JD, De La Vega P, Holder AA, Batalov S, Carucci DJ et al (2003) Discovery of gene function by expression profiling of the malaria parasite life cycle. Science 301(5639):1503–1508
85. Hall N, Karras M, Raine JD, Carlton JM, Kooij TW, Berriman M, Florens L, Janssen CS, Pain A, Christophides GK et al (2005) A comprehensive survey of the *Plasmodium* life cycle by genomic, transcriptomic, and proteomic analyses. Science 307(5706):82–86
86. Carlton JM, Adams JH, Silva JC, Bidwell SL, Lorenzi H, Caler E, Crabtree J, Angiuoli SV, Merino EF, Amedeo P et al (2008) Comparative genomics of the neglected human malaria parasite *Plasmodium vivax*. Nature 455(7214):757–763
87. Khan SM, Franke-Fayard B, Mair GR, Lasonder E, Janse CJ, Mann M, Waters AP (2005) Proteome analysis of separated male and female gametocytes reveals novel sex-specific *Plasmodium* biology. Cell 121(5):675–687
88. Goonewardene R, Daily J, Kaslow D, Sullivan TJ, Duffy P, Carter R, Mendis K, Wirth D (1993) Transfection of the malaria parasite and expression of firefly luciferase. Proc Natl Acad Sci U S A 90(11):5234–5236
89. Wu Y, Kirkman LA, Wellems TE (1996) Transformation of *Plasmodium falciparum* malaria parasites by homologous integration of plasmids that confer resistance to pyrimethamine. Proc Natl Acad Sci U S A 93(3):1130–1134
90. van Dijk MR, Janse CJ, Waters AP (1996) Expression of a *Plasmodium* gene introduced into subtelomeric regions of *Plasmodium berghei* chromosomes. Science 271(5249):662–665

91. van der Wel AM, Tomas AM, Kocken CH, Malhotra P, Janse CJ, Waters AP, Thomas AW (1997) Transfection of the primate malaria parasite *Plasmodium knowlesi* using entirely heterologous constructs. J Exp Med 185(8):1499–1503
92. Mota MM, Thathy V, Nussenzweig RS, Nussenzweig V (2001) Gene targeting in the rodent malaria parasite *Plasmodium yoelii*. Mol Biochem Parasitol 113(2):271–278
93. Mueller AK, Camargo N, Kaiser K, Andorfer C, Frevert U, Matuschewski K, Kappe SH (2005) *Plasmodium* liver stage developmental arrest by depletion of a protein at the parasite-host interface. Proc Natl Acad Sci U S A 102(8):3022–3027
94. Belnoue E, Voza T, Costa FT, Gruner AC, Mauduit M, Rosa DS, Depinay N, Kayibanda M, Vigario AM, Mazier D et al (2008) Vaccination with live *Plasmodium yoelii* blood stage parasites under chloroquine cover induces cross-stage immunity against malaria liver stage. J Immunol 181(12):8552–8558
95. Doll KL, Harty JT (2014) Correlates of protective immunity following whole sporozoite vaccination against malaria. Immunol Res 59(1-3):166–176
96. Clyde DF (1975) Immunization of man against falciparum and vivax malaria by use of attenuated sporozoites. Am J Trop Med Hyg 24(3):397–401
97. Clyde DF (1990) Immunity to falciparum and vivax malaria induced by irradiated sporozoites: a review of the University of Maryland studies, 1971–75. Bull World Health Organ 68(Suppl):9–12
98. Rieckmann KH (1990) Human immunization with attenuated sporozoites. Bull World Health Organ 68(Suppl):13–16
99. Hoffman SL (1997) Experimental challenge of volunteers with malaria. Ann Intern Med 127(3):233–235
100. Overstreet MG, Cockburn IA, Chen YC, Zavala F (2008) Protective CD8 T cells against *Plasmodium* liver stages: immunobiology of an 'unnatural' immune response. Immunol Rev 225:272–283
101. Stewart MJ, Vanderberg JP (1991) Malaria sporozoites release circumsporozoite protein from their apical end and translocate it along their surface. J Protozool 38(4):411–421
102. Stewart MJ, Nawrot RJ, Schulman S, Vanderberg JP (1986) *Plasmodium berghei* sporozoite invasion is blocked in vitro by sporozoite-immobilizing antibodies. Infect Immun 51(3):859–864
103. Doolan DL, Hoffman SL (1997) Pre-erythrocytic-stage immune effector mechanisms in *Plasmodium* spp. infections. Philos Trans R Soc Lond B Biol Sci 352(1359):1361–1367
104. Charoenvit Y, Collins WE, Jones TR, Millet P, Yuan L, Campbell GH, Beaudoin RL, Broderson JR, Hoffman SL (1991) Inability of malaria vaccine to induce antibodies to a protective epitope within its sequence. Science 251(4994):668–671
105. Chai SK, Clavijo P, Tam JP, Zavala F (1992) Immunogenic properties of multiple antigen peptide systems containing defined T and B epitopes. J Immunol 149(7):2385–2390
106. Chakravarty S, Cockburn IA, Kuk S, Overstreet MG, Sacci JB, Zavala F (2007) $CD8^+$ T lymphocytes protective against malaria liver stages are primed in skin-draining lymph nodes. Nat Med 13(9):1035–1041
107. Cockburn IA, Amino R, Kelemen RK, Kuo SC, Tse SW, Radtke A, Mac-Daniel L, Ganusov VV, Zavala F, Menard R (2013) In vivo imaging of $CD8^+$ T cell-mediated elimination of malaria liver stages. Proc Natl Acad Sci U S A 110(22):9090–9095
108. Cockburn IA, Tse SW, Radtke AJ, Srinivasan P, Chen YC, Sinnis P, Zavala F (2011) Dendritic cells and hepatocytes use distinct pathways to process protective antigen from *Plasmodium* in vivo. PLoS Pathog 7(3), e1001318
109. Pichugin A, Steers N, De la Vega P, Zarling S, Chalom I, Krzych U (2016) TAP-mediated processing of exoerythrocytic antigens is essential for protection induced with radiation-attenuated *Plasmodium sporozoites*. Eur J Immunol 46(4):885–896
110. Chen DH, Tigelaar RE, Weinbaum FI (1977) Immunity to sporozoite-induced malaria infection in mice. I. The effect of immunization of T and B cell-deficient mice. J Immunol 118(4):1322–1327

111. Verhave JP, Meuwissen JH, Golenser J (1978) Cell-mediated reactions and protection after immunization with sporozoites. Isr J Med Sci 14(5):611–616
112. Egan JE, Weber JL, Ballou WR, Hollingdale MR, Majarian WR, Gordon DM, Maloy WL, Hoffman SL, Wirtz RA, Schneider I et al (1987) Efficacy of murine malaria sporozoite vaccines: implications for human vaccine development. Science 236(4800):453–456
113. Schofield L, Villaquiran J, Ferreira A, Schellekens H, Nussenzweig R, Nussenzweig V (1987) Gamma interferon, CD8+ T cells and antibodies required for immunity to malaria sporozoites. Nature 330(6149):664–666
114. Weiss WR, Jiang CG (2012) Protective CD8+ T lymphocytes in primates immunized with malaria sporozoites. PLoS One 7(2), e31247
115. Ferreira A, Schofield L, Enea V, Schellekens H, van der Meide P, Collins WE, Nussenzweig RS, Nussenzweig V (1986) Inhibition of development of exoerythrocytic forms of malaria parasites by gamma-interferon. Science 232(4752):881–884
116. Radtke AJ, Tse SW, Zavala F (2015) From the draining lymph node to the liver: the induction and effector mechanisms of malaria-specific CD8+ T cells. Semin Immunopathol 37(3):211–220
117. Duffy PE, Sahu T, Akue A, Milman N, Anderson C (2012) Pre-erythrocytic malaria vaccines: identifying the targets. Expert Rev Vaccines 11(10):1261–1280
118. Nardin EH, Nussenzweig RS (1993) T cell responses to pre-erythrocytic stages of malaria: role in protection and vaccine development against pre-erythrocytic stages. Annu Rev Immunol 11:687–727
119. Tsuji M, Mombaerts P, Lefrancois L, Nussenzweig RS, Zavala F, Tonegawa S (1994) Gamma delta T cells contribute to immunity against the liver stages of malaria in alpha beta T-cell-deficient mice. Proc Natl Acad Sci U S A 91(1):345–349
120. Doolan DL, Hoffman SL (1999) IL-12 and NK cells are required for antigen-specific adaptive immunity against malaria initiated by CD8+ T cells in the *Plasmodium yoelii* model. J Immunol 163(2):884–892
121. Doolan DL, Hoffman SL (2000) The complexity of protective immunity against liver-stage malaria. J Immunol 165(3):1453–1462
122. Weiss WR, Good MF, Hollingdale MR, Miller LH, Berzofsky JA (1989) Genetic control of immunity to *Plasmodium yoelii* sporozoites. J Immunol 143(12):4263–4266
123. Oliveira GA, Kumar KA, Calvo-Calle JM, Othoro C, Altszuler D, Nussenzweig V, Nardin EH (2008) Class II-restricted protective immunity induced by malaria sporozoites. Infect Immun 76(3):1200–1206
124. Hoffman SL, Doolan DL (2000) Malaria vaccines-targeting infected hepatocytes. Nat Med 6(11):1218–1219
125. Romero P, Maryanski JL, Corradin G, Nussenzweig RS, Nussenzweig V, Zavala F (1989) Cloned cytotoxic T cells recognize an epitope in the circumsporozoite protein and protect against malaria. Nature 341(6240):323–326
126. Weiss WR, Mellouk S, Houghten RA, Sedegah M, Kumar S, Good MF, Berzofsky JA, Miller LH, Hoffman SL (1990) Cytotoxic T cells recognize a peptide from the circumsporozoite protein on malaria-infected hepatocytes. J Exp Med 171(3):763–773
127. Kumar S, Miller LH, Quakyi IA, Keister DB, Houghten RA, Maloy WL, Moss B, Berzofsky JA, Good MF (1988) Cytotoxic T cells specific for the circumsporozoite protein of *Plasmodium falciparum*. Nature 334(6179):258–260
128. Huang J, Tsao T, Zhang M, Tsuji M (2014) Circumsporozoite protein-specific K^d-restricted CD8+ T cells mediate protective antimalaria immunity in sporozoite-immunized MHC-I-K^d transgenic mice. Mediators Inflamm 2014:728939
129. Mishra S, Rai U, Shiratsuchi T, Li X, Vanloubbeeck Y, Cohen J, Nussenzweig RS, Winzeler EA, Tsuji M, Nussenzweig V (2011) Identification of non-CSP antigens bearing CD8 epitopes in mice immunized with irradiated sporozoites. Vaccine 29(43):7335–7342
130. Gruner AC, Mauduit M, Tewari R, Romero JF, Depinay N, Kayibanda M, Lallemand E, Chavatte JM, Crisanti A, Sinnis P et al (2007) Sterile protection against malaria is independent of immune responses to the circumsporozoite protein. PLoS One 2(12), e1371

131. Mauduit M, Gruner AC, Tewari R, Depinay N, Kayibanda M, Chavatte JM, Franetich JF, Crisanti A, Mazier D, Snounou G et al (2009) A role for immune responses against non-CS components in the cross-species protection induced by immunization with irradiated malaria sporozoites. PLoS One 4(11), e7717
132. Tsuji M, Romero P, Nussenzweig RS, Zavala F (1990) $CD4^+$ cytolytic T cell clone confers protection against murine malaria. J Exp Med 172(5):1353–1357
133. Migliorini P, Betschart B, Corradin G (1993) Malaria vaccine: immunization of mice with a synthetic T cell helper epitope alone leads to protective immunity. Eur J Immunol 23(2):582–585
134. Renia L, Grillot D, Marussig M, Corradin G, Miltgen F, Lambert PH, Mazier D, Del Giudice G (1993) Effector functions of circumsporozoite peptide-primed $CD4^+$ T cell clones against *Plasmodium yoelii* liver stages. J Immunol 150(4):1471–1478
135. Zavala F, Cochrane AH, Nardin EH, Nussenzweig RS, Nussenzweig V (1983) Circumsporozoite proteins of malaria parasites contain a single immunodominant region with two or more identical epitopes. J Exp Med 157(6):1947–1957
136. Zavala F, Tam JP, Hollingdale MR, Cochrane AH, Quakyi I, Nussenzweig RS, Nussenzweig V (1985) Rationale for development of a synthetic vaccine against *Plasmodium falciparum* malaria. Science 228(4706):1436–1440
137. Nardin EH, Nussenzweig V, Nussenzweig RS, Collins WE, Harinasuta KT, Tapchaisri P, Chomcharn Y (1982) Circumsporozoite proteins of human malaria parasites *Plasmodium falciparum* and *Plasmodium vivax*. J Exp Med 156(1):20–30
138. Herrington DA, Clyde DF, Losonsky G, Cortesia M, Murphy JR, Davis J, Baqar S, Felix AM, Heimer EP, Gillessen D et al (1987) Safety and immunogenicity in man of a synthetic peptide malaria vaccine against *Plasmodium falciparum* sporozoites. Nature 328(6127):257–259
139. Good MF, Berzofsky JA, Maloy WL, Hayashi Y, Fujii N, Hockmeyer WT, Miller LH (1986) Genetic control of the immune response in mice to a *Plasmodium falciparum* sporozoite vaccine. Widespread nonresponsiveness to single malaria T epitope in highly repetitive vaccine. J Exp Med 164(2):655–660
140. Calvo-Calle JM, Oliveira GA, Watta CO, Soverow J, Parra-Lopez C, Nardin EH (2006) A linear peptide containing minimal T- and B-cell epitopes of *Plasmodium falciparum* circumsporozoite protein elicits protection against transgenic sporozoite challenge. Infect Immun 74(12):6929–6939
141. Offeddu V, Thathy V, Marsh K, Matuschewski K (2012) Naturally acquired immune responses against *Plasmodium falciparum* sporozoites and liver infection. Int J Parasitol 42(6):535–548
142. Rogers WO, Malik A, Mellouk S, Nakamura K, Rogers MD, Szarfman A, Gordon DM, Nussler AK, Aikawa M, Hoffman SL (1992) Characterization of *Plasmodium falciparum* sporozoite surface protein 2. Proc Natl Acad Sci U S A 89(19):9176–9180
143. Nardin EH, Nussenzweig RS, Altszuler R, Herrington D, Levine M, Murphy J, Davis J, Bathurst I, Barr P, Romero P et al (1990) Cellular and humoral immune responses to a recombinant *P. falciparum* CS protein in sporozoite-immunized rodents and human volunteers. Bull World Health Organ 68(Suppl):85–87
144. Nardin EH (1990) T cell responses in a sporozoite-immunized human volunteer and a chimpanzee. Immunol Lett 25(1-3):43–47
145. Moreno A, Clavijo P, Edelman R, Davis J, Sztein M, Herrington D, Nardin E (1991) Cytotoxic $CD4^+$ T cells from a sporozoite-immunized volunteer recognize the *Plasmodium falciparum* CS protein. Int Immunol 3(10):997–1003
146. de la Cruz VF, Lal AA, McCutchan TF (1987) Sequence variation in putative functional domains of the circumsporozoite protein of *Plasmodium falciparum*. Implications for vaccine development. J Biol Chem 262(25):11935–11939
147. Moreno A, Clavijo P, Edelman R, Davis J, Sztein M, Sinigaglia F, Nardin E (1993) $CD4^+$ T cell clones obtained from *Plasmodium falciparum* sporozoite-immunized volunteers recognize polymorphic sequences of the circumsporozoite protein. J Immunol 151(1):489–499

148. Hill AV, Allsopp CE, Kwiatkowski D, Anstey NM, Twumasi P, Rowe PA, Bennett S, Brewster D, McMichael AJ, Greenwood BM (1991) Common West African HLA antigens are associated with protection from severe malaria. Nature 352(6336):595–600
149. Allsopp CE, Harding RM, Taylor C, Bunce M, Kwiatkowski D, Anstey N, Brewster D, McMichael AJ, Greenwood BM, Hill AV (1992) Interethnic genetic differentiation in Africa: HLA class I antigens in The Gambia. Am J Hum Genet 50(2):411–421
150. Doolan DL, Houghten RA, Good MF (1991) Location of human cytotoxic T cell epitopes within a polymorphic domain of the *Plasmodium falciparum* circumsporozoite protein. Int Immunol 3(6):511–516
151. Aidoo M, Lalvani A, Allsopp CE, Plebanski M, Meisner SJ, Krausa P, Browning M, Morris-Jones S, Gotch F, Fidock DA et al (1995) Identification of conserved antigenic components for a cytotoxic T lymphocyte-inducing vaccine against malaria. Lancet 345(8956):1003–1007
152. Wizel B, Houghten RA, Parker KC, Coligan JE, Church P, Gordon DM, Ballou WR, Hoffman SL (1995) Irradiated sporozoite vaccine induces HLA-B8-restricted cytotoxic T lymphocyte responses against two overlapping epitopes of the *Plasmodium falciparum* sporozoite surface protein 2. J Exp Med 182(5):1435–1445
153. Doolan DL, Southwood S, Freilich DA, Sidney J, Graber NL, Shatney L, Bebris L, Florens L, Dobano C, Witney AA et al (2003) Identification of *Plasmodium falciparum* antigens by antigenic analysis of genomic and proteomic data. Proc Natl Acad Sci U S A 100(17):9952–9957
154. Kariu T, Ishino T, Yano K, Chinzei Y, Yuda M (2006) CelTOS, a novel malarial protein that mediates transmission to mosquito and vertebrate hosts. Mol Microbiol 59(5):1369–1379
155. Trieu A, Kayala MA, Burk C, Molina DM, Freilich DA, Richie TL, Baldi P, Felgner PL, Doolan DL (2011) Sterile protective immunity to malaria is associated with a panel of novel *P. falciparum* antigens. Mol Cell Proteomics 10(9), M111.007948
156. Doolan DL, Mu Y, Unal B, Sundaresh S, Hirst S, Valdez C, Randall A, Molina D, Liang X, Freilich DA et al (2008) Profiling humoral immune responses to *P. falciparum* infection with protein microarrays. Proteomics 8(22):4680–4694
157. Aguiar JC, Bolton J, Wanga J, Sacci JB, Iriko H, Mazeika JK, Han ET, Limbach K, Patterson NB, Sedegah M et al (2015) Discovery of novel *Plasmodium falciparum* pre-erythrocytic antigens for vaccine development. PLoS One 10(8), e0136109
158. Garcia CR, Manzi F, Tediosi F, Hoffman SL, James ER (2013) Comparative cost models of a liquid nitrogen vapor phase (LNVP) cold chain-distributed cryopreserved malaria vaccine vs. a conventional vaccine. Vaccine 31(2):380–386
159. March S, Ng S, Velmurugan S, Galstian A, Shan J, Logan DJ, Carpenter AE, Thomas D, Sim BK, Mota MM et al (2013) A microscale human liver platform that supports the hepatic stages of *Plasmodium falciparum* and *vivax*. Cell Host Microbe 14(1):104–115
160. Sheehy SH, Spencer AJ, Douglas AD, Sim BK, Longley RJ, Edwards NJ, Poulton ID, Kimani D, Williams AR, Anagnostou NA et al (2013) Optimising controlled human malaria infection studies using cryopreserved parasites administered by needle and syringe. PLoS One 8(6), e65960
161. Hodgson SH, Juma E, Salim A, Magiri C, Kimani D, Njenga D, Muia A, Cole AO, Ogwang C, Awuondo K et al (2014) Evaluating controlled human malaria infection in Kenyan adults with varying degrees of prior exposure to *Plasmodium falciparum* using sporozoites administered by intramuscular injection. Front Microbiol 5:686
162. Gomez-Perez GP, Legarda A, Munoz J, Sim BK, Ballester MR, Dobano C, Moncunill G, Campo JJ, Cistero P, Jimenez A et al (2015) Controlled human malaria infection by intramuscular and direct venous inoculation of cryopreserved *Plasmodium falciparum* sporozoites in malaria-naive volunteers: effect of injection volume and dose on infectivity rates. Malar J 14:306
163. Nganou-Makamdop K, Ploemen I, Behet M, Van Gemert GJ, Hermsen C, Roestenberg M, Sauerwein RW (2012) Reduced *Plasmodium berghei* sporozoite liver load associates with low protective efficacy after intradermal immunization. Parasite Immunol 34(12):562–569

164. Ploemen IH, Chakravarty S, van Gemert GJ, Annoura T, Khan SM, Janse CJ, Hermsen CC, Hoffman SL, Sauerwein RW (2013) *Plasmodium* liver load following parenteral sporozoite administration in rodents. Vaccine 31(34):3410–3416
165. Ishizuka AS, Lyke KE, DeZure A, Berry AA, Richie TL, Mendoza FH, Enama ME, Gordon IJ, Chang LJ, Sarwar UN et al (2016) Protection against malaria at 1 year and immune correlates following PfSPZ vaccination. Nat Med 22:614–623
166. Good MF (2013) Immunology. Pasteur approach to a malaria vaccine may take the lead. Science 341(6152):1352–1353
167. Mo AX, Pesce J, Hall BF (2015) Exploring immunological mechanisms of the whole sporozoite vaccination against *P. falciparum* malaria. Vaccine 33(25):2851–2857
168. Hoffman SL, Vekemans J, Richie TL, Duffy PE (2015) The march toward malaria vaccines. Vaccine 33(Suppl 4):D13–D23
169. Jobe O, Lumsden J, Mueller AK, Williams J, Silva-Rivera H, Kappe SH, Schwenk RJ, Matuschewski K, Krzych U (2007) Genetically attenuated *Plasmodium berghei* liver stages induce sterile protracted protection that is mediated by major histocompatibility complex Class I-dependent interferon-gamma-producing $CD8^+$ T cells. J Infect Dis 196(4):599–607
170. Vaughan AM, Wang R, Kappe SH (2010) Genetically engineered, attenuated whole-cell vaccine approaches for malaria. Hum Vaccin 6(1):107–113
171. Khan SM, Janse CJ, Kappe SH, Mikolajczak SA (2012) Genetic engineering of attenuated malaria parasites for vaccination. Curr Opin Biotechnol 23(6):908–916
172. Matuschewski K, Ross J, Brown SM, Kaiser K, Nussenzweig V, Kappe SH (2002) Infectivity-associated changes in the transcriptional repertoire of the malaria parasite sporozoite stage. J Biol Chem 277(44):41948–41953
173. van Schaijk BC, Janse CJ, van Gemert GJ, van Dijk MR, Gego A, Franetich JF, van de Vegte-Bolmer M, Yalaoui S, Silvie O, Hoffman SL et al (2008) Gene disruption of *Plasmodium falciparum* p52 results in attenuation of malaria liver stage development in cultured primary human hepatocytes. PLoS One 3(10), e3549
174. Annoura T, van Schaijk BC, Ploemen IH, Sajid M, Lin JW, Vos MW, Dinmohamed AG, Inaoka DK, Rijpma SR, van Gemert GJ et al (2014) Two *Plasmodium* 6-Cys family-related proteins have distinct and critical roles in liver-stage development. FASEB J 28(5):2158–2170
175. Bijker EM, Borrmann S, Kappe SH, Mordmuller B, Sack BK, Khan SM (2015) Novel approaches to whole sporozoite vaccination against malaria. Vaccine 33(52):7462–7468
176. Aly AS, Lindner SE, MacKellar DC, Peng X, Kappe SH (2011) SAP1 is a critical post-transcriptional regulator of infectivity in malaria parasite sporozoite stages. Mol Microbiol 79(4):929–939
177. Aly AS, Mikolajczak SA, Rivera HS, Camargo N, Jacobs-Lorena V, Labaied M, Coppens I, Kappe SH (2008) Targeted deletion of SAP1 abolishes the expression of infectivity factors necessary for successful malaria parasite liver infection. Mol Microbiol 69(1):152–163
178. Silvie O, Goetz K, Matuschewski K (2008) A sporozoite asparagine-rich protein controls initiation of *Plasmodium* liver stage development. PLoS Pathog 4(6), e1000086
179. Rijpma SR, van der Velden M, Gonzalez-Pons M, Annoura T, van Schaijk BC, van Gemert GJ, van den Heuvel JJ, Ramesar J, Chevalley-Maurel S, Ploemen IH et al (2016) Multidrug ATP-binding cassette transporters are essential for hepatic development of *Plasmodium sporozoites*. Cell Microbiol 18(3):369–383
180. Hafalla JC, Rai U, Morrot A, Bernal-Rubio D, Zavala F, Rodriguez A (2006) Priming of $CD8^+$ T cell responses following immunization with heat-killed *Plasmodium sporozoites*. Eur J Immunol 36(5):1179–1186
181. Matuschewski K, Hafalla JC, Borrmann S, Friesen J (2011) Arrested *Plasmodium* liver stages as experimental anti-malaria vaccines. Hum Vaccin 7(Suppl):16–21
182. Ngonseu E, Chatterjee S, Wery M (1998) Blocked hepatic-stage parasites and decreased susceptibility to *Plasmodium berghei* infections in BALB/c mice. Parasitology 117(Pt 5):419–423

183. Mueller AK, Deckert M, Heiss K, Goetz K, Matuschewski K, Schluter D (2007) Genetically attenuated *Plasmodium berghei* liver stages persist and elicit sterile protection primarily via CD8 T cells. Am J Pathol 171(1):107–115
184. Tarun AS, Dumpit RF, Camargo N, Labaied M, Liu P, Takagi A, Wang R, Kappe SH (2007) Protracted sterile protection with *Plasmodium yoelii* pre-erythrocytic genetically attenuated parasite malaria vaccines is independent of significant liver-stage persistence and is mediated by CD8$^+$ T cells. J Infect Dis 196(4):608–616
185. Douradinha B, Doolan DL (2011) Harnessing immune responses against *Plasmodium* for rational vaccine design. Trends Parasitol 27(6):274–283
186. Trimnell A, Takagi A, Gupta M, Richie TL, Kappe SH, Wang R (2009) Genetically attenuated parasite vaccines induce contact-dependent CD8$^+$ T cell killing of *Plasmodium yoelii* liver stage-infected hepatocytes. J Immunol 183(9):5870–5878
187. Cooney LA, Gupta M, Thomas S, Mikolajczak S, Choi KY, Gibson C, Jang IK, Danziger S, Aitchison J, Gardner MJ et al (2013) Short-lived effector CD8 T cells induced by genetically attenuated malaria parasite vaccination express CD11c. Infect Immun 81(11):4171–4181
188. Vaughan AM, O'Neill MT, Tarun AS, Camargo N, Phuong TM, Aly AS, Cowman AF, Kappe SH (2009) Type II fatty acid synthesis is essential only for malaria parasite late liver stage development. Cell Microbiol 11(3):506–520
189. Murray SA, Mohar I, Miller JL, Brempelis KJ, Vaughan AM, Kappe SH, Crispe IN (2015) CD40 is required for protective immunity against liver stage *Plasmodium* infection. J Immunol 194(5):2268–2279
190. Sack BK, Keitany GJ, Vaughan AM, Miller JL, Wang R, Kappe SH (2015) Mechanisms of stage-transcending protection following immunization of mice with late liver stage-arresting genetically attenuated malaria parasites. PLoS Pathog 11(5), e1004855
191. Keitany GJ, Sack B, Smithers H, Chen L, Jang IK, Sebastian L, Gupta M, Sather DN, Vignali M, Vaughan AM et al (2014) Immunization of mice with live-attenuated late liver stage-arresting *Plasmodium yoelii* parasites generates protective antibody responses to preerythrocytic stages of malaria. Infect Immun 82(12):5143–5153
192. Wang R, Arevalo-Herrera M, Gardner MJ, Bonelo A, Carlton JM, Gomez A, Vera O, Soto L, Vergara J, Bidwell SL et al (2005) Immune responses to *Plasmodium vivax* pre-erythrocytic stage antigens in naturally exposed Duffy-negative humans: a potential model for identification of liver-stage antigens. Eur J Immunol 35(6):1859–1868
193. Chen L, Keitany GJ, Peng X, Gibson C, Mohar I, Vignali M, Crispe IN, Huang F, Wang R (2014) Identification of pre-erythrocytic malaria antigens that target hepatocytes for killing in vivo and contribute to protection elicited by whole-parasite vaccination. PLoS One 9(7), e102225
194. Haussig JM, Matuschewski K, Kooij TW (2011) Inactivation of a *Plasmodium* apicoplast protein attenuates formation of liver merozoites. Mol Microbiol 81(6):1511–1525
195. Hafalla JC, Bauza K, Friesen J, Gonzalez-Aseguinolaza G, Hill AV, Matuschewski K (2013) Identification of targets of CD8$^+$ T cell responses to malaria liver stages by genome-wide epitope profiling. PLoS Pathog 9(5), e1003303
196. Haussig JM, Burgold J, Hafalla JC, Matuschewski K, Kooij TW (2014) Signatures of malaria vaccine efficacy in ageing murine immune memory. Parasite Immunol 36(5):199–206
197. Kumar KA, Baxter P, Tarun AS, Kappe SH, Nussenzweig V (2009) Conserved protective mechanisms in radiation and genetically attenuated *uis3(−)* and *uis4(−) Plasmodium sporozoites*. PLoS One 4(2), e4480
198. van Schaijk BC, Kumar TR, Vos MW, Richman A, van Gemert GJ, Li T, Eappen AG, Williamson KC, Morahan BJ, Fishbaugher M et al (2014) Type II fatty acid biosynthesis is essential for *Plasmodium falciparum* sporozoite development in the midgut of Anopheles mosquitoes. Eukaryot Cell 13(5):550–559
199. Nganou-Makamdop K, Sauerwein RW (2013) Liver or blood-stage arrest during malaria sporozoite immunization: the later the better? Trends Parasitol 29(6):304–310
200. Sauerwein RW, Bijker EM, Richie TL (2010) Empowering malaria vaccination by drug administration. Curr Opin Immunol 22(3):367–373

201. Golenser J, Heeren J, Verhave JP, Kaay HJ, Meuwissen JH (1977) Crossreactivity with sporozoites, exoerythrocytic forms and blood schizonts of *Plasmodium berghei* in indirect fluorescent antibody tests with sera of rats immunized with sporozoites or infected blood. Clin Exp Immunol 29(1):43–51
202. Slater AF (1993) Chloroquine: mechanism of drug action and resistance in *Plasmodium falciparum*. Pharmacol Ther 57(2-3):203–235
203. Lewis MD, Pfeil J, Heiss K, Mueller AK (2014) $CD8^+$ T cells mediate robust stage-specific immunity to *P. berghei* under chemoprophylaxis and this protective environment is not down-regulated by the presence of blood-stage infection. PLoS One 9(2), e88117
204. Bijker EM, Nganou-Makamdop K, van Gemert GJ, Zavala F, Cockburn I, Sauerwein RW (2015) Studying the effect of chloroquine on sporozoite-induced protection and immune responses in *Plasmodium berghei* malaria. Malar J 14:130
205. Pfeil J, Sepp KJ, Heiss K, Meister M, Mueller AK, Borrmann S (2014) Protection against malaria by immunization with non-attenuated sporozoites under single-dose piperaquine-tetraphosphate chemoprophylaxis. Vaccine 32(45):6005–6011
206. Friesen J, Borrmann S, Matuschewski K (2011) Induction of antimalaria immunity by pyrimethamine prophylaxis during exposure to sporozoites is curtailed by parasite resistance. Antimicrob Agents Chemother 55(6):2760–2767
207. Friesen J, Matuschewski K (2011) Comparative efficacy of pre-erythrocytic whole organism vaccine strategies against the malaria parasite. Vaccine 29(40):7002–7008
208. Peng X, Keitany GJ, Vignali M, Chen L, Gibson C, Choi K, Huang F, Wang R (2014) Artesunate versus chloroquine infection-treatment-vaccination defines stage-specific immune responses associated with prolonged sterile protection against both pre-erythrocytic and erythrocytic *Plasmodium yoelii* infection. J Immunol 193(3):1268–1277
209. Bijker EM, Teirlinck AC, Schats R, van Gemert GJ, van de Vegte-Bolmer M, van Lieshout L, IntHout J, Hermsen CC, Scholzen A, Visser LG et al (2014) Cytotoxic markers associate with protection against malaria in human volunteers immunized with *Plasmodium falciparum* sporozoites. J Infect Dis 210(10):1605–1615
210. Inoue M, Tang J, Miyakoda M, Kaneko O, Yui K, Culleton R (2012) The species specificity of immunity generated by live whole organism immunisation with erythrocytic and pre-erythrocytic stages of rodent malaria parasites and implications for vaccine development. Int J Parasitol 42(9):859–870
211. Nahrendorf W, Spence PJ, Tumwine I, Levy P, Jarra W, Sauerwein RW, Langhorne J (2015) Blood-stage immunity to *Plasmodium chabaudi* malaria following chemoprophylaxis and sporozoite immunization. Elife 4, e05165
212. Schats R, Bijker EM, van Gemert GJ, Graumans W, van de Vegte-Bolmer M, van Lieshout L, Haks MC, Hermsen CC, Scholzen A, Visser LG et al (2015) Heterologous protection against malaria after immunization with *Plasmodium falciparum* sporozoites. PLoS One 10(5), e0124243
213. Bijker EM, Sauerwein RW (2012) Enhancement of naturally acquired immunity against malaria by drug use. J Med Microbiol 61(Pt 7):904–910
214. Bastiaens GJ, van Meer MP, Scholzen A, Obiero JM, Vatanshenassan M, van Grinsven T, Sim BK, Billingsley PF, James ER, Gunasekera A et al (2015) Safety, immunogenicity, and protective efficacy of intradermal immunization with aseptic, purified, cryopreserved *Plasmodium falciparum* sporozoites in volunteers under chloroquine prophylaxis: a randomized controlled trial. Am J Trop Med Hyg 94(3):663–673
215. Doll KL, Butler NS, Harty JT (2014) CD8 T cell independent immunity after single dose infection-treatment-vaccination (ITV) against *Plasmodium yoelii*. Vaccine 32(4):483–491
216. Nganou-Makamdop K, van Gemert GJ, Arens T, Hermsen CC, Sauerwein RW (2012) Long term protection after immunization with *P. berghei* sporozoites correlates with sustained IFNγ responses of hepatic $CD8^+$ memory T cells. PLoS One 7(5), e36508
217. Nahrendorf W, Scholzen A, Sauerwein RW, Langhorne J (2015) Cross-stage immunity for malaria vaccine development. Vaccine 33(52):7513–7517

218. Nahrendorf W, Scholzen A, Bijker EM, Teirlinck AC, Bastiaens GJ, Schats R, Hermsen CC, Visser LG, Langhorne J, Sauerwein RW (2014) Memory B-cell and antibody responses induced by *Plasmodium falciparum* sporozoite immunization. J Infect Dis 210(12):1981–1990
219. Teirlinck AC, McCall MB, Roestenberg M, Scholzen A, Woestenenk R, de Mast Q, van der Ven AJ, Hermsen CC, Luty AJ, Sauerwein RW (2011) Longevity and composition of cellular immune responses following experimental *Plasmodium falciparum* malaria infection in humans. PLoS Pathog 7(12), e1002389
220. Pombo DJ, Lawrence G, Hirunpetcharat C, Rzepczyk C, Bryden M, Cloonan N, Anderson K, Mahakunkijcharoen Y, Martin LB, Wilson D et al (2002) Immunity to malaria after administration of ultra-low doses of red cells infected with *Plasmodium falciparum*. Lancet 360(9333):610–617
221. Felgner PL, Roestenberg M, Liang L, Hung C, Jain A, Pablo J, Nakajima-Sasaki R, Molina D, Teelen K, Hermsen CC et al (2013) Pre-erythrocytic antibody profiles induced by controlled human malaria infections in healthy volunteers under chloroquine prophylaxis. Sci Rep 3:3549
222. Behet MC, Foquet L, van Gemert GJ, Bijker EM, Meuleman P, Leroux-Roels G, Hermsen CC, Scholzen A, Sauerwein RW (2014) Sporozoite immunization of human volunteers under chemoprophylaxis induces functional antibodies against pre-erythrocytic stages of *Plasmodium falciparum*. Malar J 13:136
223. Singh AP, Buscaglia CA, Wang Q, Levay A, Nussenzweig DR, Walker JR, Winzeler EA, Fujii H, Fontoura BM, Nussenzweig V (2007) *Plasmodium* circumsporozoite protein promotes the development of the liver stages of the parasite. Cell 131(3):492–504
224. Hollingdale MR, Leland P, Leef JL, Leef MF, Beaudoin RL (1983) Serological reactivity of in vitro cultured exoerythrocytic stages of *Plasmodium berghei* in indirect immunofluorescent or immunoperoxidase antibody tests. Am J Trop Med Hyg 32(1):24–30
225. Davies DH, Duffy P, Bodmer JL, Felgner PL, Doolan DL (2015) Large screen approaches to identify novel malaria vaccine candidates. Vaccine 33(52):7496–7505
226. Teirlinck AC, Roestenberg M, van de Vegte-Bolmer M, Scholzen A, Heinrichs MJ, Siebelink-Stoter R, Graumans W, van Gemert GJ, Teelen K, Vos MW et al (2013) NF135.C10: a new *Plasmodium falciparum* clone for controlled human malaria infections. J Infect Dis 207(4):656–660
227. Sato A, McNulty L, Cox K, Kim S, Scott A, Daniell K, Summerville K, Price C, Hudson S, Kiakos K et al (2005) A novel class of in vivo active anticancer agents: achiral seco-amino- and seco-hydroxycyclopropylbenz[e]indolone (seco-CBI) analogues of the duocarmycins and CC-1065. J Med Chem 48(11):3903–3918
228. Purcell LA, Yanow SK, Lee M, Spithill TW, Rodriguez A (2008) Chemical attenuation of *Plasmodium berghei* sporozoites induces sterile immunity in mice. Infect Immun 76(3):1193–1199
229. Purcell LA, Wong KA, Yanow SK, Lee M, Spithill TW, Rodriguez A (2008) Chemically attenuated *Plasmodium sporozoites* induce specific immune responses, sterile immunity and cross-protection against heterologous challenge. Vaccine 26(38):4880–4884
230. Lewis MD, Behrends J, Sa ECC, Mendes AM, Lasitschka F, Sattler JM, Heiss K, Kooij TW, Prudencio M, Bringmann G et al (2015) Chemical attenuation of *Plasmodium* in the liver modulates severe malaria disease progression. J Immunol 194(10):4860–4870
231. Bergmann-Leitner ES, Mease RM, De La Vega P, Savranskaya T, Polhemus M, Ockenhouse C, Angov E (2010) Immunization with pre-erythrocytic antigen CelTOS from *Plasmodium falciparum* elicits cross-species protection against heterologous challenge with *Plasmodium berghei*. PLoS One 5(8), e12294
232. Janse CJ, Ramesar J, Waters AP (2006) High-efficiency transfection and drug selection of genetically transformed blood stages of the rodent malaria parasite *Plasmodium berghei*. Nat Protoc 1(1):346–356
233. Salman AM, Mogollon CM, Lin JW, van Pul FJ, Janse CJ, Khan SM (2015) Generation of transgenic rodent malaria parasites expressing human malaria parasite proteins. Methods Mol Biol 1325:257–286

234. Lin JW, Annoura T, Sajid M, Chevalley-Maurel S, Ramesar J, Klop O, Franke-Fayard BM, Janse CJ, Khan SM (2011) A novel 'gene insertion/marker out' (GIMO) method for transgene expression and gene complementation in rodent malaria parasites. PLoS One 6(12), e29289
235. Chattopadhyay R, Conteh S, Li M, James ER, Epstein JE, Hoffman SL (2009) The effects of radiation on the safety and protective efficacy of an attenuated *Plasmodium yoelii* sporozoite malaria vaccine. Vaccine 27(27):3675–3680
236. Sauerwein RW, Roestenberg M, Moorthy VS (2011) Experimental human challenge infections can accelerate clinical malaria vaccine development. Nat Rev Immunol 11(1):57–64
237. Scholzen A, Sauerwein RW (2016) Immune activation and induction of memory: lessons learned from controlled human malaria infection with *Plasmodium falciparum*. Parasitology 143(2):224–235

Immune Responses to the RTS,S/AS01 Malaria Vaccine Candidate: Lessons from Human Immunology, Parasitologic and Clinical Evaluations

Johan Vekemans

Contents

1 Background 140
2 Immunobiology: General Considerations 141
3 Humoral Immunity 144
4 T-Cell Immunity 147
5 Immune Memory 147
6 Impact of Vaccination on Immunity to the Blood Stage of the Parasite Life Cycle 149
7 Vaccine-Induced Immunity and Parasite Genetic Diversity 150
8 Translational Science 150
References 151

Abbreviations

AI	Avidity index
CHMI	Controlled human malaria infection
CS	Circumsporozoite protein
EPI	Expanded Program on Immunization
HBsAg	Hepatitis B virus surface antigen
P. falciparum	*Plasmodium falciparum*
VE	Vaccine efficacy

J. Vekemans (✉)
GSK Vaccines, 89 Rue de l'Institut, 1330 Rixensart, Belgique
e-mail: johan.vekemans@gmail.com

M.M. Mota, A. Rodriguez (eds.), *Malaria*, DOI 10.1007/978-3-319-45210-4_7

1 Background

After over three decades of research and availability of results from a pivotal phase 3 trial [1], the European Medicines Agency issued a favorable scientific opinion regarding RTS,S/AS01 vaccination for prevention of malaria in infants and young children from 6 weeks to 17 months of age (http://www.ema.europa.eu/docs/en_GB/document_library/Press_release/2015/07/WC500190447.pdf). The World Health Organization recommended the start of large pilot implementation studies for further evaluation of the risk-benefit profile when used as a four-dose regimen in 5–17-month-old children (http://www.who.int/immunization/research/development/malaria_vaccine_qa/en/).

Phase 3 evaluation was conducted in research centers across Africa with different malaria transmission patterns. 8922 children 5–17 months old and 6537 infants 6–12 weeks old were randomized to receive either four doses of RTS,S on a 0-, 1-, 2-, and 20-month schedule, three doses on a 0-, 1-, and 2-month schedule, or control vaccines. In children 5–17 months old at first vaccination, vaccine efficacy (VE) provided by three doses during the first year of follow-up was approximately 50 %. VE waned over the 48-month course of the trial. Overall, VE against clinical malaria was 36 % (95 % CI 32–41) for the four-dose group and 28 % (95 % CI 23–33) for the three-dose group. Moderate VE against severe malaria, severe malarial anemia, hospitalization for malaria, and requirement for blood transfusion was also shown when four doses were administered. The number of cases averted varied according to exposure, age category, and whether a fourth dose was administered. Depending on study sites and the level of exposure, 205–6565 cases of malaria were averted per 1000 children vaccinated with the four-dose regimen in the 5–17-month age category. In infants 6–12 weeks old who received RTS,S/AS01 together with vaccines from the Expanded Program on Immunization (EPI), VE levels were generally lower [1].

The RTS,S vaccine antigen target is the *Plasmodium falciparum* (*P. falciparum*) circumsporozoite protein (CS). CS is abundantly expressed on the surface of the sporozoite, which emerges from the maturing *Plasmodium* oocyst in the mosquito midgut to migrate to the salivary glands. Upon infectious mosquito biting of the human host, dozens to a few 100 sporozoites are injected into the dermis, of which a fraction only will reach the circulation and, within minutes, infect hepatocytes. Within infected hepatocytes, early liver forms will develop into hepatic schizonts which within the next 6–10 days will burst to release thousands of merozoites and initiation of the blood stage of the infection. CS remains expressed on early liver forms. The 58 kDa CS protein includes a characteristic species-specific B-cell immunodominant repeat central region with approximately 41 repeats (range 37–49) of NANP amino acid sequences and a smaller number of NVDP sequences. The highly conserved N-terminus non-repetitive flanking region is involved in cell invasion through heparin sulfate proteoglycan binding (region I) and contains a proteolytic cleavage site sequence and PEXEL motifs. The C-terminus non-repetitive flanking region contains a thrombospondin-like type I repeat domain with cell adhesion properties (region II), a canonical glycosylphosphatidylinositol anchor addition sequence, and three known T-cell epitopes: a highly variable CD4+ T-cell epitope, a highly variable CD8+ T-cell epitope, and a "promiscuous" conserved CD4+ T-cell epitope [2–5].

RTS,S is a chimeric virus-like particle protein construct. 19 NANP repeats of the central region and the C-terminal flanking region (amino acids 207–395) of CS (3D7 clone derived from the NF54 strain) are fused to the hepatitis B virus surface antigen, HBsAg. The fusion protein is co-expressed in yeast with non-fused HBsAg, yielding spontaneously assembling particles with overall 25 % of the CS-HBsAg fusion protein and 75 % free HBsAg. Relative to early anti-CS vaccine candidates targeting the humoral immunodominant central repeat region only, which failed to induce significant protection, the addition of the C-terminal flanking region to the repeat region, the particulate structure, and the use of adjuvants to potentiate the immune response appear to have been critical steps to reach protective levels of immunity [6].

The adjuvant system selected, AS01, is a liposomal formulation and includes two immunostimulants, 3-*O*-desacyl-4′-monophosphoryl lipid A (a nontoxic derivative of the lipopolysaccharide from *Salmonella minnesota* shown to be a Toll-like receptor 4 agonist) and QS-21 Stimulon® (a natural saponin molecule extracted from the bark of the South American tree *Quillaja saponaria* Molina, fraction 21 (licensed by GSK from Antigenics Inc.), shown to be an inflammasome activator). These act synergistically to stimulate the innate immune system and activate antigen-presenting dendritic cells and invigorate humoral and type 1 CD4+ T-cell response [7]. Controlled human malaria infection (CHMI) studies have been instrumental in demonstrating the relative merit of various adjuvant formulations [8, 9]. RTS,S/AS02 (an oil-in-water formulation with the same immune enhancers) was initially selected for further development, before demonstration of superior immunogenicity and efficacy of RTS,S/AS01 in CHMI studies and in adult and pediatric studies in Africa [9–13]. An adjuvant justification study showed the superior immunogenicity of AS-formulated vaccines over RTS,S alone [14]. Individual RTS,S studies providing key immunological insight are presented in (Tables 1 and 2).

2 Immunobiology: General Considerations

There are three anatomical sites where the vaccine-induced immune effectors could control parasites, when considering the stage-specific nature of CS expression: the skin, the blood, and the liver. Little is known about the role of the skin compartment in RTS,S-induced immunity. During transit in the blood, antibody killing through various mechanisms [15] or functional interference could prevent liver cell invasion by sporozoites. There is no demonstrated role for antibodies against infected liver cells, but interaction with resident T cells or NK cells can be hypothesized, especially when considering that CS is being shed from the sporozoite surface throughout its motility pathway [16]. Vaccine-induced activated T cells may in theory play a killing effector function against infected hepatocytes, but this has not been demonstrated.

Table 1 Individual RTS,S studies in adults providing critical immunological insight

Formulation	Country	Schedule	Sample	Assays	References
Controlled human malaria infection studies in malaria-naïve adults					
RTS,S/AS04 RTS,S/Alum	USA	0, 2, 6 months	Serum PBMC	Serology, LP, ICS, CTL, functional assays	Gordon et al. [25]
RTS,S/AS02 RTS,S/AS03 RTS,S/AS04	USA	0, 1, 7 months	Serum PBMC	Serology (titers, isotypes, opsonization), LP, supernatant cytokine production, ELISPOT, ICS, CTL, functional assays	Stoute et al. [8, 61] Schwenk et al. [15] Sun et al. [39]
RTS,S/AS02	USA	0, 1, 3 months, 0, 7, 28 days	Serum PBMC	Serology, LP, ELISPOT	Kester et al. [62]
RTS,S/AS01 RTS,S/AS02	USA	0, 1, 2 months	Serum PBMC	Serology, LP, ELISPOT, ICS, CTL, gene expression, functional assays	Kester et al. [9] Lumsden et al. [34] Schwenk et al. [40] Vahey et al. [59]
Ad35-CS RTS,S/AS01	USA	0, 1, 2 months	Serum PBMC	Serology, ICS, ELISPOT, others ongoing	Ockenhouse [29]
RTS,S/AS01	USA	0, 1, 7 months (fractional third dose)	Ongoing	Ongoing	NCT01857869
RTS,S/AS01 ChAd/ ME-TRAP	UK	0, 1, 2 months	Ongoing	Ongoing	NCT01883609
RTS,S/AS01 ChAd/ ME-TRAP	UK	0, 1, 2 months (fractional third dose)	Ongoing	Ongoing	NCT02252640
Immunogenicity studies in malaria-naïve adults without controlled human malaria infection					
RTS,S/AS02	Belgium	0, 1, 6 months	Serum PBMC	Serology, LP, CTL, ELISPOT	Lalvani et al. [48]
RTS,S/AS01 RTS,S/AS02 RTS,S in saline	Belgium	0, 1, 2 months	Serum PBMC	Serology (titer, avidity), ICS	Leroux et al. [14]
Studies in malaria-exposed adults					
RTS,S/AS02	Gambia	0, 1, 5 months	Serum PBMC	Serology, LP, ELISPOT, parasite genetics	Pinder et al. [47], Alloueche et al. [55]
RTS,S/AS02	Kenya	0, 1, 7 months	Serum	Serology	Stoute et al. [63]
RTS,S/AS01 RTS,S/AS02	Kenya	0, 1, 2 months	Serum PBMC Whole blood	Serology, ICS, parasite genetics	Polhemus et al. [21] Waitumbi et al. [56]

LP lymphoproliferation, *ICS* intracellular cytokine staining, *CTL* lymphocyte cytotoxicity

Table 2 Individual RTS,S pediatric studies in malaria-endemic countries, providing critical immunological insight

Formulation	Age	Study design	Country	Schedule	Sample	Assay	References
RTS,S/AS02	1–4 years	Phase 2 Safety, efficacy, immunogenicity	Mozambique	0, 1, 2 months	Serum Whole blood	Serology Blood-stage immunity Parasite genetics	Campo et al. [49] Enosse et al. [57]
RTS,S/AS02	6–10 weeks	Phase 1/2 Safety, efficacy, immunogenicity	Mozambique	0, 1, 2 months (EPI staggered)	Serum Whole blood	Serology Intracellular cytokine staining	Aponte et al. [30] Barbosa et al. [46]
RTS,S/AS02	8–12 weeks	Phase 2 Safety, efficacy, immunogenicity	Tanzania	0, 1, 2 months (EPI coadmin)	Serology	Serology	Abdulla et al. [31]
RTS,S/AS01 RTS,S/AS02	18 months–4 years	Phase 2 Safety, immunogenicity	Gabon	0, 1, 2 months	Serum PBMC	Serology Intracellular cytokine staining B-cell memory	Lell et al. [11] Agnandji et al. [41]
RTS,S/AS01 RTS,S/AS02	5–17 months	Phase 2 Safety, immunogenicity	Ghana	0, 1, 2 months 0, 1 month 0, 1, 7 months	Serum Whole blood	Serology Intracellular cytokine staining	Owusu-Agiey et al. [10] Ansong et al. [42]
RTS,S/AS01	5–17 months	Phase 2 Efficacy, safety, immunogenicity	Kenya	0, 1, 2 months	Serum PBMC Whole blood	Serology (titer, avidity) Intracellular cytokine staining ELISPOT NK cell immunity Blood-stage immunity	Olotu et al. [23, 35, 37, 43] Ndungu et al. [44] Horowitz et al. [45] Bejon et al. [50] Warimwe et al. [60]
RTS,S/AS01	6–12 weeks	Phase 2 Safety, efficacy, immunogenicity	Gabon Ghana Tanzania	0, 1, 2 months (EPI coadmin)	Serum	Serology Avidity	Agnandji et al. [28] Asante et al. [33] Ajua et al. [36]
RTS,S/AS01	6–12 weeks 5–17 months	Phase 3 Efficacy, safety, immunogenicity	7 countries in Africa	0, 1, 2 months (infants: EPI coadmin)	Serum PBMC	Serology Parasite genetics	RTS,S Clinical Trials Partnership [1, 22] Neafsey et al. [58]
RTS,S/AS01	Neonates Infants	Phase 3 Safety, immunogenicity	Malawi	Several schedules (EPI coadmin)	Serum	Serology	NCT01231503
RTS,S/AS01	6 weeks–5 months (HIV infected)	Phase 3 Safety, efficacy, immunogenicity	Kenya	0, 1, 2 months	Serum	Serology	NCT01148459

The demonstration that a specific immune assay can be used as a regulatory valid predictive correlate of protection constitutes an inspiring but challenging goal of immunological vaccine research. When considering Systems Biology assessments, semiquantitative multiparametric outputs and model analysis of the relationship with outcome are sources of increasing complexity. In the condition of natural malaria exposure, while immune effector functions can be measured at different timepoints postvaccination, it is rarely contemporaneous with exposure, and the impossibility to differentiate protected from non-exposed subjects limits analyses of correlates of protection [17]. Things are different in the CHMI model, where healthy adult volunteer's exposure to drug-sensitive strains of *P. falciparum*-infected lab-reared mosquitoes is completely controlled.

There are various possible methodologies of analysis of CHMI outcome. Analysis of the proportion of subjects protected is the most clinically relevant. But considering that post-challenge delay in time-to-patent infection is a quantitative indicator of pre-erythrocytic immunity affecting the number of parasites reaching the blood stage (the liver-to-blood inoculum), log-rank survival statistics is best to compare physiologic outcome, and time to event can be used as a proxy of pre-erythrocytic immunity. Analyses using a biologically motivated mathematical model of sporozoite infection fitted to time-to-parasitemia data from RTS,S CHMI trials estimated a 96.1 % (95 % CI, 93.4–97.8 %) reduction in the liver-to-blood parasite inoculum, indicating a small number of parasites (often the progeny of a single surviving sporozoite) are responsible for breakthrough blood-stage infections [18].

In the RTS,S program, homologous challenge approximately 3 weeks after vaccination has been used to assess vaccine-induced protection. Rechallenge of initially protected subjects, a few months later, provided insight into durability of protection [8, 9].

3 Humoral Immunity

While high-dose experimental exposure to irradiated sporozoites can lead to sterile protection (immunity preventing blood-stage infection) [19], exposure in conditions of natural infection leads to very little detectable anti-CS immunity and does not seem to provide preerythrocytic sterile immunity [20]. Low levels of anti-CS antibodies are found in semi-immune adults [21]. The rationale for anti-CS vaccination strategies is therefore not to imitate something happening in nature.

RTS,S/AS01 vaccination leads to high levels of circulating anti-CS antibodies, and despite waning, concentration remains higher in vaccinated subjects after years of follow-up than in naturally exposed subjects [22, 23]. Antibodies against the CS repeat region (R32LR antigen, synthetic NANP repeats) were measured by a validated ELISA developed by GSK and expressed as ELISA optical units per ml [24], except for early studies that were tested with a CS ELISA developed at the Walter Reed Army Institute of Research using a reference serum, expressing results as μg/

ml [25]. The exact determinants of the magnitude of the anti-CS humoral response are unknown, but a number of factors have been studied.

In virtually all the age groups studied, vaccinated subjects became seropositive following two doses of RTS,S/AS01, with an increase in concentration after the third dose. The analysis of antibody kinetics showed a peak approximately 3 weeks after the last dose, followed by a biphasic, initially rapid, then slower, decay [26, 27]. As compared to a 0-, 1-, and 2-month schedule, spacing of the third dose as part of a 0-, 1-, and 7-month schedule led to a reduced post-dose three titers in two studies [10, 28]. The highest anti-CS antibody responses to RTS,S/AS01 have been observed in children aged 5–17 months old at the first vaccination. In the phase 3 study, peak anti-CS GMC overall was of 621 EU/mL (range across sites, 348–787 EU/mL) in this age group, but lower in younger infants, with overall GMC of 211 EU/mL (range across sites, 117–335 EU/mL) [22]. Post-vaccination antibody concentrations were also lower in older children [11] and adults [9, 14, 21, 29].

The role of pre-vaccination exposure remains unclear. Post-vaccination titers were higher in malaria-naïve American adults than in malaria-experienced Kenyan adults, suggesting that past malaria exposure may generate an immunological imprinting which reduces the vaccine response [9, 21, 30], but this hypothesis is not supported by the fact that pre-vaccination anti-CS antibody concentration has been associated with higher responses to vaccination in 5–17 months children and adults, rather suggesting natural priming [13, 26]. When considering the role of exposure on the longevity of the immune response, there is no evidence that re-exposure to experimental sporozoite inoculation or to natural infection in malaria-endemic areas leads to any significant boosting of anti-CS antibody levels.

In one phase 2 study in 1–4-year-old children, of which about half had been vaccinated with hepatitis B in the past, post-vaccination anti-CS antibody concentrations tended to be higher in hepatitis B-vaccinated children [11], as if the RTS,S antigen had activated hepatitis B-specific immune memory and recruited T-cell help, with a positive impact on the CS-specific response. The association between pre-vaccination anti-HBs and postvaccination anti-CS titers has also been found in a combined analysis of phase 2 studies, but not in the phase 3 trial [13, 26]. Within the 5–17-month age range, younger children seem to have higher anti-CS responses [26]. This observation is compatible with a potential role of past, recent hepatitis B vaccination.

As compared to 5–17-month-old children, immunogenicity in infants 6–12 weeks old at first vaccination is lower, with lower protection against malaria [22, 26]. Age-related immune immaturity may play a role. In addition, two factors have clearly been shown to reduce immunogenicity in these young infants. Co-administration with other EPI vaccines appears to reduce RTS,S immunogenicity. Infants vaccinated with RTS,S/AS02 in co-administration with EPI vaccines in one study in Mozambique had lower anti-CS antibody responses as compared to infants of the same age in another study in Tanzania who received staggered immunizations [30, 31]. In addition, maternally derived anti-CS antibodies have been associated to lower anti-CS responses, through mechanisms that have not been characterized [22, 26]. In the phase 3 trial, infants 6 weeks old at first vaccination had a lower anti-CS response 1 month post dose 3 compared to infants 7–12 weeks old at first vaccination, and infants who were seropositive for anti-CS antibody at baseline had a lower anti-CS antibody response at 1 month post dose 3 [22, 26]. In contrast, there was no significant association between baseline anti-hepatitis B surface antigen antibodies and anti-CS immunogenicity [26].

Children infected with HIV were shown to have reduced anti-CS antibody responses, as compared to children not infected with HIV [26]. In children 6 weeks to 17 months of age with high antiretroviral therapy coverage, the estimated VE against malaria, over 1 year, was 37.2 % (95 % CI 26.5–68.8 %) [32].

The relationship between anti-CS responses and protection against infection has been fairly well established, first in the CHMI model, then in the field. No antibody threshold is predictive of protection at the individual level, but a correlation between peak antibody level and protection has been consistently shown in CHMI studies [9, 13, 30]. In conditions of natural malaria exposure, the association between peak anti-CS antibodies and protection was confirmed in studies with active monitoring of infection and disease, with presumably high endpoint capture [21, 31, 33]. Inconsistent results have been seen in studies including passive case detection over longer follow-up time [22, 33, 34], which may be related to increased heterogeneity due to other factors such as health-seeking behavior and specificity of case definitions. Exploratory modeling analysis suggested a nonlinear continuous relationship between antibodies and protection [26, 27]. An anti-CS antibody titer of 121 EU/mL was estimated to prevent 50 % of infections [26]. Another study showed a sharp change in protection over a narrow window of antibody concentrations with 40 EU/mL estimated to be the best discriminative threshold [35].

The role of antibodies targeting other regions of the CS protein has not been fully characterized. Intra-subject correlation between the different arms or targets of the immune response may obscure our ability to independently assess the relationship with protection [34]. Altogether, no other effector has been associated to protection more closely than anti-CS antibodies targeting the repeat region.

The avidity of antibodies against the CS repeat region was assessed by measuring the avidity index (AI); the ratio of titers observed with and without chaotropic reagent. The AI was evaluated in infants [36], children 5–17 months old [37], and malaria-naïve adults [14, 30]. Post-vaccination AI in infants vaccinated with RTS,S/AS01 according to a 0-, 1-, and 2-month and a 0-, 1-, and 7-month schedule was similar. While there was no association between 1 month post dose 3 AI and efficacy, intriguingly the change in AI between post-second and third RTS,S/AS01 vaccination was associated with a reduced risk of malaria [37]. Another nested case-control analysis of 5–17-month-old children found higher AI in children with high malaria exposure compared to those with low exposure, but no association between AI and protection [38]. In a study of various RTS,S formulations, the adjuvant was not found to be a driver of increased antibody avidity [14]. The possibility to increase qualitative aspects of the humoral response through changes in vaccine dose and schedule is currently under evaluation.

4 T-Cell Immunity

The induction of T-cell activation following RTS,S vaccination has been shown using a variety of methods including proliferation and cytotoxicity assays, analysis of cytokine production following *in vitro* antigen restimulation in culture supernatant, short or long ELISPOT assays, or surface and intracellular cytokine staining [38]. CD4⁺ T-cell responses seem to peak after dose 2 in naïve adults [30]. Associations between a number of these assays and protection against CHMI have been shown [8, 9, 36, 39, 40]. In several studies but not all, the frequency on day of challenge of CS peptide-reactive CD4⁺ T cells producing any combination of two or more of the following biomarkers, IL-2, TNF-α or IFN-γ, and CD40L, was significantly higher in protected subjects as compared to non-protected subjects [9, 13, 30].

Modeling analysis showed that considering both anti-CS antibodies and polyfunctional CD4⁺ T cells led to the best estimates of relationship between immunogenicity and protection, with no indication of a synergistic effect [18]. The role of antibodies is predominant, as shown by the finding that the replacement of one first dose of RTS,S/AS01 by a recombinant adenovirus expressing the CS target antigen, which promoted the CD4⁺ T-cell response but led to a reduced anti-CS antibody response, resulted in a lower point estimate of VE against CHMI [30].

IL2-dominated CD4⁺ responses with induction of TNF-α and IFN-γ have also been demonstrated in children 18 months to 4 years and 5–17 months living in malaria-endemic areas, using intracellular cytokine staining of antigen-stimulated whole blood or PBMC samples [41, 42]. In one pediatric efficacy study, peak CD4⁺ T-cell response was associated with protection against malaria [43, 44]. One pediatric study evaluating the role of schedule suggested upon comparison of a 0- and 1-; a 0-, 1-, and 2-; or a 0-, 1-, and 7-month regimen that T-cell immunogenicity was lower after two doses than after three doses and higher on a 0-, 1-, and 7-month schedule than on a 0-, 1-, and 2-month schedule [43]. The exact role of activated CS-specific CD4⁺ T cells remains unclear. While CD4-mediated killing in lymphoid tissue or in the liver is a possibility—considering that while hepatocytes don't express MHC Class II, there are numerous other cell types that do—this has not been demonstrated. CS-specific CD4⁺T cells may play a role restricted to a helper function, assisting B-cell maturation or activation of other cell types. One study suggested a possible role for CD4-derived IL-2-mediated NK cell activation [45].

CD8 responses to RTS,S have been reported in two studies [40, 46], but not in many others [8, 9, 30, 47, 48], and AS01-adjuvanted protein vaccines CD8⁺ effectors in circulating blood.

5 Immune Memory

Several observations indicate that RTS,S/AS01 vaccination induces a response with features of immunologic memory and long-term effects. On immunological ground, characterization of CD45RO⁺ and CCR7 expression by CS-specific CD4⁺ T cells following RTS,S vaccination suggested that both central memory and effector memory cells are induced by vaccination and associated to protection [36]. Isotype switching to IgG1-dominated responses [8, 9], affinity maturation [37, 38], and the demonstrated generation of memory B cells detected 12 months after vaccination [42] are also classical features of vaccine-induced humoral immunity maturation processes and memory generation. On clinical grounds, several studies have demonstrated ongoing cumulative clinical benefit upon long follow-up time periods [1, 23]. In children 5–17 months old at first vaccination, cross-sectional surveys at several timepoints throughout the phase 3 trial showed a statistically significant reduction of prevalent parasitemia up to month 32 in the subjects having received three doses and up to the end of study (average 48 months) in children vaccinated with four doses [1].

There is nevertheless a clear indication that vaccine-induced protection wanes over time. In one representative CHMI study, about half of the subjects initially protected at 3 weeks after vaccination were no longer protected after a second challenge 6 months later [9]. In the phase 3 trial, analysis of VE in the 5–17-month age category by 6-month time periods showed declining VE post dose 3 in successive 6-month periods from 67.6 % (95 % CI 63.8–71.0) initially to 38.9 % (95 % CI 33.2, 44.0), 27.9 % (95 % CI 20.2–34.9), 13.9 % (95 % CI 4.7–22.1), and 12.5 % (95 % CI 1.1–22.6) finally to 0.1 % (95 % CI 9.9–9.1) between 30 months following the first three doses and the end of the trial (http://www.who.int/immunization/sage/meetings/2015/october/1_Final_malaria_vaccine_background_paper_v2015_09_30.pdf). A similar pattern of waning over time was also seen in the younger age category, with generally lower point estimates of VE. While these estimates need to be interpreted with caution, because after initial randomization the acquisition of immunity resulting from natural exposure is increased in the control group relative to the malaria vaccine group, and the two groups are therefore no longer strictly comparable, it clearly documents the overall waning process.

One of the central characteristics of adaptative immune memory responses is boostability. The added benefit of the fourth dose is clearly demonstrated, driving up VE estimates over the whole study duration and the late time periods, increasing the number of cases averted [1]. Nevertheless, the 42.9 % (95 % CI 36.4–48.7) VE against malaria over the first 6 months post dose 4 is lower than the VE estimate over 6 months following primary immunization [32]. This may be related to the different malaria exposure between the vaccinated and control group, but could also be related to a lower response to the fourth dose as compared to the primary immunization regimen. In line with that hypothesis, the peak antibody response post dose 4 is lower than the peak antibody response post dose 3 [32]. Boostability is demonstrated, but the data suggest boostability may diminish over time or upon successive doses [26].

The poor immunogenicity of polysaccharidic repeat motives of encapsulated bacteria, characterized by poor memory induction, with minimal isotype switching and antibody maturation processes that can be overcome by protein conjugation methodologies, is well characterized [32]. Current data does not allow to conclude as to whether there is anything similar when considering the immune response to CS as included in RTS,S/AS01, with its characteristic central repeat region, but this can be hypothesized. Modeling analysis suggests that the waning VE mirrors the predicted decay of antibodies over time [26, 27]. The transit time of sporozoites through the circulation after natural exposure is likely too short to allow an adaptive immune response to build up to control infection. This may be a key difference with classical vaccine responses to bacterial and viral infections which typically leads to pathogen replication and prolonged antigen exposure and immune effector expansion from the memory pool. Further evaluation of boostability over a higher number of doses may provide more insight into the detailed nature of the memory immune response to RTS,S/AS01.

6 Impact of Vaccination on Immunity to the Blood Stage of the Parasite Life Cycle

Early in the RTS,S development program, it was hypothesized that the reduction of the parasite numbers at the preerythrocytic stage, leading to a lower absolute number of parasites responsible for the "out-of-the-liver" blood-stage inoculum, documented by an increase in post-CHMI time to patent blood-stage infection, may give the immune system more time to respond to the blood-stage infection and reduce the probability of disease progression. This hypothesis has however not been supported through phase 3 evaluation which showed point estimates of VE against severe malaria similar or lower than point estimates of VE against non-severe malaria [1]. No study showed lower parasitemia levels in breakthrough malaria cases in vaccinated subjects as compared to unvaccinated subjects.

In the absence of CS expression during blood-stage infection, a direct protective effect of vaccination on the parasite growth in the blood would not be expected. Rather, RTS,S vaccination induces pre-erythrocytic immunity which decreases the probability of initiation of blood-stage infection. As repeated natural exposure to blood-stage infection leads to immunity targeting the blood stage and a state of partial protection limiting the risk of disease progression and severe outcomes upon infection, RTS,S/AS01 vaccination reduces the speed of acquisition of blood-stage immunity. This has been demonstrated in two pediatric studies where antibodies targeting the blood stage were reduced in RTS,S-vaccinated subjects [49, 50].

Partial reduction of the probability of blood-stage infection in the presence of pre-erythrocytic vaccine-induced immunity would be expected to induce a delay in median age of infection, malaria, and severe malaria, and that has been shown [51]. Under continuous follow-up of the vaccinated and non-vaccinated group, this would be expected to lead to delayed follow-up time periods where the measured risk of severe malaria is increased in vaccinated subjects as compared to non-vaccinated subjects, even if the overall cumulative effect on severe malaria is positive or neutral. The only situation where this would result into an increased risk to subjects would be if the outcome of infection is worse in older children than in younger children. Although the disease presentation pattern may differ according to age, with severe anemia being more often observed in younger children, and cerebral malaria being more observed in older children, there is no evidence that disease outcome is worse in older children [52, 53]. Phase 3 evaluation of RTS,S/AS01 showed, indeed, in children from the 5–17-month age category having received three doses of RTS,S upon comparison of incidence of severe malaria during a delayed follow-up time period, the point estimate of VE against severe malaria is negative—hence, the incidence of malaria is higher in the vaccinated group as compared to the unvaccinated group. In the children not vaccinated with the fourth dose, this led to an overall VE against malaria over the whole follow-up period which was not statistically significant. This was not observed in the group of children who received the fourth dose at study month 20, which showed an overall VE against severe malaria of 32 % (95 % CI 14–47) [1].

7 Vaccine-Induced Immunity and Parasite Genetic Diversity

Even though, as mentioned above, repeated malaria infections under conditions of natural exposure do not induce strong anti-CS responses and epidemiological studies suggested little pre-erythrocytic sterilizing immunity, CS does display some sequence diversity, especially within the C-terminal region, suggesting the existence of selection pressure mechanisms [54]. Early VE studies including a limited number of subjects did not suggest any differential efficacy according to CS sequence polymorphism [55–57]. In contrast, parasite genetic analysis phase 3 evaluation suggested some allelic specificity in vaccine-induced protection. The study confirmed the important general genetic diversity of the circulating malaria strains in all the settings, with strong regional differences. On a positive note, it was clearly demonstrated that VE was detected in all settings, in face of all the genetic diversity. The exploratory study also suggested a possible marginal difference in VE levels according to the degree of sequence homology with the vaccine parent strain, when considering 5–17-month-old children, but not 6–12-week-old infants [58]. Whether vaccine implementation may select for vaccine-resistant variants will need to be further evaluated. This question may be mostly relevant when considering the contribution of vaccines to the malaria elimination strategy as the induction of partial protection in children, who constitute a limited proportion of those contributing to transmission, may not be sufficient to impact the overall pool of circulating strains.

8 Translational Science

High-throughput microarray technology has been used to assess gene expression patterns associated to protection against CHMI. In one study, early post-vaccination expression of genes in the immunoproteasome pathway and late expression of genes associated with programmed cell death were associated with protection against CHMI [59]. An exploratory analysis of a pediatric phase 2 study suggested an association between the peripheral blood monocyte-to-lymphocyte ratio at study enrollment and efficacy of RTS,S/AS01 [60]. Many initiatives are ongoing, to further characterize immune protective mechanisms. These include further analysis of gene expression using microarray and deep sequencing, detailed evaluation of polyfunctional T cells, characterization of activated T-follicular helper cells, and evaluation of early activation of innate immunity. Detailed humoral immunity characterization is ongoing, with plasmablast analysis involving deep sequencing of genes coding for variable regions of immunoglobulins, assessment of TDR length and affinity maturation, evaluation of specific anti-CS candidate monoclonal antibodies in animal models, as well as characterization of memory B-cell phenotypes.

References

1. RTS,S Clinical Trials Partnership (2015) Efficacy and safety of RTS, S/AS01 malaria vaccine with or without a booster dose in infants and children in Africa: final results of a phase 3, individually randomised, controlled trial. Lancet 386(9988):31–45
2. Coppi A, Natarajan R, Pradel G, Bennett BL, James ER, Roggero MA, Corradin G, Persson C, Tewari R, Sinnis P (2011) The malaria circumsporozoite protein has two functional domains, each with distinct roles as sporozoites journey from mosquito to mammalian host. J Exp Med 208(2):341–56
3. Singh AP, Buscaglia CA, Wang Q, Levay A, Nussenzweig DR, Walker JR, Winzeler EA, Fujii H, Fontoura BM, Nussenzweig V (2007) *Plasmodium* circumsporozoite protein promotes the development of the liver stages of the parasite. Cell 131(3):492–504
4. Ferguson DJ, Balaban AE, Patzewitz EM, Wall RJ, Hopp CS, Poulin B, Mohmmed A, Malhotra P, Coppi A, Sinnis P, Tewari R (2014) The repeat region of the circumsporozoite protein is critical for sporozoite formation and maturation in *Plasmodium*. PLoS One 9(12), e113923
5. Plassmeyer ML, Reiter K, Shimp RL Jr, Kotova S, Smith PD, Hurt DE, House B, Zou X, Zhang Y, Hickman M, Uchime O, Herrera R, Nguyen V, Glen J, Lebowitz J, Jin AJ, Miller LH, MacDonald NJ, Wu Y, Narum DL (2009) Structure of the *Plasmodium falciparum* circumsporozoite protein, a leading malaria vaccine candidate. J Biol Chem 284(39):26951–63
6. Cohen J, Nussenzweig V, Nussenzweig R, Vekemans J, Leach A (2010) From the circumsporozoite protein to the RTS, S/AS candidate vaccine. Hum Vaccin 6(1):90–6
7. Didierlaurent AM, Collignon C, Bourguignon P, Wouters S, Fierens K, Fochesato M, Dendouga N, Langlet C, Malissen B, Lambrecht BN, Garçon N, Van Mechelen M, Morel S (2014) Enhancement of adaptive immunity by the human vaccine adjuvant AS01 depends on activated dendritic cells. J Immunol 193(4):1920–30
8. Stoute JA, Slaoui M, Heppner DG, Momin P, Kester KE, Desmons P, Wellde BT, Garçon N, Krzych U, Marchand M et al (1997) A preliminary evaluation of a recombinant circumsporozoite protein vaccine against *Plasmodium falciparum* malaria. N Engl J Med 336:86–91
9. Kester KE, Cummings JF, Ofori-Anyinam O, Ockenhouse CF, Krzych U, Moris P, Schwenk R, Nielsen RA, Debebe Z, Pinelis E et al (2009) Randomized, double-blind, phase 2a trial of falciparum malaria vaccines RTS, S/AS01B and RTS, S/AS02A in malaria-naive adults: safety, efficacy, and immunologic associates of protection. J Infect Dis 200:337–346
10. Owusu-Agyei S, Ansong D, Asante K, Kwarteng Owusu S, Owusu R, Wireko Brobby NA, Dosoo D, Osei Akoto A, Osei-Kwakye K, Adjei EA, Boahen KO, Sylverken J, Adjei G, Sambian D, Apanga S, Kayan K, Vekemans J, Ofori-Anyinam O, Leach A, Lievens M, Demoitie MA, Dubois MC, Cohen J, Ballou WR, Savarese B, Chandramohan D, Gyapong JO, Milligan P, Antwi S, Agbenyega T, Greenwood B, Evans J (2009) Randomized controlled trial of RTS, S/AS02D and RTS, S/AS01E malaria candidate vaccines given according to different schedules in Ghanaian children. PLoS One 4(10), e7302, Erratum in: PLoS One. 2010;5(11)

11. Lell B, Agnandji S, von Glasenapp I, Haertle S, Oyakhiromen S, Issifou S, Vekemans J, Leach A, Lievens M, Dubois MC, Demoitie MA, Carter T, Villafana T, Ballou WR, Cohen J, Kremsner PG (2009) A randomized trial assessing the safety and immunogenicity of AS01 and AS02 adjuvanted RTS, S malaria vaccine candidates in children in Gabon. PLoS One 4(10), e7611
12. Bejon P, White MT, Olotu A, Bojang K, Lusingu JP, Salim N, Otsyula NN, Agnandji ST, Asante KP, Owusu-Agyei S, Abdulla S, Ghani AC (2013) Efficacy of RTS, S malaria vaccines: individual-participant pooled analysis of phase 2 data. Lancet Infect Dis 13(4):319–27, Erratum in: Lancet Infect Dis. 2013 Sep;13(9):735
13. White MT, Bejon P, Olotu A, Griffin JT, Bojang K, Lusingu J, Salim N, Abdulla S, Otsyula N, Agnandji ST, Lell B, Asante KP, Owusu-Agyei S, Mahama E, Agbenyega T, Ansong D, Sacarlal J, Aponte JJ, Ghani AC (2014) A combined analysis of immunogenicity, antibody kinetics and vaccine efficacy from phase 2 trials of the RTS,S malaria vaccine. BMC Med 12:117
14. Leroux-Roels G, Leroux-Roels I, Clement F, Ofori-Anyinam O, Lievens M, Jongert E, Moris P, Ballou WR, Cohen J (2014) Evaluation of the immune response to RTS, S/AS01 and RTS, S/AS02 adjuvanted vaccines: randomized, double-blind study in malaria-naïve adults. Hum Vaccin Immunother 10(8):2211–9
15. Schwenk R, Asher LV, Chalom I, Lanar D, Sun P, White K, Keil D, Kester KE, Stoute J, Heppner DG, Krzych U (2003) Opsonization by antigen-specific antibodies as a mechanism of protective immunity induced by *Plasmodium falciparum* circumsporozoite protein-based vaccine. Parasite Immunol 25(1):17–25
16. Vanderberg JP (2014) Imaging mosquito transmission of *Plasmodium* sporozoites into the mammalian host: immunological implications. Parasitol Int 63(1):150–64
17. White MT, Griffin JT, Drakeley CJ, Ghani AC (2010) Heterogeneity in malaria exposure and vaccine response: implications for the interpretation of vaccine efficacy trials. Malar J 9:82
18. White MT, Bejon P, Olotu A, Griffin JT, Riley EM, Kester KE, Ockenhouse CF, Ghani AC (2013) The relationship between RTS, S vaccine-induced antibodies, $CD4^+$ T cell responses and protection against *Plasmodium falciparum* infection. PLoS One 8(4), e61395
19. Hoffman SL, Goh LM, Luke TC, Schneider I, Le TP, Doolan DL, Sacci J, de la Vega P, Dowler M, Paul C, Gordon DM, Stoute JA, Church LW, Sedegah M, Heppner DG, Ballou WR, Richie TL (2002) Protection of humans against malaria by immunization with radiation-attenuated *Plasmodium falciparum* sporozoites. J Infect Dis 185(8):1155–64
20. Tran TM, Li S, Doumbo S, Doumtabe D, Huang CY, Dia S, Bathily A, Sangala J, Kone Y, Traore A, Niangaly M, Dara C, Kayentao K, Ongoiba A, Doumbo OK, Traore B, Crompton PD (2013) An intensive longitudinal cohort study of Malian children and adults reveals no evidence of acquired immunity to *Plasmodium falciparum* infection. Clin Infect Dis 57(1):40–7
21. Polhemus ME, Remich SA, Ogutu BR, Waitumbi JN, Otieno L, Apollo S, Cummings JF, Kester KE, Ockenhouse CF, Stewart A, Ofori-Anyinam O, Ramboer I, Cahill CP, Lievens M, Dubois MC, Demoitie MA, Leach A, Cohen J, Ballou WR, Heppner DG Jr (2009) Evaluation of RTS, S/AS02A and RTS, S/AS01B in adults in a high malaria transmission area. PLoS One 4(7), e6465
22. RTS,S Clinical Trials Partnership (2014) Efficacy and safety of the RTS, S/AS01 malaria vaccine during 18 months after vaccination: a phase 3 randomized, controlled trial in children and young infants at 11 African sites. PLoS Med 11(7), e1001685
23. Olotu A, Fegan G, Wambua J, Nyangweso G, Awuondo KO, Leach A, Lievens M, Leboulleux D, Njuguna P, Peshu N, Marsh K, Bejon P (2013) Four-year efficacy of RTS, S/AS01E and its interaction with malaria exposure. N Engl J Med 368(12):1111–20
24. Clement F, Dewar V, Van Braeckel E, Desombere I, Dewerchin M, Swysen C, Demoitié MA, Jongert E, Cohen J, Leroux-Roels G, Cambron P (2012) Validation of an enzyme-linked immunosorbent assay for the quantification of human IgG directed against the repeat region of the circumsporozoite protein of the parasite *Plasmodium falciparum*. Malar J 11:384
25. Gordon DM, McGovern TW, Krzych U, Cohen JC, Schneider I, LaChance R, Heppner DG, Yuan G, Hollingdale M, Slaoui M, Hauser P, Voet P, Sadoff JV, Ballou WR (1995) Safety,

immunogenicity, and efficacy of a recombinantly produced *Plasmodium falciparum* circumsporozoite protein-hepatitis B surface antigen subunit vaccine. J Infect Dis 171(6):1576–85
26. White MT, Verity R, Griffin JT, Asante KP, Owusu-Agyei S, Greenwood B, Drakeley C, Gesase S, Lusingu J, Ansong D, Adjei S, Agbenyega T, Ogutu B, Otieno L, Otieno W, Agnandji ST, Lell B, Kremsner P, Hoffman I, Martinson F, Kamthunzu P, Tinto H, Valea I, Sorgho H, Oneko M, Otieno K, Hamel MJ, Salim N, Mtoro A, Abdulla S, Aide P, Sacarlal J, Aponte JJ, Njuguna P, Marsh K, Bejon P, Riley EM, Ghani AC (2015) Immunogenicity of the RTS, S/AS01 malaria vaccine and implications for duration of vaccine efficacy: secondary analysis of data from a phase 3 randomised controlled trial. Lancet Infect Dis 15(12):1450–8
27. Penny MA, Pemberton-Ross P, Smith TA (2015) The time-course of protection of the RTS, S vaccine against malaria infections and clinical disease. Malar J 14(1):437
28. Agnandji ST, Asante KP, Lyimo J, Vekemans J, Soulanoudjingar SS, Owusu R, Shomari M, Leach A, Fernandes J, Dosoo D, Chikawe M, Issifou S, Osei-Kwakye K, Lievens M, Paricek M, Apanga S, Mwangoka G, Okissi B, Kwara E, Minja R, Lange J, Boahen O, Kayan K, Adjei G, Chandramohan D, Jongert E, Demoitié MA, Dubois MC, Carter T, Vansadia P, Villafana T, Sillman M, Savarese B, Lapierre D, Ballou WR, Greenwood B, Tanner M, Cohen J, Kremsner PG, Lell B, Owusu-Agyei S, Abdulla S (2010) Evaluation of the safety and immunogenicity of the RTS, S/AS01E malaria candidate vaccine when integrated in the expanded program of immunization. J Infect Dis 202(7):1076–87, Erratum in: J Infect Dis. 2011 May 1;203(9):1344
29. Ockenhouse CF, Regules J, Tosh D, Cowden J, Kathcart A, Cummings J, Paolino K, Moon J, Komisar J, Kamau E, Oliver T, Chhoeu A, Murphy J, Lyke K, Laurens M, Birkett A, Lee C, Weltzin R, Wille-Reece U, Sedegah M, Hendriks J, Versteege I, Pau MG, Sadoff J, Vanloubbeeck Y, Lievens M, Heerwegh D, Moris P, Guerra Mendoza Y, Jongert E, Cohen J, Voss G, Ballou WR, Vekemans J (2015) Ad35.CS.01-RTS,S/AS01 heterologous prime boost vaccine efficacy against sporozoite challenge in healthy malaria-naïve adults. PLoS One 10(7), e0131571
30. Aponte JJ, Aide P, Renom M, Mandomando I, Bassat Q, Sacarlal J, Manaca MN, Lafuente S, Barbosa A, Leach A, Lievens M, Vekemans J, Sigauque B, Dubois MC, Demoitié MA, Sillman M, Savarese B, McNeil JG, Macete E, Ballou WR, Cohen J, Alonso PL (2007) Safety of the RTS, S/AS02D candidate malaria vaccine in infants living in a highly endemic area of Mozambique: a double blind randomised controlled phase I/IIb trial. Lancet 370(9598):1543–51
31. Abdulla S, Oberholzer R, Juma O, Kubhoja S, Machera F, Membi C, Omari S, Urassa A, Mshinda H, Jumanne A, Salim N, Shomari M, Aebi T, Schellenberg DM, Carter T, Villafana T, Demoitié MA, Dubois MC, Leach A, Lievens M, Vekemans J, Cohen J, Ballou WR, Tanner M (2008) Safety and immunogenicity of RTS, S/AS02D malaria vaccine in infants. N Engl J Med 359(24):2533–44
32. Avci FY (2013) Novel strategies for development of next-generation glycoconjugate vaccines. Curr Top Med Chem 13(20):2535–40
33. Asante KP, Abdulla S, Agnandji S, Lyimo J, Vekemans J, Soulanoudjingar S, Owusu R, Shomari M, Leach A, Jongert E, Salim N, Fernandes JF, Dosoo D, Chikawe M, Issifou S, Osei-Kwakye K, Lievens M, Paricek M, Möller T, Apanga S, Mwangoka G, Dubois MC, Madi T, Kwara E, Minja R, Hounkpatin AB, Boahen O, Kayan K, Adjei G, Chandramohan D, Carter T, Vansadia P, Sillman M, Savarese B, Loucq C, Lapierre D, Greenwood B, Cohen J, Kremsner P, Owusu-Agyei S, Tanner M, Lell B (2011) Safety and efficacy of the RTS, S/AS01E candidate malaria vaccine given with expanded-programme-on-immunisation vaccines: 19 month follow-up of a randomised, open-label, phase 2 trial. Lancet Infect Dis 11(10):741–9
34. Lumsden JM, Schwenk RJ, Rein LE, Moris P, Janssens M, Ofori-Anyinam O, Cohen J, Kester KE, Heppner DG, Krzych U (2011) Protective immunity induced with the RTS, S/AS vaccine is associated with IL-2 and TNF-α producing effector and central memory CD4 T cells. PLoS One 6(7), e20775
35. Olotu A, Lusingu J, Leach A, Lievens M, Vekemans J, Msham S, Lang T, Gould J, Dubois MC, Jongert E, Vansadia P, Carter T, Njuguna P, Awuondo KO, Malabeja A, Abdul O, Gesase S, Mturi N, Drakeley CJ, Savarese B, Villafana T, Lapierre D, Ballou WR, Cohen J, Lemnge MM, Peshu N, Marsh K, Riley EM, von Seidlein L, Bejon P (2011) Efficacy of RTS, S/AS01E

malaria vaccine and exploratory analysis on anti-circumsporozoite antibody titres and protection in children aged 5–17 months in Kenya and Tanzania: a randomised controlled trial. Lancet Infect Dis 11(2):102–9

36. Ajua A, Lell B, Agnandji ST, Asante KP, Owusu-Agyei S, Mwangoka G, Mpina M, Salim N, Tanner M, Abdulla S, Vekemans J, Jongert E, Lievens M, Cambron P, Ockenhouse CF, Kremsner PG, Mordmüller B (2015) The effect of immunization schedule with the malaria vaccine candidate RTS, S/AS01E on protective efficacy and anti-circumsporozoite protein antibody avidity in African infants. Malar J 14:72
37. Olotu A, Clement F, Jongert E, Vekemans J, Njuguna P, Ndungu FM, Marsh K, Leroux-Roels G, Bejon P (2014) Avidity of anti-circumsporozoite antibodies following vaccination with RTS, S/AS01E in young children. PLoS One 9(12), e115126
38. Casares S, Brumeanu TD, Richie TL (2010) The RTS,S malaria vaccine. Vaccine 28(31):4880–94
39. Sun P, Schwenk R, White K, Stoute JA, Cohen J, Ballou WR, Voss G, Kester KE, Heppner DG, Krzych U (2003) Protective immunity induced with malaria vaccine, RTS, S, is linked to *Plasmodium falciparum* circumsporozoite protein-specific $CD4^+$ and $CD8^+$ T cells producing IFN-gamma. J Immunol 171(12):6961–7
40. Schwenk R, Lumsden JM, Rein LE, Juompan L, Kester KE, Heppner DG, Krzych U (2011) Immunization with the RTS, S/AS malaria vaccine induces IFN-γ^+CD4 T cells that recognize only discrete regions of the circumsporozoite protein and these specificities are maintained following booster immunizations and challenge. Vaccine 29(48):8847–54
41. Agnandji ST, Fendel R, Mestré M, Janssens M, Vekemans J, Held J, Gnansounou F, Haertle S, von Glasenapp I, Oyakhirome S, Mewono L, Moris P, Lievens M, Demoitie MA, Dubois PM, Villafana T, Jongert E, Olivier A, Cohen J, Esen M, Kremsner PG, Lell B, Mordmüller B (2011) Induction of *Plasmodium falciparum*-specific $CD4^+$ T cells and memory B cells in Gabonese children vaccinated with RTS, S/AS01(E) and RTS, S/AS02(D). PLoS One 6(4), e18559
42. Ansong D, Asante KP, Vekemans J, Owusu SK, Owusu R, Brobby NA, Dosoo D, Osei-Akoto A, Osei-Kwakye K, Asafo-Adjei E, Boahen KO, Sylverken J, Adjei G, Sambian D, Apanga S, Kayan K, Janssens MH, Lievens MJ, Olivier AC, Jongert E, Dubois P, Savarese BM, Cohen J, Antwi S, Greenwood BM, Evans JA, Agbenyega T, Moris PJ, Owusu-Agyei S (2011) T cell responses to the RTS, S/AS01(E) and RTS, S/AS02(D) malaria candidate vaccines administered according to different schedules to Ghanaian children. PLoS One 6(4), e18891
43. Olotu A, Moris P, Mwacharo J, Vekemans J, Kimani D, Janssens M, Kai O, Jongert E, Lievens M, Leach A, Villafana T, Savarese B, Marsh K, Cohen J, Bejon P (2011) Circumsporozoite-specific T cell responses in children vaccinated with RTS, S/AS01E and protection against *P. falciparum* clinical malaria. PLoS One 6(10), e25786
44. Ndungu FM, Mwacharo J, Kimani D, Kai O, Moris P, Jongert E, Vekemans J, Olotu A, Bejon P (2012) A statistical interaction between circumsporozoite protein-specific T cell and antibody responses and risk of clinical malaria episodes following vaccination with RTS, S/AS01E. PLoS One 7(12), e52870
45. Horowitz A, Hafalla JC, King E, Lusingu J, Dekker D, Leach A, Moris P, Cohen J, Vekemans J, Villafana T, Corran PH, Bejon P, Drakeley CJ, von Seidlein L, Riley EM (2012) Antigen-specific IL-2 secretion correlates with NK cell responses after immunization of Tanzanian children with the RTS, S/AS01 malaria vaccine. J Immunol 188(10):5054–62
46. Barbosa A, Naniche D, Aponte JJ, Manaca MN, Mandomando I, Aide P, Sacarlal J, Renom M, Lafuente S, Ballou WR, Alonso PL (2009) *Plasmodium falciparum*-specific cellular immune responses after immunization with the RTS, S/AS02D candidate malaria vaccine in infants living in an area of high endemicity in Mozambique. Infect Immun 77(10):4502–9
47. Pinder M, Reece WH, Plebanski M, Akinwunmi P, Flanagan KL, Lee EA, Doherty T, Milligan P, Jaye A, Tornieporth N, Ballou R, McAdam KP, Cohen J, Hill AV (2004) Cellular immunity induced by the recombinant *Plasmodium falciparum* malaria vaccine, RTS, S/AS02, in semi-immune adults in The Gambia. Clin Exp Immunol 135(2):286–93

48. Lalvani A, Moris P, Voss G, Pathan AA, Kester KE, Brookes R, Lee E, Koutsoukos M, Plebanski M, Delchambre M, Flanagan KL, Carton C, Slaoui M, Van Hoecke C, Ballou WR, Hill AV, Cohen J (1999) Potent induction of focused Th1-type cellular and humoral immune responses by RTS, S/SBAS2, a recombinant *Plasmodium falciparum* malaria vaccine. J Infect Dis 180(5):1656–64
49. Campo JJ, Aponte JJ, Skinner J, Nakajima R, Molina DM, Liang L, Sacarlal J, Alonso PL, Crompton PD, Felgner PL, Dobaño C (2015) RTS, S vaccination is associated with serologic evidence of decreased exposure to *Plasmodium falciparum* liver- and blood-stage parasites. Mol Cell Proteomics 14(3):519–31
50. Bejon P, Cook J, Bergmann-Leitner E, Olotu A, Lusingu J, Mwacharo J, Vekemans J, Njuguna P, Leach A, Lievens M, Dutta S, von Seidlein L, Savarese B, Villafana T, Lemnge MM, Cohen J, Marsh K, Corran PH, Angov E, Riley EM, Drakeley CJ (2011) Effect of the pre-erythrocytic candidate malaria vaccine RTS, S/AS01E on blood stage immunity in young children. J Infect Dis 204(1):9–18
51. O'Meara WP, Bejon P, Mwangi TW, Okiro EA, Peshu N, Snow RW, Newton CR, Marsh K (2008) Effect of a fall in malaria transmission on morbidity and mortality in Kilifi. Kenya Lancet 372(9649):1555–62
52. von Seidlein L, Olaosebikan R, Hendriksen IC, Lee SJ, Adedoyin OT, Agbenyega T, Nguah SB, Bojang K, Deen JL, Evans J, Fanello CI, Gomes E, Pedro AJ, Kahabuka C, Karema C, Kivaya E, Maitland K, Mokuolu OA, Mtove G, Mwanga-Amumpaire J, Nadjm B, Nansumba M, Ngum WP, Onyamboko MA, Reyburn H, Sakulthaew T, Silamut K, Tshefu AK, Umulisa N, Gesase S, Day NP, White NJ, Dondorp AM (2012) Predicting the clinical outcome of severe falciparum malaria in African children: findings from a large randomized trial. Clin Infect Dis 54(8):1080–90
53. Dondorp AM, Lee SJ, Faiz MA, Mishra S, Price R, Tjitra E, Than M, Htut Y, Mohanty S, Yunus EB, Rahman R, Nosten F, Anstey NM, Day NP, White NJ (2008) The relationship between age and the manifestations of and mortality associated with severe malaria. Clin Infect Dis 47(2):151–7
54. Gandhi K, Thera MA, Coulibaly D, Traoré K, Guindo AB, Ouattara A, Takala-Harrison S, Berry AA, Doumbo OK, Plowe CV (2014) Variation in the circumsporozoite protein of *Plasmodium falciparum*: vaccine development implications. PLoS One 9(7), e101783
55. Alloueche A, Milligan P, Conway DJ, Pinder M, Bojang K, Doherty T, Tornieporth N, Cohen J, Greenwood BM (2003) Protective efficacy of the RTS, S/AS02 *Plasmodium falciparum* malaria vaccine is not strain specific. Am J Trop Med Hyg 68(1):97–101
56. Waitumbi JN, Anyona SB, Hunja CW, Kifude CM, Polhemus ME, Walsh DS, Ockenhouse CF, Heppner DG, Leach A, Lievens M, Ballou WR, Cohen JD, Sutherland CJ (2009) Impact of RTS, S/AS02(A) and RTS, S/AS01(B) on genotypes of *P. falciparum* in adults participating in a malaria vaccine clinical trial. PLoS One 4(11), e7849
57. Enosse S, Dobaño C, Quelhas D, Aponte JJ, Lievens M, Leach A, Sacarlal J, Greenwood B, Milman J, Dubovsky F, Cohen J, Thompson R, Ballou WR, Alonso PL, Conway DJ, Sutherland CJ (2006) RTS, S/AS02A malaria vaccine does not induce parasite CSP T cell epitope selection and reduces multiplicity of infection. PLoS Clin Trials 1(1), e5
58. Neafsey DE, Juraska M, Bedford T, Benkeser D, Valim C, Griggs A, Lievens M, Abdulla S, Adjei S, Agbenyega T, Agnandji ST, Aide P, Anderson S, Ansong D, Aponte JJ, Asante KP, Bejon P, Birkett AJ, Bruls M, Connolly KM, D'Alessandro U, Dobaño C, Gesase S, Greenwood B, Grimsby J, Tinto H, Hamel MJ, Hoffman I, Kamthunzi P, Kariuki S, Kremsner PG, Leach A, Lell B, Lennon NJ, Lusingu J, Marsh K, Martinson F, Molel JT, Moss EL, Njuguna P, Ockenhouse CF, Ogutu BR, Otieno W, Otieno L, Otieno K, Owusu-Agyei S, Park DJ, Pellé K, Robbins D, Russ C, Ryan EM, Sacarlal J, Sogoloff B, Sorgho H, Tanner M, Theander T, Valea I, Volkman SK, Yu Q, Lapierre D, Birren BW, Gilbert PB, Wirth DF (2015) Genetic diversity and protective efficacy of the RTS, S/AS01 malaria vaccine. N Engl J Med 373(21):2025–37
59. Vahey MT, Wang Z, Kester KE, Cummings J, Heppner DG Jr, Nau ME, Ofori-Anyinam O, Cohen J, Coche T, Ballou WR, Ockenhouse CF (2010) Expression of genes associated with

immunoproteasome processing of major histocompatibility complex peptides is indicative of protection with adjuvanted RTS, S malaria vaccine. J Infect Dis 201(4):580–9
60. Warimwe GM, Fletcher HA, Olotu A, Agnandji ST, Hill AV, Marsh K, Bejon P (2013) Peripheral blood monocyte-to-lymphocyte ratio at study enrollment predicts efficacy of the RTS, S malaria vaccine: analysis of pooled phase II clinical trial data. BMC Med 11:184
61. Stoute JA, Kester KE, Krzych U, Wellde BT, Hall T, White K, Glenn G, Ockenhouse CF, Garcon N, Schwenk R, Lanar DE, Sun P, Momin P, Wirtz RA, Golenda C, Slaoui M, Wortmann G, Holland C, Dowler M, Cohen J, Ballou WR (1998) Long-term efficacy and immune responses following immunization with the RTS, S malaria vaccine. J Infect Dis 178(4):1139–44
62. Kester KE, Cummings JF, Ockenhouse CF, Nielsen R, Hall BT, Gordon DM, Schwenk RJ, Krzych U, Holland CA, Richmond G, Dowler MG, Williams J, Wirtz RA, Tornieporth N, Vigneron L, Delchambre M, Demoitie MA, Ballou WR, Cohen J, Heppner DG Jr, RTS, S Malaria Vaccine Evaluation Group (2008) Phase 2a trial of 0, 1, and 3 month and 0, 7, and 28 day immunization schedules of malaria vaccine RTS, S/AS02 in malaria-naïve adults at the Walter Reed Army Institute of Research. Vaccine 26(18):2191–202
63. Stoute JA, Heppner DG Jr, Mason CJ, Siangla J, Opollo MO, Kester KE, Vigneron L, Voss G, Walter MJ, Tornieporth N, Cohen JD, Ballou WR (2006) Phase 1 safety and immunogenicity trial of malaria vaccine RTS, S/AS02A in adults in a hyperendemic region of western Kenya. Am J Trop Med Hyg 75(1):166–70

Viral Vector Vaccines for Liver-Stage Malaria

Cristina Fernández-Arias and Moriya Tsuji

Contents

1 Introduction 157
2 Prime and Homologous Prime-Boost Regimen 159
2.1 Poxviruses 159
2.2 Adenoviruses 160
2.3 Alphaviruses 161
2.4 Flaviviruses 161
3 Heterologous Prime-Boost Regimen 162
3.1 Heterologous Prime-Boost Immunization Studies Using DNA Vaccines as the Priming Vehicle Followed by Recombinant Viral Vector Boosting 163
3.2 Heterologous Prime-Boost Immunization Studies Using Recombinant Viral Vectors as Both Priming and Boosting Vehicle 165
References 166

1 Introduction

Parasites of the *Plasmodium* genus that are the causative agents of malaria are intracellular pathogens. An effective malaria vaccine is likely to require the induction of cell-mediated immunity, particularly during the liver stages of the parasite. Hence, a successful malaria vaccine should stimulate a strong protective $CD8^+$ T-cell response [1].

DNA vaccines, recombinant protein vaccines, and viral vector vaccines all appear to be suitable vaccine platforms that could efficiently elicit cell-mediated immunity, and, in fact, these vaccines have produced promising results in rodent models. The most traditional approach for malaria vaccines is based on recombinant proteins.

C. Fernández-Arias • M. Tsuji (✉)
HIV and Malaria Vaccine Program, Aaron Diamond AIDS Research Center,
Affiliate of The Rockefeller University, New York, USA
e-mail: mtsuji@adarc.org

M.M. Mota, A. Rodriguez (eds.), *Malaria*, DOI 10.1007/978-3-319-45210-4_8

However, the inoculation of soluble proteins and peptides alone is not sufficient to trigger antigen-specific $CD8^+$ T-cell responses. These molecules need to be administered together with an adjuvant to efficiently induce cell-mediated immune responses, particularly when a Th1-biased immune response is desired. Other methods to deliver proteins for efficient induction of T-cell responses include liposomes [2], bacterial toxins [3], and virus-like particles (VLPs), such as yeast-derived TyVLPs [4]. DNA vaccines also induce potent T-cell-mediated protection in mice [5] but fail to induce strong cellular immune responses in humans [6].

In this regard, viral vectors are capable of inducing strong T-cell and antibody responses in the absence of an adjuvant [7]. The first reported use of a viral vector appeared in 1984, where the authors observed that chimpanzees vaccinated with intact recombinant vaccinia viruses (VACVs) were protected against hepatitis B following challenge with *Hepatitis B virus* [8]. Immediately afterward, the same group, in collaboration with a group from New York University, showed that vaccination of rabbits with a recombinant VACV expressing the circumsporozoite protein (CSP) of the nonhuman primate malaria parasite, *Plasmodium knowlesi*, produces an antibody response [9].

Viral vectors are known to possess a built-in adjuvant effect by way of activating toll-like receptors (TLRs) and inflammasomes upon infecting the target host cells, which could ultimately lead to induction of strong innate immune responses. Furthermore, viral vectors possess other advantages, such as their consistent and inexpensive purification process and their capability to deliver more than one gene, thus inducing a broad immune response [10]. Lastly, each vector has specific properties and induces its own unique immune response.

However, viral vectors also pose problems, which must be considered. One of the primary issues regarding the clinical use of viral vectors is the potential pre-existing immunity against the vectors in the human population [11]. The neutralizing anti-viral vector antibodies mounted in humans exposed to the vector virus could lead to a significant reduction in the efficacy of viral-vectored vaccines. However, the most serious problem that needs to be addressed regarding the use of viral-vectored vaccines is the potential integration of the vector into the genome of host cells, which can result in induction of cancerous cells [12]. In order to avoid this issue, investigators genetically modify the viruses, rendering most of them replication defective, thus reducing or eliminating their pathogenicity.

Poxviruses and adenoviruses (Ad) are the most widely used vectors owing to their well-described capacity to induce strong $CD8^+$ T-cell responses. Other viruses used in the development of malaria vaccines are alphaviruses, measles virus, yellow fever (YF) virus, and vesicular stomatitis virus. Viral-vectored vaccines are highly efficacious in human malaria vaccine trials. Currently, the goal is to broaden the use of simian Ad and modified VACV Ankara (MVA) vectors for vaccination against other diseases such as tuberculosis, human immunodeficiency virus (HIV), and Ebola [13].

2 Prime and Homologous Prime-Boost Regimen

2.1 Poxviruses

The *Poxviridae* family is comprised of double-stranded DNA (dsDNA) viruses. Attenuated poxvirus became essential in the development of vaccines after Edward Jenner established the first system of human vaccination over 200 years ago. Cowpox and horsepox viruses were widely used for the development of vaccines until the appearance of VACV, which allowed for the eventual eradication of smallpox in December 1979. As described above, VACV was the first viral vector to be produced and tested as a malaria vaccine [9].

Poxvirus vectors are very stable in lyophilized form and are both easy and cheap to manufacture. They can also accommodate large DNA inserts without destabilizing the viral vector. As mentioned above, however, the major obstacle hindering their extensive use as viral vectors is the potential severe clinical side effects. Attempts to address this issue include the use of attenuated strains, such as MVA, and a highly attenuated VACV, NYVAC [14], to eliminate pathogenic genes and reduce their replicative capacity. However, these recombinant poxviruses do not induce levels of $CD8^+$ T cells sufficient to guarantee protection against malaria in murine models, when used singly or in repeated immunization (homologous boosting) [15, 16]. For instance, immunization with a VACV expressing the CSP of the rodent malaria parasite, *Plasmodium berghei*, reduces parasite load in the liver but confers a low degree of sterile protection [17]. Similarly, immunization with MVA expressing CSP and thrombospondin-related adhesive protein (TRAP) induces a modest level of protection in a *P. berghei* murine model [15].

Another poxvirus used in Phase 2b clinical trials is the NYVAC-Pf7 virus, an attenuated VACV vector expressing seven different recombinant proteins including the primary anti-invasive targets, merozoite surface protein-1 (MSP-1), and CSP. Vaccination with NYVAC-Pf7 results in a delay in the appearance of malaria symptoms, as well as induction of stronger immune responses than a VACV-based vector expressing only CSP [18]. However, none of these methods confer complete protection.

Similar to MVA, the FP9 strain of fowlpox virus has been used as a viral vector in an attenuated form. Murine dendritic cells (DCs), a subset of professional antigen-presenting cells, infected with this vector display activated specific $CD8^+$ T cells and upregulated major histocompatibility complex (MHC) and co-stimulatory molecules [19]. Human DCs express the transgene for up to 20 days, suggesting that FP9 may have less cytopathogenic effects than MVA, and allow for longer antigen expression. This FP9 has been used primarily in combination with MVA in a prime-boost immunization regimen as a malaria vaccine, as described below [20–22].

2.2 Adenoviruses

Adenoviridae is a family of dsDNA viruses that can infect both dividing and nondividing cells in a wide range of hosts. To date, they have been the most exploited vectors for vaccine development. Similar to poxviruses, Ads can be manufactured safely and inexpensively, and, because these vectors possess a tropism for epithelial cells, they can be administered in a systemic or mucosal manner. Ads also infect DCs, which confers upon the virus the capability to induce strong immune responses. Ad-infected DCs upregulate co-stimulatory molecules and increase the production of cytokines and chemokines, thus contributing to more effective antigen presentation to T cells. Ads also have a potent built-in adjuvant effect, mediated by the inherent stimulation of the innate and adaptive immune system. This stimulation of the innate immune system occurs through both TLR-dependent and TLR-independent fashions [23]. Although a replication-defective Ads reduces its virulence, the use of Ads as viral vectors in malaria vaccines requires further improvements, such as significant reductions in their hepatic toxicity [24] and modulation of the induced host immune response.

Among the 51 Ad serotypes, the conventional Ad vectors that are most widely used, including those for human clinical trials, are constructed based on the subgroup C Ad serotype 5 (Ad5). The first Ad-based malaria vaccine was based on Ad5, and its immunogenicity and protective efficacy was tested in mice [25]. In the study, immunization with the recombinant Ad5 expressing the CSP of the rodent malaria parasite, *Plasmodium yoelii* (Ad5PyCSP), confers CSP-specific cytotoxic T lymphocyte (CTL)-mediated protection from challenge with *P. yoelii* parasites [26]. The Ad-induced protection is primarily mediated by $CD8^+$ T cells [27] and is independent of IFN-γ after a single immunizing dose [28]. The administration of a recombinant Ad5 expressing *Plasmodium falciparum* CSP (Ad5PfCSP) produces CSP-specific humoral and cell-mediated immune responses comparable to the adjuvanted malaria subunit vaccine, RTS,S/AS01B [29].

As described earlier, one of the key drawbacks of using viral vectors is the presence of pre-existing immunity in humans, and Ad is no exception. Pre-existing immunity against Ad, particularly Ad5, reduces the immunogenicity of these Ad-vectored vaccines in animal models [11, 30]; pre-existing anti-Ad5 antibodies inhibit Ad5 vector-mediated transduction. This constitutes a problem for the practical use of these vectors, as the seroprevalence of Ad5 in Africa is approximately 95 %. In order to address this issue, a new Ad vector based on serotype 35 (Ad35) has been shown to act as an effective gene delivery vehicle [31, 32]. The seroprevalence of Ad35 is significantly lower than that of Ad5 [33], and pre-existing immunity to Ad5 does not inhibit the immunogenicity of Ad35-derived vaccines.

Ad35, the full-length CSP-expressing replication-deficient recombinant human Ad3 (Ad35.CS.01), displays high immunogenicity and confers protection in mice [34]. Ad35 vectors are very efficient in homologous prime-boost studies in nonhuman primates [35]. In addition, in a Phase 1 dose-escalation study conducted with Ad35.CS.01 in 2013, healthy adult subjects received three doses intramuscularly at

0-, 1-, and 6-month intervals. The Ad35.CS.01 vaccine was more immunogenic at the highest dosages [36]. When a single immunization dose with recombinant (r) Ad35 expressing liver stage antigen 1 (LSA-1) is employed, the Ad35 vaccine induces a strong antigen-specific IFN-γ $CD8^+$ T-cell response but no measurable antibody response. In contrast, vaccination with a recombinant LSA-1 protein with an adjuvant induces an almost negligible level of cellular responses but does illicit strong antibody responses [37].

Ad vectors from nonhuman primates have been tested to overcome pre-existing immunity against Ad5. These Ads include chimpanzee Ad 6, 7, 9, and 63 vectors (AdC6, AdC7, AdC9, AdC63) [38–40]. Most recently, AdC63 successfully induced partial protection in humans in Africa, as described in the heterologous immunization section below [41].

In addition to using Ads of different serotypes, a few attempts have been made to circumvent pre-existing anti-Ad5 immunity by modifying the capsid proteins of a recombinant Ad5 vaccine expressing a malaria antigen. In the first study, the hypervariable region 1 (HVR 1) of the Ad capsid was replaced by a B-cell epitope derived from *P. yoelii* CSP, while the whole PyCSP was expressed as a transgene [42]. This capsid-modified Ad5 vaccine not only circumvents pre-existing anti-Ad5 immunity but also improves immunogenicity and protective efficacy. The second group developed a capsid-modified Ad5 vaccine by replacing HVRs of Ad5 with those of Ad43. This capsid-modified Ad5 vaccine was highly immunogenic even in the presence of pre-existing anti-Ad5 immunity [43] Lastly, the most recent study showed that a recombinant Ad5, which displays a B-cell epitope from *P. falciparum* CSP on the HVR 1 of Ad5, induces a potentially protective humoral response in monkeys [44].

2.3 Alphaviruses

Viruses in the *Alphaviridae* family possess positive-sense single-stranded RNA genomes. The most commonly used delivery vectors are based on three encapsulated alphaviruses: Semliki Forest virus, Sindbis virus, and Venezuelan equine encephalitis virus. Replication-defective alphavirus vectors, also known as replicon particles, can induce strong humoral and cellular immune responses. Sindbis virus expressing a $CD8^+$ epitope of *P. yoelii* CSP is also an efficient vector for inducing a strong primary CSP-specific response, as well as protective anti-malaria immunity, after a single immunizing dose [45].

2.4 Flaviviruses

Flaviviruses consist of 70 serologically cross-reactive viruses, several of which may cause serious illnesses in humans, including Japanese encephalitis virus, YF virus, and dengue virus. The prototype flavivirus is YF virus. The YF 17D strain is a licensed, live attenuated vaccine strain used as a vector for the development of vaccines against other flaviviruses, as well as other diseases such as malaria, Japanese encephalitis, West Nile, and the four serotypes of dengue virus [46].

YF 17D expressing a CTL epitope of *P. yoelii* reduces parasite load in a rodent malaria model [47]. In addition, when the repeat sequence of *P. falciparum* CSP is inserted in the F/G loop of the E protein, the resulting virus is capable of inducing anti-CSP antibodies in a rodent model [48].

3 Heterologous Prime-Boost Regimen

A heterologous prime-boost regimen of immunization consists of the combined use of two different vaccines, both encoding the same antigen. In some cases, this strategy is more immunogenic than a single immunization or a homologous prime-boost regimen. Furthermore, although homologous prime-boost immunization is very effective at generating antibody responses, it is generally inefficient at boosting cellular immunity, which is a key element in protection against intracellular pathogens. In contrast, heterologous prime-boost strategies have been successfully used to enhance cellular immunity against pathogens such as *Mycobacterium tuberculosis*, HIV, *Plasmodium*, *Schistosoma mansoni*, *Leishmania*, herpes simplex virus, and hepatitis B and C viruses.

One of the models used for heterologous prime-boost strategies is comprised of a first inoculation with a priming agent, generally by means of a DNA vaccine, followed by inoculation of a boosting agent. Among the most commonly used boosting agents are recombinant viral vectors and recombinant proteins. The rationale for this strategy is that the initial priming results in elicitation of a primary antigen-specific T-cell response, some of which subsequently become antigen-specific memory T cells. When a boosting agent is given, these memory T cells expand, forming a larger pool of immune memory. One of the advantages of using DNA vaccines as priming agents is that upon their inoculation (normally intramuscularly), the DNA is internalized by antigen-presenting cells, which present antigen encoded by the DNA in the context of both MHC class I and II to T cells. This process ultimately allows for DNA vaccines to induce activation of both cytotoxic and helper T cells.

Heterologous prime-boost vaccines overcome some issues that may appear in other vaccine strategies. One of these issues is the weak immunogenicity of plasmid DNA and peptide-based vaccines. Even after homologous prime-boost immunization, these vaccines, in most cases, are unable to induce a sufficient immune response. As for the recombinant viral vectors that are highly immunogenic, when used alone or in homologous prime-boost regimens, much of the immunogenicity generated by these recombinant viruses is targeted at vector components instead of the desired antigens. In this regard, heterologous prime-boost immunization regimens could be utilized to overcome these issues. However, we must be aware of how priming and boosting agents are chosen, for example, some vaccine vectors, such as poxviruses and Ads, which succeed in priming the immune responses, fail to boost them [49]. In many cases, this can be explained as simply arising from immunodominance-related effects. Thus, the immunogenicity of recombinant poxviruses [50] or Ads is substantially greater than that of plasmid DNA or peptide-based vaccines. Therefore, it seems there is a consensus regarding the use of a weak immunogen as a priming agent and a strong immunogen as a boosting agent, when heterologous prime-boost immunization regimens are employed.

3.1 Heterologous Prime-Boost Immunization Studies Using DNA Vaccines as the Priming Vehicle Followed by Recombinant Viral Vector Boosting

Priming with a single dose of plasmid DNA followed by a single boost with a recombinant MVA both expressing *P. berghei* CSP and TRAP induces complete protection in almost 100 % of mice challenged with *P. berghei* sporozoite not only in BALB/c mice but also in highly susceptible C57BL/6 mice. Protection is associated with very high levels of splenic peptide-specific IFN-γ-secreting $CD8^+$ T cells. Interestingly, reversing the order of immunization abrogates this protection [15].

Similarly enhanced T-cell responses resulting in high levels of protection were observed by Sedegah et al. and Gilber et al. [4, 51]. Immunization with either TyVLPs encoding a major $CD8^+$ T-cell epitope or plasmid DNA encoding the entire *P. berghei* CSP, followed by boosting with recombinant MVA carrying the same antigen, induces a fivefold to tenfold increase in the level of CSP-specific $CD8^+$ T-cell response, as compared to either the DNA or the recombinant MVA vector alone in homologous immunization regimens. A greater T-cell response is associated with an increase from 0–20 % to 80–100 % in observed efficacy against *P. berghei* sporozoite challenge [4]. However, concurrent immunization with DNA and MVA fails to produce this enhancement. As a matter of fact, a minimum interval of 9 days between prime and boost immunizations is required to produce a significant increase in immunogenicity and protective efficacy. These and other studies underline the importance of immunization order, indicating that priming and boosting roles cannot be interchanged between DNA and MVA vectors, as we described earlier.

Subsequent works have shown that including additional boosting agents does not necessarily lead to increased protection. For instance, priming with a novel strain, FP9, of an attenuated fowlpox virus expressing *P. berghei* (Pb) CSP, followed by boosting with MVA expressing the same PbCSP, could induce substantial protection against *P. berghei* challenge. However, the sequential triple immunization with a DNA vaccine, FP9, and MVA vaccine fails to improve the immunogenicity or protection over the FP9-MVA heterologous prime-boost immunization regimen [20]. In a different line of inquiry, a study published in 1999 [52] found that different routes of administration produce the same results. In particular, intradermal and intramuscular routes of DNA priming induce a similar level of protective $CD8^+$ T-cell responses against *P. berghei* sporozoite challenge in mice when used in combination with recombinant MVA as a boosting agent. However, the intradermal prime-boost strategy requires very low amounts of DNA, signifying an important reduction in cost, which could make DNA vaccination affordable for use in developing countries.

A slightly different approach to improve the efficacy of a malaria vaccine was conducted [53] in which a candidate malaria vaccine expressing six pre-erythrocytic antigens linked together to produce a 3240-amino acid polyprotein (L3SEPTL) was constructed. Immunization with plasmid DNA expressing the polyprotein failed to prime a recombinant MVA virus boost. However, priming with DNAs expressing the single antigens contained in L3SEPTL, followed by boosting with MVAs, induced strong specific $CD8^+$ T-cell responses against TRAP and LSA-1. However, a heterologous prime-boost regimen using MVA and FP9 expressing L3SEPTL-induced IFN-γ-secreting $CD8^+$ T cells against each of the six antigens [53]. This approach was taken based on the rationale that the use of polyprotein constructs may increase the number of potential target epitopes, which would confer an important advantage for their use in immunogenetically diverse human populations. However, subsequent studies have highlighted some concerns with this approach. In a Phase 1 clinical trial [54, 55], 15 volunteers were immunized with three doses of plasmid DNA encoding both *P. falciparum* CSP and apical membrane antigen 1 (AMA1). This priming phase was followed 4 months later by a single boost with human Ad5 expressing the same antigens (AdPCA). The results of this study showed that four volunteers (27 %) developed sterile immunity due to the presence of $CD8^+$ T-cell-associated IFN-γ activities against AMA1, but not against CSP. The authors of this work hypothesized that vaccine-induced effector memory $CD8^+$ T cells recognizing a single MHC-I epitope could confer sterile immunity to *P. falciparum* in humans. The main conclusion of their work is that a better understanding of which epitopes within malaria antigens can confer sterile and effective immunity is needed [56].

Design of vaccine approaches that elicit responses to effective epitopes will increase the potency of next-generation gene-based vaccines. It is noteworthy that the Ad5 vaccine alone (AdCA) failed to induce protection despite eliciting cellular responses that were often higher than those induced by the heterologous prime-boost immunization regimen. This work again emphasizes that the induction of potent T-cell responses alone may not be a good indicator for the success of heterologous prime-boost immunization strategies.

In some cases, the use of recombinant viruses does not improve the efficacy of the vaccine. For example, RTS,S/AS01, the most advanced candidate malaria vaccine in late-stage Phase 3 testing in infants and young children in Sub-Saharan Africa [57], showed that a heterologous prime-boost immunization regimen comprising a first dose of Ad35.CS.01, followed by two doses of RTS,S/AS01, did not induce increased protection as compared to three doses of RTS,S/AS01.

There are some studies that have tested recombinant virus malaria vaccines in nonhuman primates. For example, rhesus macaques were protected against lethal *P. knowlesi* malaria challenge by immunization with heterologous DNA priming with a combination of the cytokines granulocyte-macrophage colony-stimulating factor, interleukin-4, and tumor necrosis factor alpha, followed by a boost with a mixture of four recombinant attenuated poxviruses encoding four *P. knowlesi*. Following a challenge with 100 infectious *P. knowlesi* sporozoites, 2 of 11 immunized monkeys were sterilely protected, and seven of the nine infected monkeys resolved their parasitemias spontaneously [58–60].

3.2 Heterologous Prime-Boost Immunization Studies Using Recombinant Viral Vectors as Both Priming and Boosting Vehicle

We have seen in the previous section that prime-boost heterologous immunization using a DNA vector plus a recombinant virus increases the efficacy of malaria vaccines. In contrast, the first study employing a heterologous prime-boost immunization regimen consisting of a viral vector prime and viral vector boost was reported by Li et al. [17], in which DNA priming was substituted by immunization with a recombinant influenza virus expressing an epitope of the *P. yoelii* CSP. This was followed by a boosting immunization using a recombinant VACV expressing the same epitope. In addition to a significant increase in the protection of mice against *P. yoelii* challenge [17, 61], this immunization regimen also increased the frequency of CSP-specific $CD8^+$ T cells by 20–30 times, compared to immunization with viral vector alone [62].

Following this line of research, Gilbert et al. showed in 2002 that an Ad vector can not only be used as an efficient boosting agent but also provide a strong priming vaccine vector. In this study, the authors observed effective protection using a recombinant Ad5 expressing the CSP of *P. berghei* for priming and a recombinant MVA for boosting. Furthermore, they found no significant difference in efficacy between intradermal and intramuscular routes of administration of the viral vaccine. A similar study found that an Ad expressing *P. yoelii* CSP prime, followed by a boost with recombinant VACV expressing the same protein, induced complete protection against *P. yoelii* challenge in mice [63].

Recombinant FP9 was described as being more immunogenic than DNA during the priming phase, inducing a higher level of activated $CD8^+$ T cells and better protection against *P. berghei* challenge [20]. Heterologous immunization with recombinant FP9 and MVA encoding the same *P. berghei* CSP succeeded in not only inducing a potent $CD8^+$ T-cell response against the PbCSP but also in eliciting substantial protection against challenge with *P. berghei* [20]. This heterologous immunization regimen was moved to a Phase I trial in Gambia and induced a high level of effector T-cell responses against *P. falciparum* CSP in vaccines [64]. The same group has also constructed an FP9 vector and MVA vector both expressing the multi-epitope (ME)-TRAP, as described previously. This heterologous prime-boost immunization regimen was shown to induce effector T-cell responses but ultimately failed to induce protection among children in Kenya in a Phase 2b trial [23, 65]. As for the use of this strategy in humans, several studies using vaccines that induce strong T-cell responses are only partially effective in controlling human malaria infection [66] and are highly ineffective in field studies [23, 67].

However, when AdC63 and MVA vectors both expressing ME-TRAP were used as a heterologous prime-boost immunization regimen in a Phase I trial conducted in Oxford, it induced strong T-cell responses and sterile protection against malaria in 3 out of 21 vaccinees and delayed the onset of parasitemia in 5 out of 21 vaccinees [68]. In addition, a more recent study with 121 healthy adults in Kenya found that the same vaccination regimen induced partial protection in 57 % of vaccinees in controlled human malaria infection studies [69].

Although the field of a viral-vectored malaria vaccine has advanced substantially during the past 3 decades, there is still no vaccine that can exert a significant level of protective efficacy in the most important target populations, children and infants, living in malaria-endemic areas. In order to improve the viral-vectored malaria vaccine, we need to take drastic approaches to make significant progress toward a successful malaria vaccine. These approaches should include: (1) identification of a more potent viral vector, (2) discovery of a new protective malaria antigen, and (3) identification of an effective adjuvant.

References

1. Tsuji M (2010) A retrospective evaluation of the role of T cells in the development of malaria vaccine. Exp Parasitol 126(3):421–425
2. Lipford GB et al (1994) Vaccination with immunodominant peptides encapsulated in Quil A-containing liposomes induces peptide-specific primary CD8+ cytotoxic T cells. Vaccine 12(1):73–80
3. Donnelly JJ et al (1993) Targeted delivery of peptide epitopes to class I major histocompatibility molecules by a modified *Pseudomonas* exotoxin. Proc Natl Acad Sci 90(8):3530–3534
4. Gilbert SC, Plebanski M et al (1997) A protein particle vaccine containing multiple malaria epitopes. Nat Biotechnol 15(12):1280–1284
5. Sedegah M et al (1994) Protection against malaria by immunization with plasmid DNA encoding circumsporozoite protein. Proc Natl Acad Sci U S A 91(21):9866–9870
6. Moore AC et al (2004) Progress in DNA-based heterologous prime-boost immunization strategies for malaria. Immunol Rev 199:126–143
7. Draper SJ et al (2010) Viruses as vaccine vectors for infectious diseases and cancer. Nat Rev Microbiol 8(1):62–73
8. Moss B et al (1984) Live recombinant vaccinia virus protects chimpanzees against hepatitis B. Nature 311:67–69
9. Smith GL et al (1984) *Plasmodium knowlesi* sporozoite antigen: expression by infectious recombinant vaccinia virus. Science 224(4647):397–399
10. Souza L et al (2005) Recombinant viruses as vaccines against viral disease. Braz J Med Biol Res 38(04):509–522 (Review)
11. Yang ZY et al (2003) Overcoming immunity to a viral vaccine by DNA priming before vector boosting. J Virol 77(1):799–803
12. McAllister RM (1965) Viruses and cancer. Calif Med 102:344–352
13. Ewer KJ et al (2015) Progress with viral vectored malaria vaccines: a multi-stage approach involving "unnatural immunity" Malaria. Vaccine 33(52):7444–7451
14. Tartaglia J et al (1992) NYVAC: a highly attenuated strain of vaccinia virus. Virology 188(1):217–232
15. Schneider J et al (1998) Enhanced immunogenicity for CD8+ T cell induction and complete protective efficacy of malaria DNA vaccination by boosting with modified vaccinia virus Ankara. Nat Med 4(4):397–402

16. Sedegah M et al (1990) Evaluation of vaccines designed to induce protective cellular immunity against the *Plasmodium yoelii* circumsporozoite protein: vaccinia, pseudorabies, and *Salmonella* transformed with circumsporozoite gene. Bull World Health Organ 68(Suppl):109–114
17. Li S et al (1993) Priming with recombinant influenza virus followed by administration of recombinant vaccinia virus induces $CD8^+$ T-cell-mediated protective immunity against malaria. Proc Natl Acad Sci U S A 90(11):5214–5218
18. Ockenhouse CF et al (1998) Phase I/IIa safety, immunogenicity, and efficacy trial of NYVAC-Pf7, a pox-vectored, multiantigen, multistage vaccine candidate for *Plasmodium falciparum* malaria. J Infect Dis 177(6):1664–1673
19. Brown M et al (2000) Dendritic cells infected with recombinant fowlpox virus vectors are potent stimulators of transgene-specific class I restricted T lymphocyte activity. Gene Ther 7(19):1680–1689
20. Anderson RJ et al (2004) Enhanced $CD8^+$ T cell immune responses and protection elicited against *Plasmodium berghei* malaria by prime boost immunization regimens using a novel attenuated fowlpox virus. J Immunol 172(5):3094–3100
21. Prieur E et al (2004) A *Plasmodium falciparum* candidate vaccine based on a six-antigen polyprotein encoded by recombinant poxviruses. Proc Natl Acad Sci U S A 101(1):290–295
22. Webster DP et al (2006) Safety of recombinant fowlpox strain FP9 and modified vaccinia virus Ankara vaccines against liver-stage *P. falciparum* malaria in non-immune volunteers. Vaccine 24(15):3026–3034
23. Bejon P et al (2006) A phase 2b randomised trial of the candidate malaria vaccines FP9 ME-TRAP and MVA ME-TRAP among children in Kenya. PLoS Clin Trials 1(6), e29
24. Zhu J et al (2007) Innate immune response to adenoviral vectors is mediated by both Toll-like receptor-dependent and -independent pathways. J Virol 81(7):3170–3180
25. Yang Y et al (1994) Cellular immunity to viral antigens limits E1-deleted adenoviruses for gene therapy. Proc Natl Acad Sci U S A 91(10):4407–4411
26. Rodrigues EG et al (1997) Single immunizing dose of recombinant adenovirus efficiently induces $CD8^+$ T cell-mediated protective immunity against malaria. J Immunol 158(3):1268–1274
27. Rodrigues EG et al (1998) Efficient induction of protective anti-malaria immunity by recombinant adenovirus. Vaccine 16(19):1812–1817
28. Rodrigues EG et al (2000) Interferon-gamma-independent $CD8^+$ T cell-mediated protective anti-malaria immunity elicited by recombinant adenovirus. Parasite Immunol 22(3):157–160
29. Shott JP et al (2008) Adenovirus 5 and 35 vectors expressing *Plasmodium falciparum* circumsporozoite surface protein elicit potent antigen-specific cellular IFN-gamma and antibody responses in mice. Vaccine 26(23):2818–2823
30. Zaiss AK et al (2009) The influence of innate and pre-existing immunity on adenovirus therapy. J Cell Biochem 108(4):778–790
31. Seshidhar Reddy P et al (2003) Development of adenovirus serotype 35 as a gene transfer vector. Virology 311(2):384–393
32. McVey D et al (2010) Characterization of human adenovirus 35 and derivation of complex vectors. Virol J 7:276
33. Nwanegbo E et al (2004) Prevalence of neutralizing antibodies to adenoviral serotypes 5 and 35 in the adult populations of The Gambia, South Africa, and the United States. Clin Diagn Lab Immunol 11(2):351–357
34. Ophorst OJ et al (2006) Immunogenicity and protection of a recombinant human adenovirus serotype 35-based malaria vaccine against *Plasmodium yoelii* in mice. Infect Immun 74(1):313–320
35. Rodríguez A et al (2009) Evaluation of a prime-boost vaccine schedule with distinct adenovirus vectors against malaria in rhesus monkeys. Vaccine 27(44):6226–6233
36. Creech CB et al (2013) Randomized, placebo-controlled trial to assess the safety and immunogenicity of an adenovirus type 35-based circumsporozoite malaria vaccine in healthy adults. Hum Vaccin Immunother 9(12):2548–2557
37. Rodríguez A et al (2008) Impact of recombinant adenovirus serotype 35 priming versus boosting of a *Plasmodium falciparum* protein: characterization of T- and B-cell responses to liver-stage antigen. Infect Immun 76(4):1709–1718

38. Reyes-Sandoval A et al (2008) Single-dose immunogenicity and protective efficacy of simian adenoviral vectors against *Plasmodium berghei*. Eur J Immunol 38(3):732–741
39. Dudareva M et al (2009) Prevalence of serum neutralizing antibodies against chimpanzee adenovirus 63 and human adenovirus 5 in Kenyan children, in the context of vaccine vector efficacy. Vaccine 27(27):3501–3504
40. O'Hara GA et al (2012) Clinical assessment of a recombinant simian adenovirus ChAd63: a potent new vaccine vector. J Infect Dis 205(5):772–781
41. Ogwang C et al (2015) Prime-boost vaccination with chimpanzee adenovirus and modified vaccinia Ankara encoding TRAP provides partial protection against *Plasmodium falciparum* infection in Kenyan adults. Sci Transl Med 7(286):286
42. Shiratsuchi T et al (2010) Replacing adenoviral vector HVR1 with a malaria B cell epitope improves immunogenicity and circumvents preexisting immunity to adenovirus in mice. J Clin Invest 120(10):3688–3701
43. Bruder JT et al (2012) Modification of Ad5 hexon hypervariable regions circumvents pre-existing Ad5 neutralizing antibodies and induces protective immune responses. PLoS One 7(4), e33920
44. Karen KA et al (2015) A replicating adenovirus capsid display recombinant elicits antibodies against *Plasmodium falciparum* sporozoites in Aotus nancymaae monkeys. Infect Immun 83(1):268–275
45. Tsuji M et al (1998) Recombinant Sindbis viruses expressing a cytotoxic T-lymphocyte epitope of a malaria parasite or of influenza virus elicit protection against the corresponding pathogen in mice. J Virol 72(8):6907–6910
46. Monath T et al (2015) Live virus vaccines based on a yellow fever vaccine backbone: standardized template with key considerations for a risk/benefit assessment. Vaccine 33(1):62–72
47. Tao D et al (2015) Yellow fever 17D as a vaccine vector for microbial CTL epitopes: protection in a rodent malaria model. J Exp Med 201(2):201–209
48. Bonaldo MC et al (2002) Surface expression of an immunodominant malaria protein B cell epitope by yellow fever virus. J Mol Biol 315(4):873–885
49. Gilbert SC et al (2002) Enhanced CD8 T-cell immunogenicity and protective efficacy in a mouse malaria model using a recombinant adenoviral vaccine in heterologous prime-boost immunisation regimes. Vaccine 20(7-8):1039–1045
50. Harrington LE et al (2002) Recombinant vaccinia virus-induced T-cell immunity: quantitation of the response to the virus vector and the foreign epitope. J Virol 76(7):3329–3337
51. Sedegah M et al (1998) Boosting with recombinant vaccinia increases immunogenicity and protective efficacy of malaria DNA vaccine. Proc Natl Acad Sci 95(13):7648–7653
52. Dégano P et al (1999) Gene gun intradermal DNA immunization followed by boosting with modified vaccinia virus Ankara: enhanced $CD8^+$ T cell immunogenicity and protective efficacy in the influenza and malaria models. Vaccine 18(7-8):623–632
53. Prieur E et al (2004) A *Plasmodium falciparum* candidate vaccine based on a six-antigen polyprotein encoded by recombinant poxviruses. Proc Natl Acad Sci 101(1):290–295
54. Chuang I et al (2013) DNA prime/Adenovirus boost malaria vaccine encoding *P. falciparum* CSP and AMA1 induces sterile protection associated with cell-mediated immunity. PLoS One 8(2), e55571
55. Sedegah M et al (2014) Sterile immunity to malaria after DNA prime/adenovirus boost immunization is associated with effector memory $CD8^+$ T cells targeting AMA1 class I epitopes. PLoS One 9(9), e106241
56. Sedegah M et al (2015) Controlled Human Malaria Infection (CHMI) differentially affects cell-mediated and antibody responses to CSP and AMA1 induced by adenovirus vaccines with and without DNA-priming. Hum Vaccin Immunother 11(11):2705–2715
57. Ockenhouse CF et al (2015) Ad35.CS.01-RTS, S/AS01 heterologous prime boost vaccine efficacy against sporozoite challenge in healthy malaria-naïve adults. PLoS One 10(7), e0131571
58. Rogers WO et al (2001) Multistage multiantigen heterologous prime boost vaccine for *Plasmodium knowlesi* malaria provides partial protection in rhesus macaques. Infect Immun 69(9):5565–5572

59. Rogers WO et al (2002) Protection of rhesus macaques against lethal *Plasmodium knowlesi* malaria by a heterologous DNA priming and poxvirus boosting immunization regimen. Infect Immun 70(8):4329–4335
60. Schneider J et al (2001) A prime-boost immunisation regimen using DNA followed by recombinant modified vaccinia virus Ankara induces strong cellular immune responses against the *Plasmodium falciparum* TRAP antigen in chimpanzees. Vaccine 19(32):4595–4602
61. Rodrigues M et al (1994) Influenza and vaccinia viruses expressing malaria $CD8^+$ T and B cell epitopes. Comparison of their immunogenicity and capacity to induce protective immunity. J Immunol 153(10):4636–4648
62. Murata K et al (1996) Characterization of in vivo primary and secondary $CD8^+$ T cell responses induced by recombinant influenza and vaccinia viruses. Cell Immunol 173(1):96–107
63. Bruña-Romero O et al (2001) Complete, long-lasting protection against malaria of mice primed and boosted with two distinct viral vectors expressing the same plasmodial antigen. Proc Natl Acad Sci 98(20):11491–11496
64. Imoukhuede EB et al (2006) Safety and immunogenicity of the malaria candidate vaccines FP9 CS and MVA CS in adult Gambian men. Vaccine 24(42–43):6526–6533
65. Bejon P et al (2007) Extended follow-up following a phase 2b randomized trial of the candidate malaria vaccines FP9 ME-TRAP and MVA ME-TRAP among children in Kenya. PLoS One 2(8), e707
66. Webster DP et al (2005) Enhanced T cell-mediated protection against malaria in human challenges by using the recombinant poxviruses FP9 and modified vaccinia virus Ankara. Proc Natl Acad Sci 102(13):4836–4841
67. Moorthy VS et al (2004) A randomised, double-blind, controlled vaccine efficacy trial of DNA/MVA ME-TRAP against malaria infection in Gambian adults. PLoS Med 1(2), e33
68. Ogwang C et al (2013) Safety and immunogenicity of heterologous prime-boost immunisation with *Plasmodium falciparum* malaria candidate vaccines, ChAd63 ME-TRAP and MVA ME-TRAP, in healthy Gambian and Kenyan adults. PLoS One 8(3), e57726
69. Ogwang C et al (2015) Prime-boost vaccination with chimpanzee adenovirus and modified vaccinia Ankara encoding TRAP provides partial protection against *Plasmodium falciparum* infection in Kenyan adults. Sci Transl Med 7(286):286re5

Epitopic Malaria Vaccines Comprised of Minimal T- and B-Cell Epitopes of the *P. falciparum* CS Protein

Elizabeth H. Nardin

Contents

1 Introduction 171
2 CS Repeat Peptide-Protein Conjugates 173
3 Branched Synthetic Peptides 175
4 Epitopic Modules and TLR Agonist Adjuvants 176
4.1 TLR7 Agonist Adjuvant 177
4.2 TLR-5 Agonist Adjuvant 178
5 Viruslike Particle (VLP) Containing CS Epitopes 178
6 Microparticle Epitopic Vaccines 181
7 Epitopic Vaccines Based on Self-Assembling Scaffolds 183
8 Perspectives 185
References 187

1 Introduction

The feasibility of a pre-erythrocyticvaccine was clearly established by the demonstration that attenuated sporozoites can elicit sterile immunity in experimental rodents, primates, and human volunteers (see Chap. "Whole-Sporozoite Malaria Vaccines", R. Sauerwein). The circumsporozoite (CS) protein was the first target of protective immunity identified by serum and cells obtained from sporozoite-immunized hosts [1, 2] (Fig. 1a). The goal of epitopic vaccines based on *P. falciparum* CS minimal T- and B-cell epitopes is to focus the host immune responses on biologically relevant targets and circumvent potential immune evasion mechanisms developed over thousands of years of coevolution of the parasite, mosquito vector, and human host. The *P. falciparum* epitopic vaccines reviewed in this chapter are based on epitopes identified using sera and cells of sporozoite-immunized hosts. The first protective immunodominant B-cell epitope was identified in the repeat

E.H. Nardin (✉)
Division of Parasitology, Department of Microbiology, New York University School of Medicine, New York, NY 10016, USA
e-mail: elizabeth.nardin@nyumc.org

M.M. Mota, A. Rodriguez (eds.), *Malaria*, DOI 10.1007/978-3-319-45210-4_9

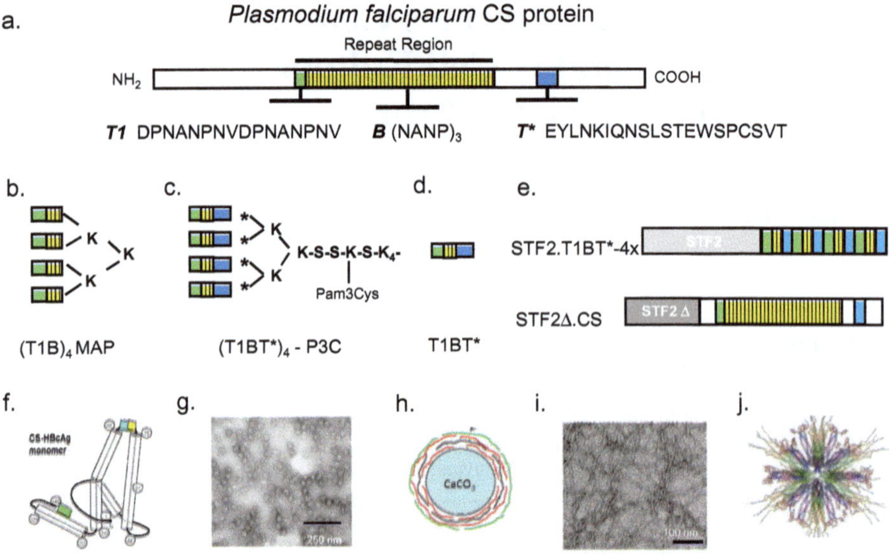

Fig. 1 Epitopic vaccines based on *P. falciparum* circumsporozoite protein. (**a**) Diagram of *P. falciparum* CS protein showing central repeat region containing B-cell epitopes in the major repeat region (NANP)*n*, T1 epitope in the alternating NANP-NVDP minor repeat region, and universal T* epitope in the C-terminus aa 326–345. Epitopic vaccines comprised of these epitopes were constructed as (**b–d**) synthetic peptides; (**e**) flagellin chimeric proteins; (**f, g**) HBcAg viruslike particles (VLP); (**h**) layer-by-layer (LbL) microparticles; and (**i, j**) self-assembling macromolecular scaffolds. Synthetic peptide vaccine candidates: (**b**) Multiple antigen peptide (MAP) tetrabranched peptide constructed by stepwise synthesis of T1 and B repeat epitopes. (**c**) Polyoxime peptide comprised of epitopic modules containing T1 and B repeats and T* universal Th epitope chemoligated (*asterisks*) to a tetrabranch core module containing TLR-2 agonist Pam3Cys; (**d**) linear 48mer synthetic peptide containing T1 and B repeats and T* universal Th epitope. Recombinant protein vaccine candidates: (**e**) flagellin (STF2) chimeric proteins containing four copies of T1BT* epitopic module or full-length CS; (**f**) monomers of hepatitis B core protein containing T1B repeats inserted in the loop region (aa 78–82) and T* Th epitope at the truncated C-terminus (aa 149); (**g**) transmission electron microscopy of VLP formed by the CS-HBcAg monomers (ICC-1132). Peptide particle vaccine candidates: (**h**) layer-by-layer (LbL) particles formed on $CaCO_3$ core by alternating layers of poly-L-lysine (*black*) and poly-L-glutamic acid (*red*) with epitopic peptide (*green*) attached to the outer layer; (**i**) Nanofibers comprised of self-assembling $(NANP)_3$-Q11 peptide; (**j**) self-assembling protein nanoparticles (SAPN) comprised of 60 protein monomers containing four NANP repeats at the C-terminus and three $CD8^+$ T-cell epitopes at the N-terminus which are surface expressed on the assembled SAPN

region of the surface CS protein, which in *P. falciparum* is comprised of NANP tetramer repeats or alternating NANP-NVDP repeats [3–5] (Fig. 1a). Anti-repeat antibodies can immobilize the sporozoite in the skin and block invasion of hepatic cells [3–6], thereby preventing the development of parasite erythrocytic stages responsible for clinical disease. The induction of high levels of sporozoite-neutralizing antibodies is T cell dependent, requiring $CD4^+$ T-cell cytokines as helper factors for B-cell differentiation [7], as well as for the development of $CD8^+$ T memory cells [8]. T-cell cytokines such as IFN-γ also function directly in protective immunity by inhibiting development of intracellular EEF [9]. To ensure immunogenicity in individuals expressing a broad range of class II haplotypes, universal $CD4^+$ Th cell epitopes in the *P. falciparum* CS protein have been identified for inclusion in epitopic vaccines [10–12].

Due to space limitations, the chapter focuses on studies that provide information on functional immunity, obtained in phase I/II clinical trials or using the rodent transgenic parasites expressing *P. falciparum* CS protein. While the *P. falciparum* sporozoite human challenge model is optimal for analysis of vaccine-induced protective immunity, the number of studies is limited due to the cost of phase II trials. A major advance in analysis of functional immunity is the development of transgenic rodent parasites that express *P. falciparum* CS protein which provide a small animal model for testing the function of antibodies elicited during phase I trials, as well as for preclinical screening of vaccine candidates. The first of these transgenic *P. berghei* parasites termed PfPb, which expresses the *P. falciparum* CS repeats plus the region I cleavage site upstream of the CS repeats, was shown to be useful for measuring protective anti-repeat antibodies in vivo and in vitro [13, 14]. As the majority of $CD4^+$ and $CD8^+$ T-cell epitopes are contained in the C-terminus, transgenic *P. berghei* expressing the *P. falciparum* C-terminus have recently been developed to analyze *P. falciparum*-specific cell-mediated immune responses [15]. Transgenic rodent parasites expressing full-length *P. falciparum* CS have also been recently optimized to consistently produce infective sporozoites for i.v. challenge studies [16, 17]. More recent studies have shown that *P. yoelii* parasites expressing full-length *P. falciparum* CS are highly infectious, and as few as five mosquito bites can elicit patent infection in mice [18]. The in vitro and in vivo assays based on transgenic rodent parasites expressing *P. falciparum* CS epitopes provide valuable reagents for down-selection of vaccine candidates for future clinical trials.

2 CS Repeat Peptide-Protein Conjugates

The phase I trial in 1987 of a CS repeat peptide-protein conjugate $(NANP)_3$-TT, comprised of three copies of the CS repeat NANP conjugated to tetanus toxoid (TT) as protein carrier, represented the first clinical trial of a synthetic peptide vaccine against an infectious disease [19]. Following three 160 μg doses of $(NANP)_3$-TT adsorbed to alum administered I.M. at monthly intervals, the majority of the volunteers (71 %) seroconverted. A small number of volunteers with the highest anti-repeat antibody titer, when challenged by bites of *P. falciparum*-infected mosquitoes, developed either sterile immunity or delayed prepatent periods based on Giemsa-stained blood smears, demonstrating that a malaria peptide vaccine could elicit protective anti repeat antibody responses.

The peptide-TT conjugate, however, was limited by low peptide density and potential toxicity of the TT carrier protein which precluded administration of higher vaccine doses. Recent studies in murine and nonhuman primate hosts have explored immunogenicity of $(NANP)_6$ repeats conjugated to the outer membrane protein complex (OMPC) of *Neisseria meningitidis* which contains human toll-like receptor

2 (TLR2) agonists [20]. OMPC is used as carrier in a licensed pediatric *Haemophilus influenzae* b (Hib) capsular polysaccharide (PS) conjugate vaccine, PedvaxHIB®, and thus has an established safety and scale-up record that is attractive for malaria vaccines aimed at pediatric populations in endemic areas which bear the major burden of malaria morbidity and mortality. The construction of a *P. falciparum* $(NANP)_6$-OMPC peptide-protein conjugate provided a particle of ~100–200 nm in diameter with a high density of repeat peptide on the surface [21]. Mice immunized with $(NANP)_6$-OMPC adsorbed to alum developed high levels of anti-repeat antibody that inhibited in vitro invasion of human hepatoma cells by PfPb transgenic *P. berghei* sporozoites that express *P. falciparum* CS repeats. The presence of serum-neutralizing antibodies detected in vitro correlated with in vivo resistance to challenge by the bites of PfPb-infected mosquitoes. Challenged mice had >90 % reduction of hepatic stage parasites as measured by real-time PCR and either sterile immunity, i.e., no detectable blood-stage parasites, or delayed prepatent periods which indicate neutralization of a majority, but not all, sporozoites.

Rhesus macaques immunized with two doses of $(NANP)_6$-OMPC/alum formulated with Iscomatrix, a particulate adjuvant comprising cholesterol, phospholipid, and saponin, developed anti-repeat antibodies that persisted for ~2 years [21]. A third dose of $(NANP)_6$-OMPC/MAA/Iscomatrix at 2 years elicited strong anamnestic antibody responses. Rhesus immune sera obtained post second and third dose of vaccine displayed high levels of sporozoite-neutralizing activity in vitro that correlated with the presence of high anti-repeat antibody titers. Of particular relevance to human vaccines was the difference in adjuvant dependency noted in the rodent versus nonhuman primates. The induction of high levels of long-lived anti-repeat antibodies in rhesus required the inclusion of the Iscomatrix co-adjuvant, while mice immunized with $(NANP)_6$-OMPC/alum developed high anti-repeat titers with or without the addition of Iscomatrix. Differences in TLR expression between species and cell subsets are critical factors in the preclinical evaluation of adjuvant formulations.

OMPC has also been shown to be an efficient carrier for a transmission-blocking vaccine candidate, a recombinant protein Pfs25H [22]. Following adsorption to alum, the protein-conjugate vaccine elicited high-titer antibody to rPfs25H in mice, rabbits, and rhesus monkeys. In vitro membrane-feeding assays demonstrated high levels of transmission-blocking activity in serum of immunized animals. Combinations of peptide-protein conjugates, CS repeat-OMPC, and Pfs25H-OMPC could provide as a multi-antigen vaccine to target both the mammalian and arthropod transmission stages of the parasite.

A multistage transmission-blocking vaccine has been constructed by conjugating CS repeats to recombinant Pfs25 protein as carrier [23]. The CS repeat/Pfs25 bicomponent vaccine, comprised of five NANP copies conjugated to the cross-linked Pfs25-AH-Pfs25 protein adsorbed to alum, elicited long-lasting antibodies to both CS repeats and Pfs25 protein in mice. Antibodies continued to rise over a period of 7 months suggesting a strong depot effect of the alum-adjuvanted vaccine and/or the cross-linked carrier protein. Critical factors regulating immunogenicity were peptide density and the use of a cross-linked but not monomeric Pfs25 protein as carrier molecule. Functional transmission-blocking antibodies that inhibited oocyst development in mosquitoes were demonstrated in an in vitro membrane-feeding assay, although the anti-repeat antibodies were not assessed in functional assays.

3 Branched Synthetic Peptides

In contrast to peptide-protein carrier vaccines, Tam and colleagues demonstrated that macromolecular branched synthetic peptides, termed multiple antigen peptide (MAP), were immunogenic without protein carriers [24]. Malaria T- and B-cell epitopes were synthesized on a branched polylysine core matrix in a stepwise fashion, and unlike peptide-carrier protein conjugates, the stoichiometry of T- and B-cell epitopes in branched peptides could be precisely controlled to optimize immunogenicity. Preclinical studies in the rodent model demonstrated that MAPs containing *P. berghei* CS repeats and a CS Th cell epitope could elicit high levels of sterile immunity following sporozoite challenge.

A *P. falciparum* MAP termed $(T1B)_4$ was designed to contain the $(NANP)_3$ B-cell epitope synthesized in tandem with a highly conserved human $CD4^+$ Th cell epitope located in the *P. falciparum* CS minor repeat, termed T1, represented by alternating NANP and NVDP repeats [25–27] (Fig. 1b). The $(T1B)_4$ MAP elicited a strong anamnestic response in *P. falciparum* sporozoite-primed mice and monkeys, indicating the potential to boost the low anti-sporozoite antibody titers found in endemic areas.

A phase I prospective study was carried out in volunteers of HLA class II genotypes predicted to be responders to CS repeats based on genetic restriction of $CD4^+$ T-cell clones from sporozoite-immunized volunteers and in vitro peptide/HLA-binding assays [28]. The murine response to the CS repeat peptide was known to be genetically restricted to a limited number of murine haplotypes [25, 29]. Volunteers of predicted responder or of random HLA class II genotypes were immunized s.c. with 500–1000 μg MAP adsorbed to alum, with or without a purified saponin derivative, QS21, as co-adjuvant. Following three doses of vaccine, a clear responder/nonresponder phenotype was observed. All of the volunteers with high antibody titers expressed predicted responder class II genotypes (DQB1*0603, DRB1*0401 or *1101). Peak GMT were an order of magnitude higher that those observed in individuals of random HLA genotypes. Anti-repeat antibodies were IgG1 and IgG3, consistent with detectable of Th1-type IFN-γ-producing $CD4^+$ T cells in individuals of responder genotypes. Noteworthy was the fact that even in the high-responder genotypes, vaccine immunogenicity was adjuvant dependent with minimal seroconversion following three doses of $(T1B)_4$ MAP/alum without the co-adjuvant QS21. The inclusion of the more potent QS21 adjuvant, however, increased reactogenicity as well as immunogenicity [30]. A second cohort of seven volunteers of responder genotypes confirmed the correlation of class II genotypes and high-responder phenotypes and demonstrated that only two doses of $(T1B)_4$ MAP vaccine was highly immunogenic with minimal reactogenicity.

The high-responder class II genotypes, however, were found in only 25–35 % of the population, and efforts were made to identify T-helper cell epitopes capable of binding to a broad range of class II molecules. Universal Th cell epitopes have been identified in bacterial and viral antigens and artificial constructs such as PADRE, a pan-DR-binding epitope [31–34]. In contrast to foreign antigens, CS-derived universal Th cell epitopes provide the advantage of priming malaria-specific T cells, and two such universal epitopes were identified using human T cells and algorithms predicting peptide/class II binding, CS.T3 [10] and T* (aka UHC) [11, 12]. Empirical studies in mice identified the *P. falciparum* CS protein T* epitope as the most promising Th cell epitope for combination with CS repeats.

The technical challenge of synthesizing a tetrabranched peptide containing a 48mer T1BT* peptide in each branch was overcome by constructing polyoximes in which chemoselective ligation was used to conjugate an aldehyde-modified 48mer T1BT* epitopic module to a reciprocal aminooxyactyl-modified tetrabranched core lipopeptide containing the TLR2 agonist lipopeptide palmitoyl-*S*-glyceryl cysteine (P3C) as endogenous adjuvant [35, 36] (Fig. 1c). The $(T1BT^*)_4$-P3C polyoxime was highly immunogenic, without addition of exogenous adjuvant, in three inbred strains of mice tested. Antibody titers persisted for over 3 months after the last immunizing dose.

A small phase I trial was carried out in ten volunteers of diverse HLA types immunized s.c. with 1 mg of $(T1BT^*)_4$-P3C polyoxime at 0, 1, and 3 months [37]. The majority of the volunteers (8/10) seroconverted following the first dose and reached peak titers of 10^3–10^4 following three immunizations. Antibodies were predominately Th1-type IgG1 and IgG3 subtypes and the majority of immunized volunteers had T*-specific Th1-type $CD4^+$ T-cell responses. $CD4^+$ T-cell clones derived from PBMC up to 10 months after peptide immunization recognized the T* epitope in the context of multiple HLA DR and DQ molecules and secreted high levels of IFN-γ and variable levels of TNF-α [38]. Although the T* epitope overlaps a polymorphic region of the *P. falciparum* CS protein, both cross-reactive and strain-specific T cells could be isolated from individuals at the same time point, suggesting a limited role these polymorphisms in parasite immune evasion [11, 38]. Of potential functional significance, a subset of the human T*-specific $CD4^+$ T-cell clones were cytotoxic and directly lysed CS peptide-pulsed target cells, as previously observed with a subset of clones derived from *P. falciparum* sporozoite-immunized volunteers [39]. Both peptide- and sporozoite-induced human $CD4^+$ CTLs formed typical immunological synapses and induced apoptosis of peptide-pulsed target cells, consistent with reports for $CD8^+$ T cells [40, 41].

4 Epitopic Modules and TLR Agonist Adjuvants

The clinical trials of branched synthetic peptides demonstrated safety and immunogenicity in human volunteers, although the ability to synthesize large quantities of branched peptide was a technical limitation. Surprisingly, a linear T1BT* peptide adjuvanted with potent oil-in-water adjuvants, Montanide ISA 51 and ISA 720, was found to elicit high titers of Th2-type IgG1 anti-repeat antibody in BALB/c and C57Bl mice, with GMT 81,920–327,680, respectively [42] (Fig. 1d). The presence of the universal T* epitope was critical for immunogenicity of the linear peptide, as a linear peptide containing only (T1B) repeats was not immunogenic. The T1BT* linear peptide in Montanide ISA 51 was also immunogenic in outbred *Aotus* monkeys and elicited high anti-repeat ELISA and IFA titers (GMT 10^4). Mice immunized with linear T1BT* peptide in Montanide ISA 720 when challenged by bites of PfPb-infected mosquitoes had >90 % reduction in parasite burden in the liver as measured by real-time PCR. Protection against sporozoite challenge was antibody mediated, as depletion of $CD4^+$ or $CD8^+$ T cells prior to PfPb sporozoite challenge did not abrogate immune resistance. The predominance of Th2-type IgG1, a non-opsonizing antibody subtype, in the vaccinated mice suggests that direct inhibition of sporozoites, rather than enhanced clearance and phagocytosis, was functioning in immune resistance.

4.1 TLR7 Agonist Adjuvant

While oil-in-water emulsions are potent adjuvants, their use in phase I trials of transmission-blocking and blood-stage vaccines has been associated with unacceptable reactogenicity [43, 44]. More precisely targeted TLR agonists can function as potent adjuvants for synthetic peptide vaccines which lack pathogen-associated molecular patterns (PAMPs) required to stimulate dendritic cells and initiate strong adaptive immune responses [45, 46].

The TLR-7 agonist imiquimod, an imidazoquinoline contained in an FDA-approved topical treatment for various dermatologic conditions, has been shown to be a potent adjuvant to elicit T cells against intracellular pathogens, tumors and model antigens [47–49]. For malaria peptide vaccines, topical imiquimod applied to the site of s.c. injected $(T1BT^*)_4$ branched peptide or T1BT* linear peptide (Fig. 1c, d) provided a potent adjuvant for induction of anti-repeat antibodies [50]. Peak titers obtained following s.c. injection of peptide followed by topical imiquimod reached 10^4–10^5 GMT, comparable to the magnitude of response elicited by s.c. injected peptide formulated in oil emulsions Montanide ISA 720, ISA 51, or Freunds adjuvant. In contrast to predominantly IgG1 antibodies elicited with oil adjuvants, a balanced IgG2/IgG1 antibody response was elicited using the topical imiquimod adjuvant. Consistent with increased IgG2 antibody response in these mice, the numbers of malaria-specific IFN-γ-secreting $CD4^+$ T cells measured in ELISPOT were a log higher than those obtained following injection of peptide in Montanide oil adjuvant formulations [42]. More importantly, the sporozoite-neutralizing activity in serum of mice immunized with CS peptide followed by topical imiquimod correlated with in vivo protection when the mice were challenged by exposure to the bites of PfPb-infected mosquitoes [50]. While the skin of mice and humans differs in cell composition and structure [51], recent phase I/II trials of i.d.

injected seasonal flu vaccine followed by topical imiquimod have demonstrated increased seroconversion, prolonged antibody persistence, and reduced flu-associated pathology in elderly individuals as well as young children [52, 53]. These studies support the potential of murine studies for the identification of novel TLR agonist adjuvant formulations for human vaccines.

4.2 TLR-5 Agonist Adjuvant

The TLR-5 agonist flagellin has been shown to be a potent adjuvant for bacterial and viral antigens [54, 55], and recombinant flagellin-influenza chimeric vaccines are currently in clinical trials [56, 57]. For analysis of epitopic malaria vaccines using flagellin as adjuvant, a chimeric recombinant protein containing multiples of the T1BT* module or nearly full-length *P. falciparum* CS protein was expressed in tandem with the TLR5 agonist flagellin from *Salmonella typhimurium* [58] (Fig. 1e). Mice were immunized s.c. and immunogenicity was compared with intranasal (i.n.) immunization as a potential route for needle-free delivery of malaria vaccine. Mice immunized s.c. with the flagellin-modified CS constructs containing four copies of the T1BT* epitopic module or full-length CS protein developed similar levels of anti-repeat IgG1 antibody and IL-5-secreting Th2 cells. Importantly, immunization via the intranasal route, but not the subcutaneous route, elicited sporozoite-neutralizing antibodies capable of inhibiting >90 % of PfPb sporozoite invasion in vitro and in vivo. Confocal microscopy of the nasopharynx-associated lymphoid tissue (NALT) in immunized mice demonstrated a predominance of germinal center (GC) B cells and increased numbers of CD11c + DCs localized beneath the epithelium and within the GC T-cell area [59]. Microfold cells, with similar morphology to those reported in gut-associated lymphoid tissue (GALT), were distributed throughout the NALT epithelial cell layer. DC dendrites were found extending from the epithelium into the nasal cavity, suggesting a potential function in capturing luminal CS antigen. In vitro analysis demonstrated that flagellin-modified CS taken up by DCs was initially localized within intracellular vesicles, with increasing cytosolic distribution over time. These findings demonstrate that functional sporozoite-neutralizing antibody can be elicited by i.n. immunization with a flagellin-modified *P. falciparum* CS protein and raise the potential of a scalable, safe, needle-free vaccine that would reduce cost of immunization in resource poor areas of the world.

5 Viruslike Particle (VLP) Containing CS Epitopes

An historic milestone was reached in 2015 when the first malaria vaccine was licensed by the European Medicines Agency (EMA). The CS-based vaccine, RTS,S, is comprised of a hepatitis B virus surface antigen (HBsAg) VLP containing the repeats and C-terminus of *P. falciparum* CS (see Chap. "Immune Responses to the RTS,S/AS01 Malaria Vaccine Candidate: Lessons from Human Immunology and Parasitologic and Clinical Evaluations", J. Vekemans). In initial phase I/IIa studies conducted at WRAIR, sterile immunity was elicited in a significant percentage of malaria-naïve individuals immunized with RTS,S in an optimal adjuvant formulation [60]. However, the EMA-licensed pediatric RTS,S vaccine protects 30–50 % of infants and children against clinical disease, and efforts to improve RTS,S vaccine efficacy are ongoing. The mechanism of immunity in children has been shown to be mediated by anti-repeat antibodies and $CD4^+$ T cells [61, 62]. $CD8^+$ T cells were not elicited by RTS,S immunization, despite the presence of multiple $CD8^+$ T-cell epitopes in the C-terminus of the *P. falciparum* CS contained in the RTS,S VLP.

Additional VLPs based on hepatitis B virus core antigen (HBcAg) have also been studied as a delivery vehicle for viral and bacterial antigens [63, 64]. When expressed in *E. coli*, the 183-aa HBcAg assembles to form 27–30 nm particles that comprise the virion nucleocapsid [65]. In contrast to HBsAg based RTS,S vaccine, which requires a mix of native HBsAg and chimeric CS/HBsAg to form stable VLP, the HBcAg allows foreign epitope insertions without loss of capsid-forming ability, thereby providing a higher density of peptide epitopes in the assembled VLP. In early studies, HBcAg VLP containing $(NANP)_4$ or the *P. berghei* $(DP4NPN)_2$ CS repeats inserted in the HBcAg immunodominant loop (aa 75–81) were shown to be highly immunogenic in mice when formulated with alum or Freunds adjuvant [66]. High levels of sterile immunity were obtained when BALB/c mice immunized with *P. berghei* CS repeats HBcAg VLP were challenged by i.v. injection of *P. berghei* sporozoites.

More recent studies examined HBc VLP containing *P. falciparum* T1 and B repeat epitopes in combination with the universal T* epitope inserted at the C-terminus of the HBc monomer [67] (Fig. 1f, g). The optimal immunogen, termed ICC-1132, was highly immunogenic in mice and in *Macaca fascicularis* (cynomolgus) monkeys. Two doses of ICC-1132 in Montanide 720 or Freunds adjuvant in mice and monkeys elicited high anti-repeat antibody in ELISA (GMT 10^6) that correlated with high IFA titers with *P. falciparum* sporozoites (10^5 titer). Murine antibodies were predominantly Th2-associated IgG1 subtype and responses were T cell dependent, as mice lacking class II molecules did not make anti-repeat antibodies. The ICC-1132 VLP also elicited potent anamnestic antibody responses in mice primed with *P. falciparum* sporozoites, suggesting potential efficacy in enhancing the sporozoite-primed immune responses of individuals living in areas where malaria is endemic.

A series of phase I trials of ICC-1132 VLP were carried out to examine safety and immunogenicity and to identify an optimal adjuvant formulation. In the first phase I trial, 20 healthy adult volunteers received 20 μg or 50 μg of alum-adsorbed ICC-1132 administered intramuscularly at 0, 2, and 6 months [68]. The majority of volunteers receiving the 50 μg dose developed modest antibodies to CS repeats, as well as to HBcAg, and malaria-specific T cells that secreted IFN-γ. A second phase I trial confirmed that alum was a suboptimal adjuvant for the HBc VLP [69]. A total of 51 malaria-naïve adults were immunized i.m. on days 0, 56, and 168. After two injections, all volunteers receiving the 50μg dose of ICC-1132 developed antibody to HBc carrier; however, only 75 % and 63 % of volunteers developed anti-repeat or anti-sporozoite antibody, respectively. Functional neutralizing antibody was low, with serum of vaccinees giving a mean 54 % reduction in PfPb sporozoite invasion of hepatoma cells in vitro.

A subsequent small single-blind, phase I trial examined a single i.m. injection of 20 or 50μg ICC-1132 formulated in the more potent water-in-oil adjuvant Montanide ISA 720 [70]. The ICC-1132 ISA 720 adjuvant formulation was more immunogenic, with the majority of volunteers developing Th1-type IgG1 and IgG3 anti-repeat antibodies after a single immunization; the magnitude of the response was comparable to antibody titers obtained following two to three immunizations with alum-adsorbed ICC-1132. PBMC stimulated with recombinant *P. falciparum* CS protein proliferated and secreted IL-2 and IFN-γ cytokines. Th1-type CS-specific $CD4^+$ T-cell lines could be established from volunteers with high levels of anti-repeat antibodies. A small phase II trial in 11 volunteers administered a single 50μg dose of ICC-1132 in ISA 720, elicited low anti-repeat antibodies in majority of volunteers (10/11), and no protection following challenge by bites of *P. falciparum*-infected mosquitoes [71].

A VLP based on woodchuck hepatitis core antigen (WHcAg) is also under development as a delivery vehicle for *P. falciparum* CS T- and B-cell epitopes [15, 72]. In murine studies, optimal immunogenicity was obtained with a WHc VLP, termed Mal-78-3T, containing the *P. falciparum* CS repeats inserted in the loop region and multiple universal T-cell epitopes, including T* (termed UTC) [12], CS.T3 [10], and TH.3R [73], attached at the C-terminus of WHc. Mice immunized intraperitoneally (i.p.) with 100μg Mal-78-3T VLP formulated in alum/QS21 or ISA 720 adjuvant, developed high levels of anti-repeat antibodies. Sterile immunity was obtained in Mal-78-3T immunized mice of three different strains following challenge by Pf/Pb sporozoites expressing *P. falciparum* CS repeats. VLP containing only the three universal $CD4^+$ T-cell epitopes, T*/UTC, CS.T3, and TH.3R, although eliciting IL-2 and IFN-γ-secreting $CD4^+$ T cells, did not protect immunized mice against challenge with a transgenic rodent parasite expressing the C-terminus of *P. falciparum* CS protein. WHc VLP containing *P. falciparum* B-cell epitopes located outside the CS repeat region, either in the C-terminus or in an N-terminus sequence that overlaps the CS cleavage site [74–76], although eliciting high antibody titers, failed to protect mice against challenge with transgenic sporozoites expressing the corresponding regions of the *P. falciparum* CS protein.

The high levels of immunogenicity of the WHc VLP were TLR-7 dependent [77, 78]. The full-length WHc protein (aa 1–184) used in construction of the VLP includes the Arg-rich C-terminus that nonspecifically binds ssRNA from *E. coli* or yeast expression systems [77, 76]. In contrast, the ICC-1132 VLP was based on a truncated HBc protein (aa 1–149) that removed the protamine-rich C-terminus to eliminate nonspecific binding of contaminating nucleic acid [67]. The binding of ssRNA was critical for immunogenicity of WHc VLP [77], however, the presence of uncharacterized bacterial and eukaryotic ssRNA raises potential regulatory issues for clinical trials.

6 Microparticle Epitopic Vaccines

Liposomes are spherical vesicles having at least one lipid bilayer which have multiple applications for delivery of drugs, compounds, and antigens [79]. In one of the earliest efforts to enhance immunogenicity of CS repeats, phase I/II trials assessed immunogenicity of alum-adsorbed liposomes containing a TLR-4 agonist monophosphoryl lipid A (MPLA) encapsulating a recombinant protein R32NS81 containing 32 copies of the NANP repeats [80]. Three doses of the liposome vaccine elicited relatively modest levels of IgG1 (4–33 μg/ml). Moderate local reactogenicity was noted with high doses of the liposomal formulation which contained up to 2200μg MPLA/dose. Sera from volunteers receiving the two highest doses of liposome vaccine inhibited *P. falciparum* sporozoite invasion of cultured hepatoma cells by an average of 92 %. More recent application of liposome-based adjuvant has been in the phase III trials of RTS,S adjuvanted with AS01 comprised of liposome, MPLA, and QS2, which has led to licensing of a pediatric malaria vaccine (see Chap. "Immune Responses to the RTS,S/AS01 Malaria Vaccine Candidate: Lessons from Human Immunology and Parasitologic and Clinical Evaluations", J. Vekemans).

A variation of liposomes has been provided by virosomes, 150nm semisynthetic unilamellar liposomal vesicles reconstituted from influenza virus membranes containing virus-derived influenza A hemagglutinin (HA) and neuraminidase (NA) glycoproteins with added cholesterol and other lipids [81]. Virosome-based vaccines for influenza and hepatitis A were licensed for human use in the 1990s. Enhanced carrier and adjuvant activity is provided by the presence of the influenza HA glycoprotein on the surface of the virosomes which facilitates receptor-mediated uptake and endosomal processing [82, 83].

For construction of a malaria virosome, a structurally constrained peptide containing five CS repeats $(NPNA)_5$ was conjugated to phosphatidylethanolamine and integrated into virosomes [84]. Following i.m. injection of the CS virosome into influenza-primed BALB/c mice, antibodies reactive with repeat peptide and *P. falciparum* sporozoites were obtained. MAB (200 μg/ml) derived from the CS virosome-immunized mice inhibited 80–100 % invasion of *P. falciparum* sporozoites into primary human hepatocytes in vitro. Purified IgG (1 mg/ml) from CS virosome-immunized rabbits inhibited 40–70 % of sporozoite invasion in vitro. Immunogenicity depended on the presence of flu-specific T- and B-cells in the primed mice, indicating that T help was provided primarily by the viral proteins contained in the virosome.

In a phase I trial, three i.m. injections of the CS virosome, comprised of 10μg CS repeat peptide incorporated into vesicles containing phospholipids and influenza A virus HA and NA glycoproteins, were administered at 0, 2, and 6 months [85, 86]. The CS virosome elicited anti-sporozoite antibodies in all volunteers, with peak antibody titers of 10^3. Total IgG (1 mg/ml) from serum of the immunized volunteers gave modest inhibition (range 18–74 %) of *P. falciparum* sporozoite invasion into primary human hepatocytes cultures.

The CS virosome was also tested in phase I/II studies in combination with a virosome containing a 49-aa peptide from the semi-conserved region of domain III of the AMA1 blood-stage antigen [87, 88]. Preclinical studies demonstrated that immunization with a combination of CS and AMA1 virosomes did not alter the magnitude of antibody responses to either of the malaria antigens, indicating that there was no epitopic competition. Volunteers immunized with CS (10 μg)/AMA1 (50 μg) virosomes, delivered at 0, 1, and 2 months, all seroconverted to anti-repeat antibody following the second immunization. All of the volunteers also developed anti-AMA1 peptide antibodies, with positive IFA to blood-stage parasites in 6/24 vaccines. However, immune serum from the vaccines did not inhibit the growth of *P. falciparum*-infected RBC in vitro. Following challenge by exposure to *P. falciparum*-infected mosquitoes, the prepatent period in the virosome-immunized volunteers was not significantly different from naïve controls, indicating limited efficacy of vaccine-induced anti-repeat antibodies in blocking sporozoite infectivity. However, significantly lower blood-stage parasite growth was observed in immunized volunteers when compared to controls suggesting functional anti-blood-stage immunity was elicited by virosome vaccination.

Similar results were obtained in a phase 1b trial in Tanzanian adults and children aged 5–9 years immunized i.m. with CS/AMA1 virosomes at 0 and 90 days [89]. The vaccine formulation utilized a lyophilized preparation of virosomes which could potentially provide a significant practical advantage in endemic areas where maintenance of cold chains is problematic. In children, the target population for a malaria vaccine, there was 87 % seroconversion to repeat peptide after two doses with peak geometric mean titers (GMT) 3275, an approximately 60-fold increase from day 0 baseline. Similarly, there was a 97 % response to AMA1 peptide with a 30-fold increase in anti-AMA1 GMT (peak 5572). In exploratory analysis, the number of clinical episodes in CS/AMA1 virosome-immunized children was half that of controls receiving the influenza virosome (Inflexal), a 50 % vaccine efficacy comparable to that obtained with RTS,S/AS01 in phase III trials [90].

Liposomes have also been used as models for artificial cells. Microparticles formed by layer-by-layer (LbL) assembly of biofilms, which were originally used to construct artificial cells for oxygen therapeutics, have recently been applied to vaccine development [91, 92]. LbL microparticles were constructed by sequential layering of positively charged poly-L-lysine and negatively charged poly-L-glutamic acid on a $CaCO_3$ core particle with antigenic peptides, modified by a polylysine tail ($K_{20}Y$), attached to the final outer layer (Fig. 1h). In murine studies, LBL particles containing an OVA peptide elicited $CD8^+$ CTL that protected against challenge with OVA-expressing *Listeria monocytogenes* [92]. For malaria vaccines, LbL microparticles containing the *P. falciparum* CS repeats alone or in combination with the CS-derived universal T* epitope were injected via the footpad (f.p.) into C57Bl mice on days 0, 21, and 42 [93]. LbL particles containing the T1BT* peptide were found to be optimal immunogens and elicited sporozoite-neutralizing antibodies that blocked in vitro invasion of transgenic PfPb sporozoites into human hepatoma cells. Following challenge by exposure to the bites of PfPb-infected mosquitoes, the parasite burden in the livers of T1BT* LbL-immunized mice was reduced to 94 %

as measured by qPCR of liver cell extracts obtained 2 days post-challenge. Protection was comparable to levels obtained following immunization with T1BT* peptide in Freunds adjuvant. The mechanism of immune resistance in vivo was antibody mediated, as depletion of T cells prior to challenge did not abrogate immune protection. In constructs containing only CS repeats, the addition of the TLR2 agonist Pam3Cys lipopeptide to the outer LbL layer enhanced antibody levels and protection after challenge, when compared to LbL containing CS repeats alone. Despite the ability of LbL microparticles containing OVA model antigens to elicit functional OVA-specific $CD8^+$ T-cell responses [92], LbL particles containing the *P. berghei* CTL epitope, although eliciting high levels of peptide-specific cytotoxic $CD8^+$ T cells, did not protect mice against sporozoite challenge.

7 Epitopic Vaccines Based on Self-Assembling Scaffolds

Self-assembling β-sheet peptides developed for tissue engineering and drug delivery have recently been used as scaffolds for vaccines [94]. The solid-phase synthesis of a beta-sheet-rich peptide QQKFQFQFEQQ, termed Q11, containing epitopes of model or viral antigens at the N-terminus was shown to self-assemble into long, unbranched 15nm-wide fibrils [95] (Fig. 1i). Immunization of mice with Q11 containing a peptide from ovalbumin, OVA $_{323–329}$-Q11, in PBS elicited antibody titers comparable to OVA peptide in Freunds adjuvant. Immunogenicity of the nanofibrils was dependent on tandem synthesis of the OVA peptide and Q11, as a mixture of peptide and Q11 did not elicit detectable anti-OVA antibody. The Q11 peptide itself was not immunogenic when administered with Freunds adjuvant. Additional murine studies with flu peptide-Q11 found that the nanofibrils did not elicit detectable inflammatory cytokines [96]. DC and macrophages at the injection site internalized the Q11 nanofibrils, but expression of CD80 and CD86 was increased only on DC. The flu-Q11 nanofibrils stimulated Tfh and B cells in GC and elicited high-affinity IgG with peak titers comparable to Freunds that were functional in an influenza HA inhibition assay in vitro.

A particular advantage of the fully synthetic nanofibrils was thermal stability [97]. A tuberculosis $ESAT_{651–670}$-Q11 was strongly immunogenic when stored as a dry powder or as aqueous nanofibers, for as long as six months at 45° C. Thermal stability would be a particular advantage for vaccines destined for use in tropical environments where malaria is endemic.

A malaria nanofibril $(NANP)_3$-Q11, comprised of three NANP repeats synthesized at the N-terminus of the Q11 β-sheet peptide, has been tested for immunogenicity in the rodent model [98]. $(NANP)_3$-Q11 self-assembled into nanofibers comparable in appearance to other peptide-Q11 constructs in TEM (Fig. 1l). C57BL/6 (H-2^b) mice immunized s.c. with two doses of $(NANP)_3$-Q11 nanofibrils developed modest anti-repeat antibody that lasted up to 40 weeks post-immunization. Importantly, the $(NANP)_3$-Q11 nanofibrils boosted anti-repeat antibody responses in mice primed either by bites of PfPb-infected mosquitoes or by s.c. injection of

$(T1BT^*)_4$-P3C polyoxime peptide. The serum of polyoxime peptide-primed mice boosted with $(NANP)_3$-Q11 nanofibrils inhibited 97 % of PfPb sporozoite invasion of human hepatoma cells in vitro. Mice immunized with a mixture of $(NANP)_3$-Q11 and OVA-Q11 had similar magnitude of anti-repeat and anti-OVA antibody titers as mice immunized with individual nanofibrils, suggesting that mixtures of nanofibrils could be used as multi-antigen vaccines.

The mechanism of adjuvant activity of the $(NANP)_3$-Q11 nanofibrils was investigated using different murine strains and knockout mice. Balb/c ($H-2^d$) mice, which do not recognize the Th epitope within CS repeats (22, 26), did not respond to immunization with $(NANP)_3$-Q11 indicating that the anti-repeat antibody response was T cell dependent. Studies in KO mice demonstrated that immunogenicity was dependent on MyD88, but not NALP3 inflammasomes. While the repetitive morphology of nanofibrils was suggestive of the TLR-5 agonist flagellin and the TLR-2 agonist curli amyloid fibrils of *E. coli* [99], there was no loss of immunogenicity in TLR-5 KO or TLR-2 KO mice. Additional studies demonstrated normal immune responses to peptide-Q11 nanofibers in mice lacking TLR-4 and TLR-9 [94]. In addition to defining the mechanism of adjuvant activity, the uncharacterized heterogeneity in the lengths of the nanofibrils and relation of this heterogeneity to immunogenicity remain to be addressed.

In addition to self-assembling peptides, vaccines based on self-assembling proteins that form nanoparticles (SAPN) have also been examined in murine studies. The SAPN are comprised of 60 monomers of a recombinant linear protein containing trimeric and pentameric coiled-coil domains separated by a flexible linker with T- and B-cell epitopes expressed at N- or C-terminus. Following expression in *E. coli*, monomers self-assemble through the interaction of the trimeric and pentameric oligomerization domains creating α-helical rodlike coiled-coils to form spherical SAPN of ~40 nm in diameter (Fig. 1j). In initial studies, monomers containing tandem repeats of the *P. berghei* CS repeat epitope $(DPPPPNPN)_2$ formed an SAPN that elicited $CD4^+$ T cell-dependent, anti-repeat antibodies in $H-2^b$, $H-2^d$, and $H-2^k$ mice without the addition of adjuvant [100]. SAPN-immunized mice were protected against challenge with *P. berghei* sporozoites up to 6 months after the last immunization.

In order to develop a *P. falciparum* SAPN, the self-assembling linear protein was modified to replace sequences corresponding to the human cartilage oligomeric matric protein (COMP) to avoid cross-reactivity with the human protein [101, 102]. A de novo designed Trp-zipper that forms a pentameric coiled-coil domain was substituted for the COMP sequence; however, the resultant SAPN lost immunogenicity due to removal of a critical $CD4^+$ Th epitope contained in the COMP sequence. Immunogenicity was recovered by the insertion of PADRE, an engineered pan-DR-binding T-cell epitope [34], in the coiled-coil trimer domain. In addition to PADRE, the monomer contained four copies of the NANP repeats at the C-terminus (PfCSP-SAPN) with or without the addition of three previously identified *P. falciparum* CS $CD8^+$ T-cell epitopes (KPKDELDY, MPNDPNRNV, YLNKIQNSL) at the N-terminus (PfCSP-KMY-SAPN). The *P. falciparum* SAPN displayed the NANP repeats and the $CD8^+$ T-cell epitopes on the surface of the particle, with the $CD4^+$ T-cell epitope PADRE at the core of the particle.

Mice were immunized either intramuscularly (i.m.) or intraperitoneally (i.p.) with SAPN in saline on days 0, 14, and 28. All strains of mice immunized with two or three doses of SAPN developed high anti-repeat antibody ELISA titers that persisted over 52 weeks. Mice immunized with PfCSP-KMY-SAPN also developed $CD8^+$ T central memory cells secreting IL-2 and IFN-γ. SAPN-immunized mice challenged by i.v. injection of transgenic rodent parasites expressing full-length *P. falciparum* CS protein showed 90–100 % protection, with 50 % of SAPN-immunized mice still protected against sporozoite challenge at week 52. Protective immunity was mediated by both sporozoite-neutralizing anti-repeat antibodies and $CD8^+$ T cells, as shown by passive transfer of $CD8^+$ T cells and reduced protection in MHC class I KO mice immunized with PfCSP-KMY-SAPN.

8 Perspectives

Epitopic immunogens have the potential to increase vaccine efficacy by focusing the host immune response on known functional T- and B-cell epitopes, thereby eliminating immune response to nonfunctional or immunoregulatory epitopes potentially present in full-length recombinant proteins or attenuated parasites. Iterative studies in recent years have emphasized the need for functional assays for evaluation of malaria vaccine candidates. The development of transgenic rodent parasites expressing the full-length or defined regions of the *P. falciparum* CS protein is a major advance for the analysis of functional immunity in a small rodent model. However, multiple strains of transgenic parasites of varying infectivity, as well as various in vitro and in vivo assays using these parasites, have been developed in different laboratories making direct comparison of results difficult. The establishment of standardized functional assays, similar to the GIA run by NIH for evaluation of antibody to *P. falciparum* blood stages, is needed to rationally evaluate and down-select vaccine candidates for pre-erythrocytic vaccine development.

The basic components of epitopic vaccines designed to elicit high levels of sporozoite-neutralizing antibody include multiple copies of the CS major NANP repeat sequence with or without the minor repeat region T1 epitope. A high density of B-cell epitopes can increase immunogenicity as shown by studies with synthetic MAPs and peptide-protein conjugates. The use of licensed vaccine components as delivery vehicles, such as the *Neisseria meningitides* OMPC carrier and virosomes used in influenza and hepatitis A-licensed vaccines, provides the added advantage of extensive information on scale-up, regulatory and safety issues obtained with these carrier moieties. The addition of a strong malaria-specific universal T-cell epitope provides additional enhancement of immunogenicity as shown by studies with linear T1BT* peptide and polyoxime branched peptides, as well as HBcAg VLP

In addition to the design of the epitopic immunogen and the choice of delivery vehicle, adjuvant formulation remains a critical factor, as synthetic epitopic vaccines containing minimal T- and B-cell epitopes lack the pathogen-associated molecular patterns (PAMPS) required to stimulate innate immune cells to initiate strong, long-lived adaptive immunity. Alum adjuvant, used in the majority of licensed vaccines, has been shown to be a poor adjuvant for malaria epitopic vaccines in phase I trials. While the use of more potent oil adjuvants such as Montanide ISA series, or the saponin derivative QS21, enhanced immunogenicity of malaria epitopic vaccines, they were also associated with increased reactogenicity [103].

Adjuvant formulations based on TLR agonists remain attractive alternatives to complex adjuvant formulations, as they provide precisely defined moieties that specifically target TLR of innate immune cells. The fact that the topical TLR-7 agonist imiquimod provided a strong adjuvant for CS peptide vaccine in mice and for seasonal flu vaccine in humans is encouraging and supports the use of rodent models to identifying TLR adjuvant formulations for human vaccines. High levels of immune responses elicited by WHc VLP were also shown to be TLR-7 dependent, with bacterial ssRNA bound to the C-terminus of the WHc protein serving as an endogenous adjuvant.

Epitopic vaccines modified to contain the TLR-5 agonist flagellin have shown that intranasal immunization can elicit immune responses comparable in magnitude to parenteral (s.c.) routes as well as eliciting higher levels of sporozoite-neutralizing activity [58, 59]. The needle-free IN route is attractive for vaccines designed for resource-limited areas where malaria is endemic and may be advantageous for reducing potential toxicity of potent TLR agonist adjuvants [104]. An interesting advance has been the development of epitopic vaccines that are immunogenic in the absence of exogenous adjuvants, as observed with nanofibrils, SAPN, and LbL particles. While immunogenicity of nanofibrils and SAPN was MyD88 dependent, the identification of specific TLR or other innate immune receptors that recognize these unique self-assembled molecular structures remains to be identified.

The choice of animal model is an additional critical factor for assessing immunogenicity of adjuvant formulations for epitopic vaccines, as differences in adjuvant dependency have been noted in murine versus nonhuman primate studies. The route of immunization is also a variable, as routes of immunization not applicable to human vaccines, e.g., footpads or intraperitoneal injections, have been used in some preclinical studies. While at the present time there is no method to determine which animal model or route of immunization will predict immunogenicity in humans, these challenges may be addressed in the future by the humanized mouse model. These mice have been used to elicit human CS-specific IgG and $CD4^+$ T-cell responses following vaccination with CS vaccines [105] and for assessment of protection against *P. falciparum* sporozoite challenge following passive transfer of immune serum [106] or human MAB derived from vaccinated volunteers [62].

The identification of optimal adjuvants and delivery systems for the CS repeat immunodominant B-cell epitope will provide the framework for the development of epitopic vaccines containing new B-cell epitopes of *P. falciparum* CS, such as the N-terminus CS cleavage site [75, 76], as well as epitopes from new antigens identified by molecular screening and bioinformatics [107–109]. The lessons learned in the development of *P. falciparum* vaccines will also be directly applicable to *P. vivax* vaccines, which have been neglected due to the lack of an in vitro culture system and human challenge model [110, 111]. The recent development of a transgenic

P. berghei strain expressing *P. vivax* CS repeats will facilitate evaluation of *P. vivax* epitopic vaccines [15, 112].

A major requirement for advancing malaria vaccine development, in addition to standardized functional assays, is the ability to conduct head-to-head comparisons. The licensing of the first malaria vaccine RTS,S, in which antibody to CS repeats is associated with protection against clinical disease [61, 62], may provide the standard for such comparative studies which are essential for down-selection of next-generation epitopic vaccine candidates designed to elicit optimal levels of sporozoite-neutralizing antibodies.

References

1. Nussenzweig V, Nussenzweig RS (1989) Rationale for the development of an engineered sporozoite malaria vaccine. Adv Immunol 45:283–334
2. Kumar KA, Sano G, Boscardin S, Nussenzweig RS, Nussenzweig MC, Zavala F, Nussenzweig V (2006) The circumsporozoite protein is an immunodominant protective antigen in irradiated sporozoites. Nature 444(7121):937–940
3. Enea V, Ellis J, Zavala F, Arnot DE, Asavanich A, Masuda A, Quakyi I, Nussenzweig RS (1984) DNA cloning of *Plasmodium falciparum* circumsporozoite gene: amino acid sequence of repetitive epitope. Science 225(4662):628–630
4. Nardin EH, Nussenzweig V, Nussenzweig RS, Collins WE, Harinasuta KT, Tapchaisri P, Chomcharn Y (1982) Circumsporozoite proteins of human malaria parasites *Plasmodium falciparum* and *Plasmodium vivax*. J Exp Med 156(1):20–30
5. Zavala F, Tam JP, Hollingdale MR, Cochrane AH, Quakyi I, Nussenzweig RS, Nussenzweig V (1985) Rationale for development of a synthetic vaccine against *Plasmodium falciparum* malaria. Science 228(4706):1436–1440
6. Vanderbert, JP, Frevert U. (2004) Intravital microscopy demonstrating antibody-mediated immobilisation of Plasmodium berghei sporozoites injected into skin by mosquitoes. Int J Parasitol. 34(9):991–6. doi:10.1016/j.ijpara.2004.05.005
7. Molano A, Park SH, Chiu YH, Nosseir S, Bendelac A, Tsuji M (2000) Cutting edge: the IgG response to the circumsporozoite protein is MHC class II-dependent and CD1d-independent: exploring the role of GPIs in NK T cell activation and antimalarial responses. J Immunol 164(10):5005–5009
8. Carvalho LH, Sano G, Hafalla JC, Morrot A, Curotto de Lafaille MA, Zavala F (2002) IL-4-secreting CD4+ T cells are crucial to the development of CD8+ T-cell responses against malaria liver stages. Nat Med 8(2):166–170
9. Ferreira A, Schofield L, Enea V, Schellekens H, van der Meide P, Collins WE, Nussenzweig RS, Nussenzweig V (1986) Inhibition of development of exoerythrocytic forms of malaria parasites by gamma-interferon. Science 232(4752):881–884
10. Sinigaglia F, Guttinger M, Kilgus J, Doran DM, Matile H, Etlinger H, Trzeciak A, Gillessen D, Pink JR (1988) A malaria T-cell epitope recognized in association with most mouse and human MHC class II molecules. Nature 336(6201):778–780
11. Moreno A, Clavijo P, Edelman R, Davis J, Sztein M, Sinigaglia F, Nardin E (1993) CD4+ T cell clones obtained from *Plasmodium falciparum* sporozoite-immunized volunteers recognize polymorphic sequences of the circumsporozoite protein. J Immunol 151(1):489–499
12. Calvo-Calle JM, Hammer J, Sinigaglia F, Clavijo P, Moya-Castro ZR, Nardin EH (1997) Binding of malaria T cell epitopes to DR and DQ molecules in vitro correlates with immunogenicity in vivo: identification of a universal T cell epitope in the *Plasmodium falciparum* circumsporozoite protein. J Immunol 159(3):1362–1373

13. Persson C, Oliveira GA, Sultan AA, Bhanot P, Nussenzweig V, Nardin E (2002) Cutting edge: a new tool to evaluate human pre-erythrocytic malaria vaccines: rodent parasites bearing a hybrid *Plasmodium falciparum* circumsporozoite protein. J Immunol 169(12):6681–6685
14. Kumar KA, Oliveira GA, Edelman R, Nardin E, Nussenzweig V (2004) Quantitative *Plasmodium* sporozoite neutralization assay (TSNA). J Immunol Methods 292(1-2):157–164. doi:10.1016/j.jim.2004.06.017
15. Whitacre DC, Espinosa DA, Peters CJ, Jones JE, Tucker AE, Peterson DL, Zavala FP, Milich DR (2015) *P. falciparum* and *P. vivax* epitope-focused VLPs elicit sterile immunity to blood stage infections. PLoS One 10(5), e0124856. doi:10.1371/journal.pone.0124856
16. Tewari R, Spaccapelo R, Bistoni F, Holder AA, Crisanti A (2002) Function of region I and II adhesive motifs of *Plasmodium falciparum* circumsporozoite protein in sporozoite motility and infectivity. J Biol Chem 277(49):47613–47618. doi:10.1074/jbc.M208453200
17. Porter MD, Nicki J, Pool CD, DeBot M, Illam RM, Brando C, Bozick B, De La Vega P, Angra D, Spaccapelo R, Crisanti A, Murphy JR, Bennett JW, Schwenk RJ, Ockenhouse CF, Dutta S (2013) Transgenic parasites stably expressing full-length *Plasmodium falciparum* circumsporozoite protein as a model for vaccine down-selection in mice using sterile protection as an endpoint. Clin Vaccine Immunol 20(6):803–810. doi:10.1128/CVI.00066-13
18. Zhang M, Kaneko I, Tsao T, Mitchell R, Nardin EH, Iwanaga S, Yuda M, Tsuji M (2016) A highly infectious Plasmodium yoelii parasite, bearing Plasmodium falciparum circumsporozoite protein. Malar J 15(1):201. doi:10.1186/s1293-016-1248-z
19. Herrington DA, Clyde DF, Losonsky G, Cortesia M, Murphy JR, Davis J, Baqar S, Felix AM, Heimer EP, Gillessen D et al (1987) Safety and immunogenicity in man of a synthetic peptide malaria vaccine against *Plasmodium falciparum* sporozoites. Nature 328(6127):257–259
20. Latz, E., Franko, J, Golenbock, DT, Schreiber, JF. (2004) Haemophilus influenzae type b-outer membrane protein complex glycoconjugate vaccine induces cytokine production by engaging human toll-like receptor 2 (TLR2) and requires the presesnce of TLR2 for optimal immunogenicity. J Immunol 172(4): 2431-8. doi 10.4049/jimmunol.172.4.2431
21. Przysiecki C, Lucas B, Mitchell R, Carapau D, Wen Z, Xu H, Wang XM, Nahas D, Wu C, Hepler R, Ottinger E, Ter Meulen J, Kaslow D, Shiver J, Nardin E (2012) Sporozoite neutralizing antibodies elicited in mice and rhesus macaques immunized with a *Plasmodium falciparum* repeat peptide conjugated to meningococcal outer membrane protein complex. Front Cell Infect Microbiol 2:146. doi:10.3389/fcimb.2012.00146
22. Wu Y, Przysiecki C, Flanagan E, Bello-Irizarry SN, Ionescu R, Muratova O, Dobrescu G, Lambert L, Keister D, Rippeon Y, Long CA, Shi L, Caulfield M, Shaw A, Saul A, Shiver J, Miller LH (2006) Sustained high-titer antibody responses induced by conjugating a malarial vaccine candidate to outer-membrane protein complex. Proc Natl Acad Sci U S A 103(48):18243–18248. doi:10.1073/pnas.0608545103
23. Kubler-Kielb J, Majadly F, Biesova Z, Mocca CP, Guo C, Nussenzweig R, Nussenzweig V, Mishra S, Wu Y, Miller LH, Keith JM, Liu TY, Robbins JB, Schneerson R (2010) A bicomponent *Plasmodium falciparum* investigational vaccine composed of protein-peptide conjugates. Proc Natl Acad Sci U S A 107(3):1172–1177. doi:10.1073/pnas.0913374107
24. Tam JP, Clavijo P, Lu YA, Nussenzweig V, Nussenzweig R, Zavala F (1990) Incorporation of T and B epitopes of the circumsporozoite protein in a chemically defined synthetic vaccine against malaria. J Exp Med 171(1):299–306
25. Munesinghe DY, Clavijo P, Calle MC, Nussenzweig RS, Nardin E (1991) Immunogenicity of multiple antigen peptides (MAP) containing T and B cell epitopes of the repeat region of the *P. falciparum* circumsporozoite protein. Eur J Immunol 21(12):3015–3020. doi:10.1002/eji.1830211217
26. de Oliveira GA, Clavijo P, Nussenzweig RS, Nardin EH (1994) Immunogenicity of an alum-adsorbed synthetic multiple-antigen peptide based on B- and T-cell epitopes of the *Plasmodium falciparum* CS protein: possible vaccine application. Vaccine 12(11):1012–1017
27. Moreno CA, Rodriguez R, Oliveira GA, Ferreira V, Nussenzweig RS, Moya Castro ZR, Calvo-Calle JM, Nardin E (1999) Preclinical evaluation of a synthetic *Plasmodium falciparum* MAP malaria vaccine in Aotus monkeys and mice. Vaccine 18(1-2):89–99

28. Nardin EH, Oliveira GA, Calvo-Calle JM, Castro ZR, Nussenzweig RS, Schmeckpeper B, Hall BF, Diggs C, Bodison S, Edelman R (2000) Synthetic peptide malaria vaccine elicits high levels of antibodies in vaccines of defined HLA genotypes. J Infect Dis 182(5):1486–1496
29. Del Giudice G, Cooper JA, Merino J, Verdini AS, Pessi A, Togna AR, Engers HD, Corradin G, Lambert PH (1986) The antibody response in mice to carrier-free synthetic polymers of *Plasmodium falciparum* circumsporozoite repetitive epitope is I-Ab- restricted: possible implications for malaria vaccines. J Immunol 137(9):2952–2955
30. Edelman R, Wasserman SS, Kublin JG, Bodison SA, Nardin EH, Oliveira GA, Ansari S, Diggs CL, Kashala OL, Schmeckpeper BJ, Hamilton RG (2002) Immediate-type hypersensitivity and other clinical reactions in volunteers immunized with a synthetic multi-antigen peptide vaccine (PfCS-MAP1NYU) against *Plasmodium falciparum* sporozoites. Vaccine 21(3-4):269–280
31. Ho PC, Mutch DA, Winkel KD, Saul AJ, Jones GL, Doran TJ, Rzepczyk CM (1990) Identification of two promiscuous T cell epitopes from tetanus toxin. Eur J Immunol 20(3): 477–483
32. Greenstein JL, Schad VC, Goodwin WH, Brauer AB, Bollinger BK, Chin RD, Kuo MC (1992) A universal T cell epitope-containing peptide from hepatitis B surface antigen can enhance antibody specific for HIV gp120. J Immunol 148(12):3970–3977
33. Valmori D, Pessi A, Bianchi E, Corradin G (1992) Use of human universally antigenic tetanus toxin T cell epitopes as carriers for human vaccination. J Immunol 149(2):717–721
34. Alexander J, Sidney J, Southwood S, Ruppert J, Oseroff C, Maewal A, Snoke K, Serra HM, Kubo RT, Sette A et al (1994) Development of high potency universal DR-restricted helper epitopes by modification of high affinity DR-blocking peptides. Immunity 1(9):751–761
35. Zeng W, Jackson DC, Rose K (1996) Synthesis of a new template with a built-in adjuvant and its use in constructing peptide vaccine candidates through polyoxime chemistry. J Pept Sci 2(1):66–72. doi:10.1002/psc.51
36. Nardin EH, Calvo-Calle JM, Oliveira GA, Clavijo P, Nussenzweig R, Simon R, Zeng W, Rose K (1998) *Plasmodium falciparum* polyoximes: highly immunogenic synthetic vaccines constructed by chemoselective ligation of repeat B-cell epitopes and a universal T-cell epitope of CS protein. Vaccine 16(6):590–600
37. Nardin EH, Calvo-Calle JM, Oliveira GA, Nussenzweig RS, Schneider M, Tiercy JM, Loutan L, Hochstrasser D, Rose K (2001) A totally synthetic polyoxime malaria vaccine containing *Plasmodium falciparum* B cell and universal T cell epitopes elicits immune responses in volunteers of diverse HLA types. J Immunol 166(1):481–489
38. Calvo-Calle JM, Oliveira GA, Nardin EH (2005) Human CD4+ T cells induced by synthetic peptide malaria vaccine are comparable to cells elicited by attenuated *Plasmodium falciparum* sporozoites. J Immunol 175(11):7575–7585
39. Moreno A, Clavijo P, Edelman R, Davis J, Sztein M, Herrington D, Nardin E (1991) Cytotoxic CD4+ T cells from a sporozoite-immunized volunteer recognize the *Plasmodium falciparum* CS protein. Int Immunol 3(10):997–1003
40. Frevert U, Nardin E (2008) Cellular effector mechanisms against *Plasmodium* liver stages. Cell Microbiol 10(10):1956–1967
41. Frevert U, Moreno A, Calvo-Calle JM, Klotz C, Nardin E (2009) Imaging effector functions of human cytotoxic CD4+ T cells specific for *Plasmodium falciparum* circumsporozoite protein. Int J Parasitol 39(1):119–132. doi:10.1016/j.ijpara.2008.06.014
42. Calvo-Calle JM, Oliveira GA, Watta CO, Soverow J, Parra-Lopez C, Nardin EH (2006) A linear peptide containing minimal T- and B cell epitopes of *Plasmodium falciparum* circumsporozoite protein elicits protection against transgenic sporozoite challenge. Infect Immun 74(12):6929–6939. doi:10.1128/IAI.01151-06
43. Audran R, Cachat M, Lurati F, Soe S, Leroy O, Corradin G, Druilhe P, Spertini F (2005) Phase I malaria vaccine trial with a long synthetic peptide derived from the merozoite surface protein 3 antigen. Infect Immun 73(12):8017–8026. doi:10.1128/IAI.73.12.8017-8026.2005
44. Wu Y, Ellis RD, Shaffer D, Fontes E, Malkin EM, Mahanty S, Fay MP, Narum D, Rausch K, Miles AP, Aebig J, Orcutt A, Muratova O, Song G, Lambert L, Zhu D, Miura K, Long C, Saul

A, Miller LH, Durbin AP (2008) Phase 1 trial of malaria transmission blocking vaccine candidates Pfs25 and Pvs25 formulated with montanide ISA 51. PLoS One 3(7), e2636
45. Black M, Trent A, Tirrell M, Olive C (2010) Advances in the design and delivery of peptide subunit vaccines with a focus on toll-like receptor agonists. Expert Rev Vaccines 9(2):157–173. doi:10.1586/erv.09.160
46. Duthie MS, Windish HP, Fox CB, Reed SG (2011) Use of defined TLR ligands as adjuvants withinhumanvaccines.ImmunolRev239(1):178–196.doi:10.1111/j.1600-065X.2010.00978.x
47. Craft N, Bruhn KW, Nguyen BD, Prins R, Lin JW, Liau LM, Miller JF (2005) The TLR7 agonist imiquimod enhances the anti-melanoma effects of a recombinant *Listeria* monocytogenes vaccine. J Immunol 175(3):1983–1990
48. Johnston D, Bystryn JC (2006) Topical imiquimod is a potent adjuvant to a weakly-immunogenic protein prototype vaccine. Vaccine 24(11):1958–1965
49. Adams S, O'Neill DW, Nonaka D, Hardin E, Chiriboga L, Siu K, Cruz CM, Angiulli A, Angiulli F, Ritter E, Holman RM, Shapiro RL, Berman RS, Berner N, Shao Y, Manches O, Pan L, Venhaus RR, Hoffman EW, Jungbluth A, Gnjatic S, Old L, Pavlick AC, Bhardwaj N (2008) Immunization of malignant melanoma patients with full-length NY-ESO-1 protein using TLR7 agonist imiquimod as vaccine adjuvant. J Immunol 181(1):776–784
50. Othoro C, Johnston D, Lee R, Soverow J, Bystryn JC, Nardin E (2009) Enhanced immunogenicity of *Plasmodium falciparum* peptide vaccines using a topical adjuvant containing a potent synthetic Toll-like receptor 7 agonist, imiquimod. Infect Immun 77(2):739–748. doi:10.1128/IAI.00974-08
51. Pasparakis M, Haase I, Nestle FO (2014) Mechanisms regulating skin immunity and inflammation. Nat Rev Immunol 14(5):289–301. doi:10.1038/nri3646
52. Hung IF, Zhang AJ, To KK, Chan JF, Li C, Zhu HS, Li P, Li C, Chan TC, Cheng VC, Chan KH, Yuen KY (2014) Immunogenicity of intradermal trivalent influenza vaccine with topical imiquimod: a double blind randomized controlled trial. Clin Infect Dis 59(9):1246–1255. doi:10.1093/cid/ciu582
53. Hung IF, Zhang AJ, To KK, Chan JF, Li P, Wong TL, Zhang R, Chan TC, Chan BC, Wai HH, Chan LW, Fong HP, Hui RK, Kong KL, Leung AC, Ngan AH, Tsang LW, Yeung AP, Yiu GC, Yung W, Lau JY, Chen H, Chan KH, Yuen KY (2015) Topical imiquimod before intradermal trivalent influenza vaccine for protection against heterologous non-vaccine and antigenically drifted viruses: a single-centre, double-blind, randomised, controlled phase 2b/3 trial. Lancet Infect Dis 16(2):209–218. doi:10.1016/S1473-3099(15)00354-0
54. Ben-Yedidia T, Arnon R (2007) Epitope-based vaccine against influenza. Expert Rev Vaccines 6(6):939–948. doi:10.1586/14760584.6.6.939
55. Mizel SB, Bates JT (2010) Flagellin as an adjuvant: cellular mechanisms and potential. J Immunol 185(10):5677–5682. doi:10.4049/jimmunol.1002156
56. Tussey L, Strout C, Davis M, Johnson C, Lucksinger G, Umlauf S, Song L, Liu G, Abraham K, White CJ (2016) Phase 1 safety and immunogenicity study of a quadrivalent seasonal flu vaccine comprising recombinant hemagglutinin-flagellin fusion proteins. Open Forum Infect Dis 3(1), ofw015. doi:10.1093/ofid/ofw015
57. Turley CB, Rupp RE, Johnson C, Taylor DN, Wolfson J, Tussey L, Kavita U, Stanberry L, Shaw A (2011) Safety and immunogenicity of a recombinant M2e-flagellin influenza vaccine (STF2.4xM2e) in healthy adults. Vaccine 29(32):5145–5152. doi:10.1016/j.vaccine.2011.05.041
58. Carapau D, Mitchell R, Nacer A, Shaw A, Othoro C, Frevert U, Nardin E (2013) Protective humoral immunity elicited by a needle-free malaria vaccine comprised of a chimeric *Plasmodium falciparum* circumsporozoite protein and a Toll-like receptor 5 agonist, flagellin. Infect Immun 81(12):4350–4362. doi:10.1128/IAI.00263-13
59. Nacer A, Carapau D, Mitchell R, Meltzer A, Shaw A, Frevert U, Nardin EH (2014) Imaging murine NALT following intranasal immunization with flagellin-modified circumsporozoite protein malaria vaccines. Mucosal Immunol 7(2):304–314. doi:10.1038/mi.2013.48
60. Stoute JA, Slaoui M, Heppner DG, Momin P, Kester KE, Desmons P, Wellde BT, Garcon N, Krzych U, Marchand M (1997) A preliminary evaluation of a recombinant circumsporozoite

protein vaccine against *Plasmodium falciparum* malaria. RTS, S Malaria Vaccine Evaluation Group. N Engl J Med 336(2):86–91. doi:10.1056/NEJM199701093360202

61. White MT, Verity R, Griffin JT, Asante KP, Owusu-Agyei S, Greenwood B, Drakeley C, Gesase S, Lusingu J, Ansong D, Adjei S, Agbenyega T, Ogutu B, Otieno L, Otieno W, Agnandji ST, Lell B, Kremsner P, Hoffman I, Martinson F, Kamthunzu P, Tinto H, Valea I, Sorgho H, Oneko M, Otieno K, Hamel MJ, Salim N, Mtoro A, Abdulla S, Aide P, Sacarlal J, Aponte JJ, Njuguna P, Marsh K, Bejon P, Riley EM, Ghani AC (2015) Immunogenicity of the RTS, S/AS01 malaria vaccine and implications for duration of vaccine efficacy: secondary analysis of data from a phase 3 randomised controlled trial. Lancet Infect Dis 15(12):1450–1458. doi:10.1016/S1473-3099(15)00239-X
62. Foquet L, Hermsen CC, van Gemert GJ, Van Braeckel E, Weening KE, Sauerwein R, Meuleman P, Leroux-Roels G (2014) Vaccine-induced monoclonal antibodies targeting circumsporozoite protein prevent *Plasmodium falciparum* infection. J Clin Invest 124(1):140–144. doi:10.1172/JCI70349
63. Schodel F, Moriarty AM, Peterson DL, Zheng JA, Hughes JL, Will H, Leturcq DJ, McGee JS, Milich DR (1992) The position of heterologous epitopes inserted in hepatitis B virus core particles determines their immunogenicity. J Virol 66(1):106–114
64. Pumpens P, Borisova GP, Crowther RA, Grens E (1995) Hepatitis B virus core particles as epitope carriers. Intervirology 38(1-2):63–74
65. Crowther RA, Kiselev NA, Bottcher B, Berriman JA, Borisova GP, Ose V, Pumpens P (1994) Three-dimensional structure of hepatitis B virus core particles determined by electron cryomicroscopy. Cell 77(6):943–950
66. Schodel F, Peterson D, Hughes J, Wirtz R, Milich D (1996) Hybrid hepatitis B virus core antigen as a vaccine carrier moiety: I. presentation of foreign epitopes. J Biotechnol 44(1-3):91–96. doi:10.1016/0168-1656(95)00118-2
67. Birkett A, Lyons K, Schmidt A, Boyd D, Oliveira GA, Siddique A, Nussenzweig R, Calvo-Calle JM, Nardin E (2002) A modified hepatitis B virus core particle containing multiple epitopes of the *Plasmodium falciparum* circumsporozoite protein provides a highly immunogenic malaria vaccine in preclinical analyses in rodent and primate hosts. Infect Immun 70(12):6860–6870
68. Nardin EH, Oliveira GA, Calvo-Calle JM, Wetzel K, Maier C, Birkett AJ, Sarpotdar P, Corado ML, Thornton GB, Schmidt A (2004) Phase I testing of a malaria vaccine composed of hepatitis B virus core particles expressing *Plasmodium falciparum* circumsporozoite epitopes. Infect Immun 72(11):6519–6527. doi:10.1128/IAI.72.11.6519-6527.2004
69. Gregson AL, Oliveira G, Othoro C, Calvo-Calle JM, Thorton GB, Nardin E, Edelman R (2008) Phase I trial of an alhydrogel adjuvanted hepatitis B core virus-like particle containing epitopes of *Plasmodium falciparum* circumsporozoite protein. PLoS One 3(2), e1556. doi:10.1371/journal.pone.0001556
70. Oliveira GA, Wetzel K, Calvo-Calle JM, Nussenzweig R, Schmidt A, Birkett A, Dubovsky F, Tierney E, Gleiter CH, Boehmer G, Luty AJ, Ramharter M, Thornton GB, Kremsner PG, Nardin EH (2005) Safety and enhanced immunogenicity of a hepatitis B core particle *Plasmodium falciparum* malaria vaccine formulated in adjuvant Montanide ISA 720 in a phase I trial. Infect Immun 73(6):3587–3597. doi:10.1128/IAI.73.6.3587-3597.2005
71. Walther M, Dunachie S, Keating S, Vuola JM, Berthoud T, Schmidt A, Maier C, Andrews L, Andersen RF, Gilbert S, Poulton I, Webster D, Dubovsky F, Tierney E, Sarpotdar P, Correa S, Huntcooke A, Butcher G, Williams J, Sinden RE, Thornton GB, Hill AV (2005) Safety, immunogenicity and efficacy of a pre-erythrocytic malaria candidate vaccine, ICC-1132 formulated in Seppic ISA 720. Vaccine 23(7):857–864. doi:10.1016/j.vaccine.2004.08.020
72. Billaud JN, Peterson D, Barr M, Chen A, Sallberg M, Garduno F, Goldstein P, McDowell W, Hughes J, Jones J, Milich D (2005) Combinatorial approach to hepadnavirus-like particle vaccine design. J Virol 79(21):13656–13666. doi:10.1128/JVI.79.21.13656-13666.2005
73. de Groot AS, Johnson AH, Maloy WL, Quakyi IA, Riley EM, Menon A, Banks SM, Berzofsky JA, Good MF (1989) Human T cell recognition of polymorphic epitopes from malaria circumsporozoite protein. J Immunol 142(11):4000–4005

74. Coppi A, Natarajan R, Pradel G, Bennett BL, James ER, Roggero MA, Corradin G, Persson C, Tewari R, Sinnis P (2011) The malaria circumsporozoite protein has two functional domains, each with distinct roles as sporozoites journey from mosquito to mammalian host. J Exp Med 208(2):341–356. doi:10.1084/jem.20101488
75. Rathore D, Nagarkatti R, Jani D, Chattopadhyay R, de la Vega P, Kumar S, McCutchan TF (2005) An immunologically cryptic epitope of *Plasmodium falciparum* circumsporozoite protein facilitates liver cell recognition and induces protective antibodies that block liver cell invasion. J Biol Chem 280(21):20524–20529. doi:10.1074/jbc.M414254200
76. Espinosa DA, Gutierrez GM, Rojas-Lopez M, Noe AR, Shi L, Tse SW, Sinnis P, Zavala F (2015) Proteolytic cleavage of the *Plasmodium falciparum* circumsporozoite protein is a target of protective antibodies. J Infect Dis 212(7):1111–1119. doi:10.1093/infdis/jiv154
77. Riedl P, Stober D, Oehninger C, Melber K, Reimann J, Schirmbeck R (2002) Priming Th1 immunity to viral core particles is facilitated by trace amounts of RNA bound to its arginine-rich domain. J Immunol 168(10):4951–4959
78. Lee BO, Tucker A, Frelin L, Sallberg M, Jones J, Peters C, Hughes J, Whitacre D, Darsow B, Peterson DL, Milich DR (2009) Interaction of the hepatitis B core antigen and the innate immune system. J Immunol 182(11):6670–6681. doi:10.4049/jimmunol.0803683
79. Alving CR, Beck Z, Matyas GR, Rao M (2016) Liposomal adjuvants for human vaccines. Expert Opin Drug Deliv 13(6):807–816. doi:10.1517/17425247.2016.1151871
80. Fries LF, Gordon DM, Richards RL, Egan JE, Hollingdale MR, Gross M, Silverman C, Alving CR (1992) Liposomal malaria vaccine in humans: a safe and potent adjuvant strategy. Proc Natl Acad Sci U S A 89(1):358–362
81. Moser C, Muller M, Kaeser MD, Weydemann U, Amacker M (2013) Influenza virosomes as vaccine adjuvant and carrier system. Expert Rev Vaccines 12(7):779–791. doi:10.1586/14760584.2013.811195
82. Arkema A, Huckriede A, Schoen P, Wilschut J, Daemen T (2000) Induction of cytotoxic T lymphocyte activity by fusion-active peptide-containing virosomes. Vaccine 18(14): 1327–1333
83. Kammer AR, Amacker M, Rasi S, Westerfeld N, Gremion C, Neuhaus D, Zurbriggen R (2007) A new and versatile virosomal antigen delivery system to induce cellular and humoral immune responses. Vaccine 25(41):7065–7074
84. Okitsu SL, Kienzl U, Moehle K, Silvie O, Peduzzi E, Mueller MS, Sauerwein RW, Matile H, Zurbriggen R, Mazier D, Robinson JA, Pluschke G (2007) Structure-activity-based design of a synthetic malaria peptide eliciting sporozoite inhibitory antibodies in a virosomal formulation. Chem Biol 14(5):577–587
85. Genton B, Pluschke G, Degen L, Kammer AR, Westerfeld N, Okitsu SL, Schroller S, Vounatsou P, Mueller MM, Tanner M, Zurbriggen R (2007) A randomized placebo-controlled phase Ia malaria vaccine trial of two virosome-formulated synthetic peptides in healthy adult volunteers. PLoS One 2(10), e1018
86. Okitsu SL, Silvie O, Westerfeld N, Curcic M, Kammer AR, Mueller MS, Sauerwein RW, Robinson JA, Genton B, Mazier D, Zurbriggen R, Pluschke G (2007) A virosomal malaria peptide vaccine elicits a long-lasting sporozoite-inhibitory antibody response in a phase 1a clinical trial. PLoS One 2(12), e1278. doi:10.1371/journal.pone.0001278
87. Mueller MS, Renard A, Boato F, Vogel D, Naegeli M, Zurbriggen R, Robinson JA, Pluschke G (2003) Induction of parasite growth-inhibitory antibodies by a virosomal formulation of a peptidomimetic of loop I from domain III of *Plasmodium falciparum* apical membrane antigen 1. Infect Immun 71(8):4749–4758
88. Thompson FM, Porter DW, Okitsu SL, Westerfeld N, Vogel D, Todryk S, Poulton I, Correa S, Hutchings C, Berthoud T, Dunachie S, Andrews L, Williams JL, Sinden R, Gilbert SC, Pluschke G, Zurbriggen R, Hill AV (2008) Evidence of blood stage efficacy with a virosomal malaria vaccine in a phase IIa clinical trial. PLoS One 3(1), e1493
89. Cech PG, Aebi T, Abdallah MS, Mpina M, Machunda EB, Westerfeld N, Stoffel SA, Zurbriggen R, Pluschke G, Tanner M, Daubenberger C, Genton B, Abdulla S (2011) Virosome-formulated *Plasmodium falciparum* AMA-1 & CSP derived peptides as malaria

vaccine: randomized phase 1b trial in semi-immune adults & children. PLoS One 6(7), e22273. doi:10.1371/journal.pone.0022273
90. RTS,S Clinical Trials Partnership (2015) Efficacy and safety of RTS, S/AS01 malaria vaccine with or without a booster dose in infants and children in Africa: final results of a phase 3, individually randomised, controlled trial. Lancet 386(9988):31–45. doi:10.1016/S0140-6736(15)60721-8
91. Haynie DT, Zhang L, Zhao W, Rudra JS (2006) Protein-inspired multilayer nanofilms: science, technology and medicine. Nanomedicine 2(3):150–157. doi:10.1016/j.nano.2006.07.008
92. Powell TJ, Palath N, DeRome ME, Tang J, Jacobs A, Boyd JG (2011) Synthetic nanoparticle vaccines produced by layer-by-layer assembly of artificial biofilms induce potent protective T-cell and antibody responses in vivo. Vaccine 29(3):558–569. doi:10.1016/j.vaccine.2010.10.001
93. Powell, TJ, Tang, J, Derome, ME, Mitchell, RA, Jacobs, A, Deng, Y, Palath, N, Cardenas, E, Boyd, JG, Nardin, E. (2013). Plasmodium falciparum synthetic LbL microparticle vaccine elicits protective neutralizing antibody and parasite-specific cellular immune responses. Vaccine 31(15): 1898-904. doi:10.1016/j.vaccine.2013.02.027
94. Wen Y, Collier JH (2015) Supramolecular peptide vaccines: tuning adaptive immunity. Curr Opin Immunol 35:73–79. doi:10.1016/j.coi.2015.06.007
95. Rudra JS, Tian YF, Jung JP, Collier JH (2010) A self-assembling peptide acting as an immune adjuvant. Proc Natl Acad Sci U S A 107(2):622–627. doi:10.1073/pnas.0912124107
96. Chen J, Pompano RR, Santiago FW, Maillat L, Sciammas R, Sun T, Han H, Topham DJ, Chong AS, Collier JH (2013) The use of self-adjuvanting nanofiber vaccines to elicit high-affinity B cell responses to peptide antigens without inflammation. Biomaterials 34(34):8776–8785. doi:10.1016/j.biomaterials.2013.07.063
97. Sun T, Han H, Hudalla GA, Wen Y, Pompano RR, Collier JH (2016) Thermal stability of self-assembled peptide vaccine materials. Acta Biomater 30:62–71. doi:10.1016/j.actbio.2015.11.019
98. Rudra JS, Mishra, S, Chong, AS, Mitchell, RA, Nardin, EH, Nussenzweig, V, Collier, JH. (2012) Self-assembled peptide nanofibers raising durable antibody responses against a malaria epitope. Biomaterials. 33(27):6476–84. doi:10.1016/j.biomaterials.2012.05.041.
99. Tukel C, Nishimori JH, Wilson RP, Winter MG, Keestra AM, van Putten JP, Baumler AJ (2010) Toll-like receptors 1 and 2 cooperatively mediate immune responses to curli, a common amyloid from enterobacterial biofilms. Cell Microbiol 12(10):1495–1505. doi:10.1111/j.1462-5822.2010.01485.x
100. Kaba SA, Brando C, Guo Q, Mittelholzer C, Raman S, Tropel D, Aebi U, Burkhard P, Lanar DE (2009) A nonadjuvanted polypeptide nanoparticle vaccine confers long-lasting protection against rodent malaria. J Immunol 183(11):7268–7277. doi:10.4049/jimmunol.0901957
101. Kaba SA, McCoy ME, Doll TA, Brando C, Guo Q, Dasgupta D, Yang Y, Mittelholzer C, Spaccapelo R, Crisanti A, Burkhard P, Lanar DE (2012) Protective antibody and CD8+ T-cell responses to the *Plasmodium falciparum* circumsporozoite protein induced by a nanoparticle vaccine. PLoS One 7(10), e48304. doi:10.1371/journal.pone.0048304
102. Guo Q, Dasgupta D, Doll TA, Burkhard P, Lanar DE (2013) Expression, purification and refolding of a self-assembling protein nanoparticle (SAPN) malaria vaccine. Methods 60(3):242–247. doi:10.1016/j.ymeth.2013.03.025
103. Langermans JA, Schmidt A, Vervenne RA, Birkett AJ, Calvo-Calle JM, Hensmann M, Thornton GB, Dubovsky F, Weiler H, Nardin E, Thomas AW (2005) Effect of adjuvant on reactogenicity and long-term immunogenicity of the malaria Vaccine ICC-1132 in macaques. Vaccine 23(41):4935–4943. doi:10.1016/j.vaccine.2005.05.036
104. Xiao Y, Liu F, Yang J, Zhong M, Zhang E, Li Y, Zhou D, Cao Y, Li W, Yu J, Yang Y, Yan H (2015) Over-activation of TLR5 signaling by high-dose flagellin induces liver injury in mice. Cell Mol Immunol 12(6):729–742. doi:10.1038/cmi.2014.110
105. Huang J, Li X, Coelho-Dos-Reis JG, Zhang M, Mitchell R, Nogueira RT, Tsao T, Noe AR, Ayala R, Sahi V, Gutierrez GM, Nussenzweig V, Wilson JM, Nardin EH, Nussenzweig RS,

Tsuji M (2015) Human immune system mice immunized with *Plasmodium falciparum* circumsporozoite protein induce protective human humoral immunity against malaria. J Immunol Methods 427:42–50. doi:10.1016/j.jim.2015.09.005

106. Sack BK, Miller JL, Vaughan AM, Douglass A, Kaushansky A, Mikolajczak S, Coppi A, Gonzalez-Aseguinolaza G, Tsuji M, Zavala F, Sinnis P, Kappe SH (2014) Model for in vivo assessment of humoral protection against malaria sporozoite challenge by passive transfer of monoclonal antibodies and immune serum. Infect Immun 82(2):808–817. doi:10.1128/IAI.01249-13
107. Westenberger SJ, McClean CM, Chattopadhyay R, Dharia NV, Carlton JM, Barnwell JW, Collins WE, Hoffman SL, Zhou Y, Vinetz JM, Winzeler EA (2010) A systems-based analysis of *Plasmodium vivax* lifecycle transcription from human to mosquito. PLoS Negl Trop Dis 4(4), e653. doi:10.1371/journal.pntd.0000653
108. Doolan DL, Mu Y, Unal B, Sundaresh S, Hirst S, Valdez C, Randall A, Molina D, Liang X, Freilich DA, Oloo JA, Blair PL, Aguiar JC, Baldi P, Davies DH, Felgner PL (2008) Profiling humoral immune responses to *P. falciparum* infection with protein microarrays. Proteomics 8(22):4680–4694. doi:10.1002/pmic.200800194
109. Trieu A, Kayala MA, Burk C, Molina DM, Freilich DA, Richie TL, Baldi P, Felgner PL, Doolan DL (2011) Sterile protective immunity to malaria is associated with a panel of novel *P. falciparum* antigens. Mol Cell Proteom 10(9), M111 007948. doi:10.1074/mcp.M111.007948
110. Carlton JM, Adams JH, Silva JC, Bidwell SL, Lorenzi H, Caler E, Crabtree J, Angiuoli SV, Merino EF, Amedeo P, Cheng Q, Coulson RM, Crabb BS, Del Portillo HA, Essien K, Feldblyum TV, Fernandez-Becerra C, Gilson PR, Gueye AH, Guo X, Kang'a S, Kooij TW, Korsinczky M, Meyer EV, Nene V, Paulsen I, White O, Ralph SA, Ren Q, Sargeant TJ, Salzberg SL, Stoeckert CJ, Sullivan SA, Yamamoto MM, Hoffman SL, Wortman JR, Gardner MJ, Galinski MR, Barnwell JW, Fraser-Liggett CM (2008) Comparative genomics of the neglected human malaria parasite *Plasmodium vivax*. Nature 455(7214):757–763. doi:10.1038/nature07327
111. Arevalo-Herrera M, Forero-Pena DA, Rubiano K, Gomez-Hincapie J, Martinez NL, Lopez-Perez M, Castellanos A, Cespedes N, Palacios R, Onate JM, Herrera S (2014) *Plasmodium vivax* sporozoite challenge in malaria-naive and semi-immune Colombian volunteers. PLoS One 9(6), e99754. doi:10.1371/journal.pone.0099754
112. Espinosa DA, Yadava A, Angov E, Maurizio PL, Ockenhouse CF, Zavala F (2013) Development of a chimeric *Plasmodium berghei* strain expressing the repeat region of the *P. vivax* circumsporozoite protein for in vivo evaluation of vaccine efficacy. Infect Immun 81(8):2882–2887. doi:10.1128/IAI.00461-13

Part III
Immune Response to Malaria Vaccines: Blood Stage Vaccines

Immune Responses to Whole-Organism Blood-Stage Malaria Vaccines

Amber I. Raja, Danielle I. Stanisic, and Michael F. Good

Contents

1 Introduction 197
2 Immune Responses to Blood-Stage Malaria Parasites 198
3 Evidence Supporting a Whole Blood-Stage Parasite Vaccine Approach 199
4 Killed Blood-Stage Parasite Vaccines 200
5 Radiation-Attenuated Blood-Stage Parasite Vaccines 202
6 Genetically Attenuated Blood-Stage Parasite Vaccines 203
7 Chemically Attenuated Blood-Stage Parasite Vaccines 204
8 Challenges of Developing Whole Blood-Stage Parasite Vaccines 205
9 Conclusion 206
References 206

1 Introduction

Malaria remains a serious global health burden, with an estimated 214 million cases and a malaria-associated death toll of approximately 438,000 in 2015 alone [1]. Current control measures against malaria such as insecticide-treated nets, indoor residual spraying, and anti-malaria drug therapies have provided some reduction in malaria-associated morbidity and mortality; however, insecticide and drug resistance continue to impede progress in the control of malaria. Re-emergence of the disease in many parts of the world [2, 3] emphasizes the need for a vaccine if the burden of malaria is to be significantly reduced.

A.I. Raja • D.I. Stanisic • M.F. Good (✉)
Institute for Glycomics, Griffith University, Gold Coast Campus, Parklands Drive, Southport, QLD 4222, Australia
e-mail: amber.raja@griffithuni.edu.au; d.stanisic@griffith.edu.au; michael.good@griffith.edu.au

M.M. Mota, A. Rodriguez (eds.), *Malaria*, DOI 10.1007/978-3-319-45210-4_10

Whole-organism vaccines have been successfully developed against many diseases, including tuberculosis, polio, measles, mumps, and rubella (reviewed in [4]). Development of a blood-stage malaria vaccine began with the whole-parasite approach in the 1940s [5, 6]. However, since the cloning and expression of *Plasmodium* antigens [7, 8], malaria vaccine development has largely focused on a limited number of recombinant subunit antigens. Selection of subunit antigens has been based on their predicted biological function, as well as immune responses showing an association with protection in immuno-epidemiological studies [9–13]. Many of these immune targets, such as antigens involved in red blood cell (RBC) invasion, are encoded by multiple alleles. Allelic polymorphism is a major stumbling block for subunit vaccine candidates aiming to provide sustained vaccine efficacy in endemic settings [14–17].

The limited efficacy of subunit vaccine candidates to date has renewed interest in the use of whole parasites. This approach maximizes the number of antigens presented to the immune system with the natural inclusion of multiple conserved epitopes, and as such parasite diversity will have minimal impact on efficacy. An enormous body of work has been undertaken to identify suitable target antigens for subunit vaccine development; however, the whole-parasite approach does not rely on any knowledge of critical antigens. This is an advantage as evidence shows that many antigens are likely to play some role in either antibody- or cell-mediated immune protection [18–20]. This chapter will focus on immune responses to killed and attenuated blood-stage malaria vaccines.

2 Immune Responses to Blood-Stage Malaria Parasites

The blood stage of the parasite life cycle is associated with the clinical manifestations of malaria. In highly endemic areas, immunity against severe malaria and death is largely established by the age of five [21]. A complex and variable range of immune responses are induced during natural malaria infection (Fig. 1), but these do not provide sterile protection to individuals. Older children and adults, who are considered to be semi-immune or immune, still become infected with *Plasmodium* but remain asymptomatic with low parasite densities in the blood [22]. For these individuals, severe malaria is rare, but mild and uncomplicated disease can still occur (reviewed in [23]).

The persistence of and suboptimal immunity to *Plasmodium* infection is thought to be largely due to antigenic variation and allelic polymorphism of antigens expressed on the surface of parasitized RBCs (pRBCs) and merozoites, respectively ([25]; reviewed in [26, 27]). Additionally, blood-stage malaria infection can cause exhaustion and apoptotic deletion of parasite-specific T cells [28–31]. Suppression of cellular immune responses impacts the generation of parasite-specific memory T cells that are required for enduring protection.

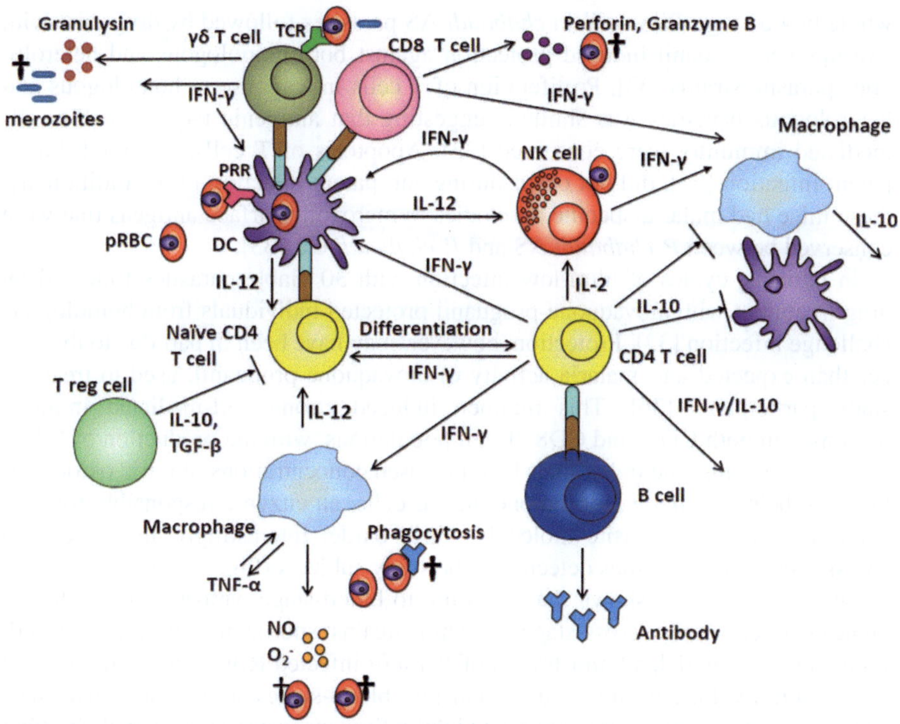

Fig. 1 Immune responses during blood-stage *Plasmodium* infection (from [24]). Antigen-presenting cells (APCs), such as dendritic cells (DCs) and macrophages, present parasite antigens and secrete IL-12 to prime CD4⁺ T cells. DCs also present antigen to CD8⁺ T cells. IFN-γ production by natural killer (NK) cells, CD8⁺ T cells, and CD4⁺ T cells induces cytokine production that aids DC maturation and macrophage activation. Activated macrophages induce phagocytosis and killing of parasites by the production of nitric oxide and reactive oxygen intermediates. CD4⁺ T cells can also engage with B cells to assist with antibody production

3 Evidence Supporting a Whole Blood-Stage Parasite Vaccine Approach

It is well known from both human and animal studies that deliberate infection followed by drug-cure can induce immune responses capable of reducing parasite burden following subsequent infections [32–35]. Protection against challenge is seen following both patent infections and sub-patent infections [33]. Immunity in both humans and rodents was observed following administration of multiple doses of blood-stage parasites with each infection treated prior to patency [32, 33].

The evidence that sub-clinical infections induce immunity provides strong support for a whole parasite vaccine approach as it suggests that only low numbers of attenuated parasites will be required for vaccination, thus reducing many logistical barriers in vaccine production. In the rodent model, sub-patent infections with whole blood-stage *Plasmodium chabaudi* AS parasites followed by drug-cure with atovaquone-proguanil induced protection against both homologous and heterologous parasite strains [33]. Proliferation of T cells in response to homologous and heterologous parasites was similar, suggesting that antigenic targets of this cell-mediated immunity were conserved [33]. Apoptosis of T cells, observed during patent infection [31], did not occur during sub-patent infection [33]. Additionally, these mice had malaria-specific antibodies to merozoite surface antigens that were conserved between *P. chabaudi* AS and *P. chabaudi* CB [33].

In humans, cycles of ultra-low infection with 30 viable parasites followed by drug treatment with atovaquone-proguanil protected individuals from homologous challenge infection [32]. Protection, however, may have been in part due to the longer than expected anti-malaria activity of atovaquone-proguanil, used to treat the study participants [36]. This regimen induced strong cell-mediated immune responses in both $CD4^+$ and $CD8^+$ T cell populations, with the production of IFN-γ (Fig. 2, [32]). Immune individuals had increased concentrations of nitric oxide synthase in their peripheral blood mononuclear cells, an enzyme responsible for production of the anti-parasite molecule, nitric oxide. Interestingly, there were no parasite-specific antibodies detected in the study subjects (Fig. 2, [32]).

Other studies have shown that exposure to blood-stage parasites under chloroquine cover can induce cross-stage protection against sporozoite challenge [34, 35]. Using a rodent model, administration of *P. yoelii*-infected RBCs under chloroquine cover conferred long-lasting protection against blood-stage and liver-stage parasites. $CD4^+$ and $CD8^+$ T cells were required to inhibit liver-stage parasites, with their effect being mediated by and dependent on nitric oxide and partially mediated through production of IFN-γ [34]. Antibodies were induced against both pre-erythrocytic and blood-stage parasites and were essential for protection [34].

Administration of multiple cycles of infection and drug treatment is not feasible as an effective vaccination approach. However, these studies highlight the potential use of whole blood-stage parasites and support the development of this vaccine approach.

4 Killed Blood-Stage Parasite Vaccines

The whole-organism blood-stage malaria vaccine approach was first investigated using killed parasites. Administration of formalin-killed and adjuvanted *Plasmodium lophurae*- and *Plasmodium knowlesi*-infected RBCs protected ducks and monkeys, respectively, from challenge infection [5, 6]. Vaccination with killed and adjuvanted *Plasmodium knowlesi*-infected RBCs induced higher titers of complement-fixing antibodies than vaccination with killed parasites without adjuvant [6]. The groups with higher antibody titers showed protection; however, there was no link between antibody titer and protection of individual monkeys [6].

The whole killed blood-stage parasite vaccine approach requires an adjuvant to help induce an effective immune response. Many early studies used killed parasites

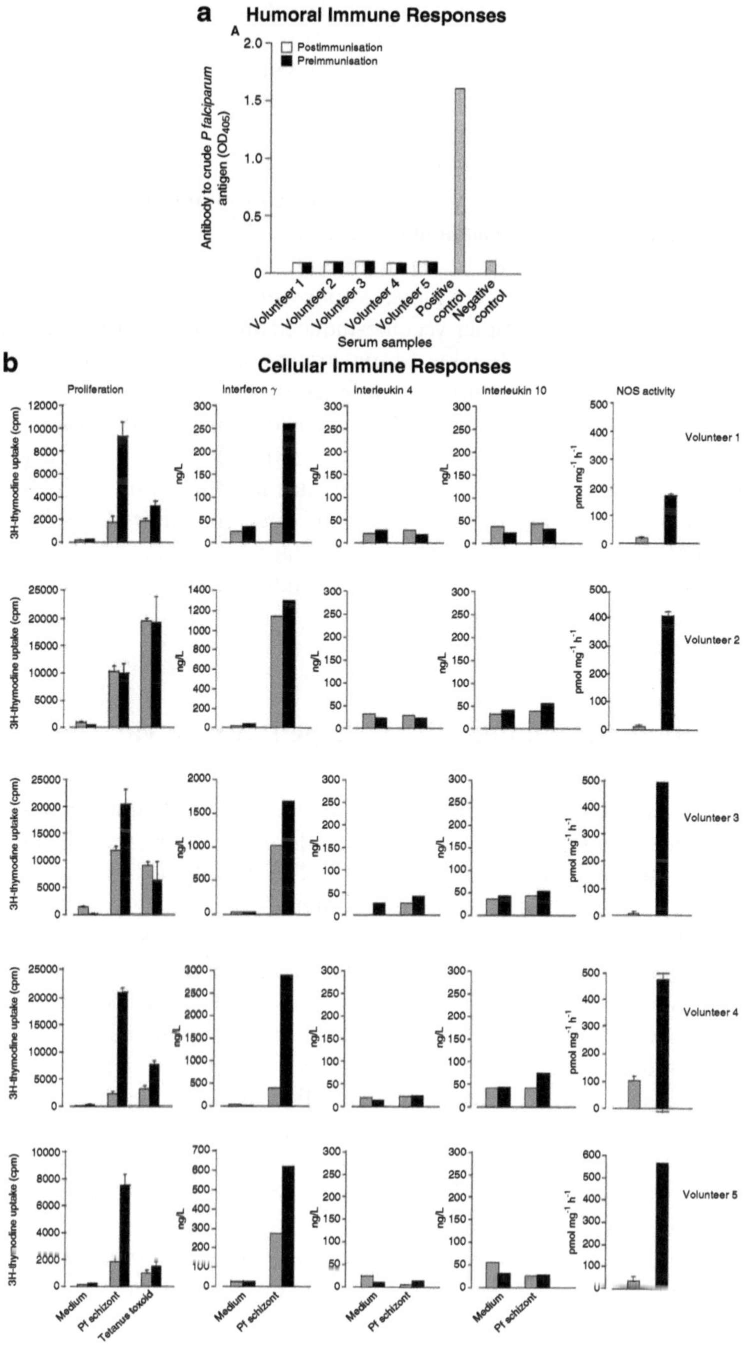

Fig. 2 Immune responses in human volunteers administered ultra-low doses of blood-stage *P. falciparum* parasites followed by drug treatment (from [32]). (**a**) Humoral immune responses assessed by ELISA to unfractionated *P. falciparum* antigens. (**b**) Cellular immune responses assessed according to proliferation of and cytokine production by peripheral blood mononuclear cells

adjuvanted with complete Freund's adjuvant; however, this is not suitable for use in humans due to safety issues (reviewed in [37]). A recent study used whole, killed blood-stage parasites with a strong T cell adjuvant (CpG-ODN) [38]. This study used a low-dose parasite approach based on previous findings that low doses of parasites induced parasite-specific T cells [33] that are deleted at higher parasite doses [31]. Mice were administered low doses (100 and 1000) of frozen and thawed infected RBCs firstly adjuvanted with CpG-ODN and alum followed by two booster doses without adjuvant [38]. Vaccination protected mice from high parasitemia and death following homologous and heterologous blood-stage challenge [38]. Both cellular and antibody responses were induced following vaccination. However, further investigations showed that neither vaccine-induced antibodies nor B cells were necessary for protection [38]. Following administration of the adjuvanted vaccine, IFN-γ, IL-12, TNF-α, and IL-10 were present in serum. Depletion of IFN-γ and IL-12 resulted in the abrogation of protection, whereas depletion of TNF-α or IL-10 had no effect on the survival of vaccinated mice [38]. Additionally, the depletion of $CD4^+$ T cells and nitric oxide also abrogated vaccine-induced protection. The low-dose vaccine was able to induce both central and effector memory $CD4^+$ T cells [38].

These studies show that whole killed blood-stage parasites can induce protective cellular immune responses. However, further studies are required to identify adjuvants that are suitable for use in humans.

5 Radiation-Attenuated Blood-Stage Parasite Vaccines

Radiation is a well-established method of attenuation [39]. Production of radiation-attenuated *Plasmodium* parasite lines was first developed using the lethal *P. berghei* NK65 [40]. After infected blood was exposed to 40 kilorad, irradiated parasites were inoculated into athymic nude and immune-competent mice. While infected immune-competent mice did not develop parasitemia, one nude mouse developed a slow but progressive parasitemia [40]. The isolated parasites, designated *P. berghei* NK65 XAT, produced a self-limiting infection of less than 6 % parasitemia in immune-competent mice [40]. This avirulent strain was maintained by passage through athymic nude mice. There was no reversion to the virulent form following more than 50 passages [41]. This attenuated line induced long-lasting strain and species-transcending protection [41]. Vaccination induced both parasite-specific cellular proliferation and antibodies [41]. However, antibody titers of mice were not linked to their survival [41]. Further studies in rodent models showed that vaccination with radiation-attenuated blood-stage *P. yoelii nigeriensis* parasites conferred protection against severe parasitemia and death following challenge infections with the original virulent blood-stage or pre-erythrocytic parasites [42]. Irradiated *P. berghei* ANKA blood-stage parasites were also able to protect mice from parasitemia and severe disease, including cerebral malaria [43]. Protection was associated with the induction of parasite-specific antibodies and an early but limited IFN-γ response [43].

Reversion of radiation-attenuated parasites to their virulent forms is the major concern for this vaccine approach, especially when considering their use in immune-compromised individuals. An early in vitro study of irradiated *P. falciparum* parasites demonstrated that the initial growth rates of surviving parasites were reduced; however, sub-inoculation of these attenuated parasites into culture led to a reversion to normal parasite growth [44]. Studies that characterize the cellular and molecular alteration of parasites following irradiation will further our understanding of the mechanism of radiation attenuation and may consequently overcome concerns related to the reversion of radiation-attenuated parasites to their virulent forms [45].

6 Genetically Attenuated Blood-Stage Parasite Vaccines

Genetic attenuation of parasites can be achieved by the disruption or deletion of genes that are essential for parasite development and replication. Blood-stage parasites lacking proteins involved in the essential purine-salvage pathway, such as purine nucleoside phosphorylase (PNP) and parasite nucleoside transporter 1 (NT1), have been studied.

PNP-deficient *P. yoelii* parasites demonstrated attenuated growth and virulence compared with their parental parasites [46]. The administration of a single dose of these PNP-deficient parasites protected mice against homologous and heterologous blood-stage challenge [46]. Although growth of these parasites was attenuated compared with the parental parasites, substantial growth of these parasites was recorded in mice following vaccination, with parasitemias of up to ~30 % [46]. The immune responses to these genetically attenuated *P. yoelii* parasites were not assessed in this study [46]. A PNP-deficient *P. falciparum* parasite line has also been generated [47]. In vitro assessment of this parasite line demonstrated severely retarded growth of parasites at physiological concentrations of hypoxanthine [47].

Plasmodium falciparum parasites lacking the *NT1* gene are incapable of using physiological concentrations of purines and demonstrated attenuated growth [48]. Normal growth rates of parasites were only restored when purines were provided at supra-physiological concentrations. *P. yoelii* parasites lacking NT1 also demonstrated severely attenuated growth when injected into mice, only growing in the presence of very high, non-physiological concentrations of purines [49]. A low-grade transient parasitemia was evident in mice injected with a single dose of 5000 NT1-deficient parasites; however, when the dose was reduced to 100 or 50, NT1-deficient parasite mice did not develop parasitemia. Mice that received the reduced dose of NT1-deficient parasites were protected against a lethal blood-stage challenge with *P. yoelii* YM. Mice vaccinated with a single dose of 100 NT1-deficient parasites demonstrated sterile protection following challenge with 25,000 *P. yoelii* YM sporozoites [49]. Alpha-beta-T cell-deficient mice and B cell-deficient mice were used to investigate the immune responses required for vaccine-induced protection. Both αβ-T cell and B cell responses were essential for vaccine-induced protection [49].

Disruption of the gene for plasmepsin-4 can generate virulence-attenuated parasites. Plasmepsin-4 contributes to hemoglobin digestion in the digestive vacuole of the parasite. Although disruption of the gene in *P. berghei* had a limited effect on the growth rate, these parasites showed significantly reduced virulence and an inability to induce experimental cerebral malaria compared to the parental parasite [50]. Mice vaccinated with these virulence-attenuated parasites were protected against both homologous and heterologous parasite challenge. Following vaccination, antibodies were induced, and transfer of IgG from mice that had cleared attenuated parasites resulted in a rapid decrease in the parasitemia and accumulation of parasites in the spleen of recipient mice infected with wild-type parasites [50]. Antibodies were suggested to enhance the clearance of infected RBCs by splenic macrophages [50].

The genetically attenuated vaccine approach will need to overcome concerns regarding reversion of attenuated parasites to their virulent wild type. One approach that is currently being utilized is the disruption or deletion of multiple genes. The disruption of both plasmepsin-4 and merozoite surface protein-7 genes generated double knockout parasites with greater virulence attenuation than either of the single knockout strains [51].

7 Chemically Attenuated Blood-Stage Parasite Vaccines

Chemical attenuation of blood-stage parasites using DNA-binding drugs is an effective method for generating a whole-parasite blood-stage vaccine in rodent models [52]. Originally developed as anti-cancer agents, centanamycin (CM) and tafuramycin-A (TF-A) belong to a family of chemical agents that irreversibly bind to poly-A regions of DNA [53]. Simple sequence repeats of adenine are abundant in the A-T-rich genome of *Plasmodium* spp. [54]. These drugs were originally investigated as anti-malaria drugs and then developed as attenuating agents for *Plasmodium* spp. initially using sporozoites [55–57]. CM and TF-A were used in vitro to attenuate blood-stage rodent *Plasmodium* spp. before injection into mice [52]. Administration of these parasites did not lead to patent parasitemia [52]. A single dose of chemically attenuated ring-stage *P. chabaudi* parasites protected mice against homologous and heterologous blood-stage parasite challenge. Protection lasted up to 6 months and was mediated by $CD4^+$ T cells in the absence of parasite-specific antibodies. Following vaccination, chemically attenuated parasites accumulated in the spleen and liver and were found inside macrophages and dendritic cells [52]. Data suggest that persistence of attenuated parasites or parasite antigens is necessary for induction of immune responses and protection (Reiman et al. submitted). Chemically attenuated ring-stage *P. chabaudi* parasites rapidly activated the immune system, with activation of both $CD4^+$ and $CD8^+$ T cells observed in the peripheral blood of vaccinated mice (Fig. 3, [52]). Strong proliferative responses were demonstrated against both homologous and heterologous parasites (Fig. 3, [52]). This chemically attenuated blood-stage vaccine approach is being assessed using other rodent models [59] and in an early-stage clinical trial for *P. falciparum*.

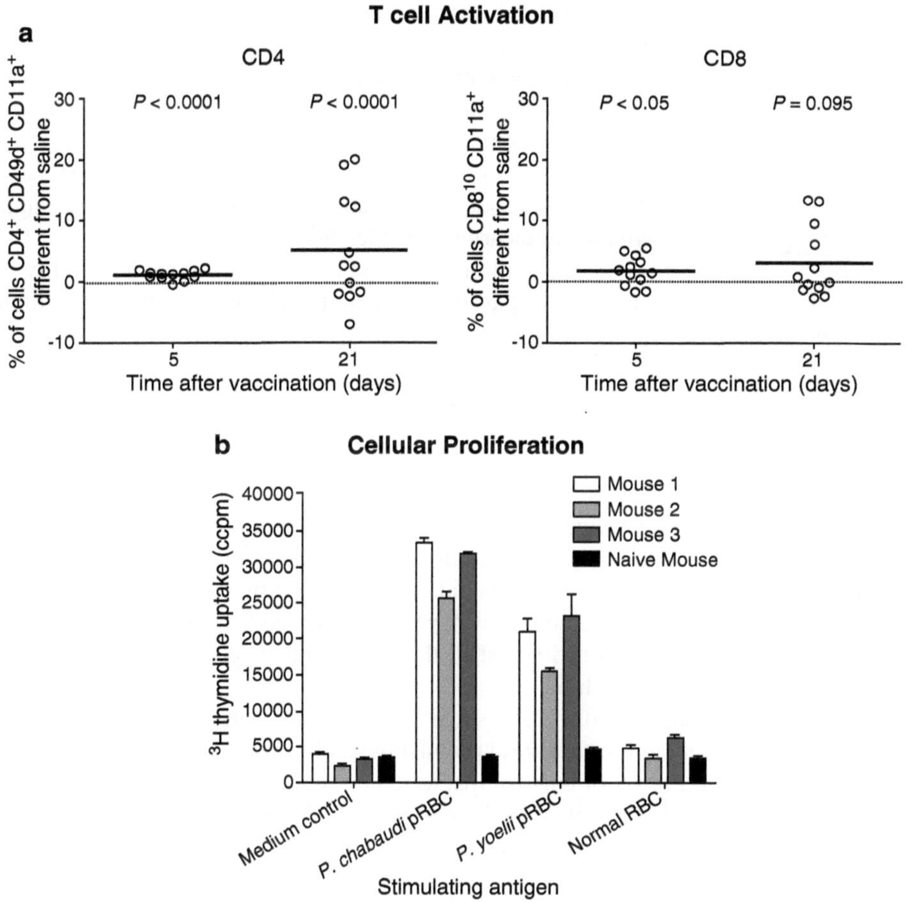

Fig. 3 Immune responses in mice following administration of chemically attenuated blood-stage *P. chabaudi* parasites (from [52]). (**a**) $CD4^+$ and $CD8^+$ T cell activation in blood. (**b**) Cellular proliferation of spleen cells using [^{3}H] thymidine uptake assay

8 Challenges of Developing Whole Blood-Stage Parasite Vaccines

The development of a whole blood-stage parasite vaccine presents a number of challenges, most prominently the use of RBCs in the vaccine formulation and the need for culturing to produce the vaccine [58]. Production will require human RBCs, as well as other blood components, and large-scale culture of parasites. The use of human blood also raises concerns regarding the induction of antibodies against RBC surface antigens (ABO and Rh blood group systems). This can be greatly limited by the use of universal donor (blood group O Rh negative) RBCs. Antibodies to minor antigens may also arise, but their occurrence will be dependent on the dose of red cells in the vaccine. Development of killed blood-stage vaccines also requires the identification of adjuvants suitable for use in humans.

Another consideration is the regulation of vaccine-induced immune responses, in particular cellular immune responses. The importance of cellular immune responses in protection has been demonstrated by a number of studies [38, 52]; however, cellular immune responses may also be pathogenic. A whole blood-stage vaccine will need to induce a balance of pro- and anti-inflammatory cellular immune responses capable of effectively clearing parasites without causing pathology. The factors regulating this balance are still not well understood. However, the ability of the immune response to contain parasite density quickly will dramatically limit pathogenic responses.

9 Conclusion

The development of a vaccine is essential for the elimination and eventual eradication of malaria. Despite many years of effort, an efficacious malaria vaccine has not yet been achieved. Subunit vaccine candidates that have progressed through to clinical trials in malaria-endemic countries have demonstrated limited efficacy [14–17] and have, therefore, renewed interest in the development of a whole blood-stage parasite vaccine against malaria.

Killed or attenuated whole blood-stage parasites have been used to develop the whole vaccine approach further, with promising results. Many animal vaccine studies have provided a proof of concept that killed or attenuated parasites can provide protection [38, 41, 43, 49, 50, 52]; however, clinical studies are now required to determine the protective role of vaccine-induced immune responses in humans.

References

1. World Health Organisation (2015) World malaria report 2015. World Health Organisation, Geneva
2. Faulde MK, Hoffmann R, Fazilat KM, Hoerauf A (2007) Malaria reemergence in northern Afghanistan. Emerg Infect Dis 13(9):1402. doi:10.3201/eid1309.061325
3. Zhou SS, Wang Y, Li Y (2011) Malaria situation in the People's Republic of China in 2010. Chin J Parasitol Parasitic Dis 29(6):401–403
4. Zepp F (2010) Principles of vaccine design—lessons from nature. Vaccine 28(Suppl 3):C14–C24. doi:10.1016/j.vaccine.2010.07.020
5. Thomson KJ, Freund J, Sommer HE, Walter AW, Pisani T (1947) Immunization of ducks against malaria by means of killed parasites with or without adjuvants. Am J Trop Med Hyg 27(2):79–105
6. Freund J, Thomson KJ, Sommer HE, Walter AW, Pisani TM (1948) Immunization of monkeys against malaria by means of killed parasites with adjuvants. Am J Trop Med Hyg 28(1):1–22
7. Kemp DJ, Coppel RL, Cowman AF, Saint RB, Brown GV, Anders RF (1983) Expression of *Plasmodium falciparum* blood-stage antigens in *Escherichia coli*: detection with antibodies from immune humans. Proc Natl Acad Sci U S A 80(12):3787–3791

8. Ellis J, Ozaki LS, Gwadz RW, Cochrane AH, Nussenzweig V, Nussenzweig RS, Godson GN (1983) Cloning and expression in *E. coli* of the malarial sporozoite surface antigen gene from *Plasmodium knowlesi*. Nature 302(5908):536–538. doi:10.1038/302536a0
9. Tongren JE, Drakeley CJ, McDonald SL, Reyburn HG, Manjurano A, Nkya WM, Lemnge MM, Gowda CD, Todd JE, Corran PH (2006) Target antigen, age, and duration of antigen exposure independently regulate immunoglobulin G subclass switching in malaria. Infect Immun 74(1):257–264. doi:10.1128/IAI.74.1.257-264.2006
10. Stanisic DI, Richards JS, McCallum FJ, Michon P, King CL, Schoepflin S, Gilson PR, Murphy VJ, Anders RF, Mueller I (2009) Immunoglobulin G subclass-specific responses against *Plasmodium falciparum* merozoite antigens are associated with control of parasitemia and protection from symptomatic illness. Infect Immun 77(3):1165–1174. doi:10.1128/IAI.01129-08
11. Richards JS, Stanisic DI, Fowkes FJI, Tavul L, Dabod E, Thompson JK, Kumar S, Chitnis CE, Narum DL, Michon P, Siba PM, Cowman AF, Mueller I, Beeson JG (2010) Association between naturally acquired antibodies to erythrocyte-binding antigens of *Plasmodium falciparum* and protection from malaria and high-density parasitemia. Clin Infect Dis 51(8):e50–e60. doi:10.1086/656413
12. Richards JS, Arumugam TU, Reiling L, Healer J, Hodder AN, Fowkes FJ, Cross N, Langer C, Takeo S, Uboldi AD (2013) Identification and prioritization of merozoite antigens as targets of protective human immunity to *Plasmodium falciparum* malaria for vaccine and biomarker development. J Immunol 191(2):795–809. doi:10.4049/jimmunol.1300778
13. Reiling L, Richards JS, Fowkes FJI, Wilson DW, Chokejindachai W, Barry AE, Tham W-H, Stubbs J, Langer C, Donelson J, Michon P, Tavul L, Crabb BS, Siba PM, Cowman AF, Mueller I, Beeson JG (2012) The *Plasmodium falciparum* erythrocyte invasion ligand Pfrh4 as a target of functional and protective human antibodies against malaria. PLoS One 7(9), e45253. doi:10.1371/journal.pone.0045253
14. Genton B, Betuela I, Felger I, Al-Yaman F, Anders RF, Saul A, Rare L, Baisor M, Lorry K, Brown GV, Pye D, Irving DO, Smith TA, Beck HP, Alpers MP (2002) A recombinant blood-stage malaria vaccine reduces *Plasmodium falciparum* density and exerts selective pressure on parasite populations in a phase 1-2b trial in Papua New Guinea. J Infect Dis 185(6):820–827
15. Ockenhouse CF, Angov E, Kester KE, Diggs C, Soisson L, Cummings JF, Stewart AV, Palmer DR, Mahajan B, Krzych U, Tornieporth N, Delchambre M, Vanhandenhove M, Ofori-Anyinam O, Cohen J, Lyon JA, Heppner DG (2006) Phase I safety and immunogenicity trial of FMP1/AS02A, a *Plasmodium falciparum* MSP-1 asexual blood stage vaccine. Vaccine 24(15):3009–3017. doi:10.1016/j.vaccine.2005.11.028
16. Stoute JA, Gombe J, Withers MR, Siangla J, McKinney D, Onyango M, Cummings JF, Milman J, Tucker K, Soisson L, Stewart VA, Lyon JA, Angov E, Leach A, Cohen J, Kester KE, Ockenhouse CF, Holland CA, Diggs CL, Wittes J, Gray Heppner D Jr (2007) Phase 1 randomized double-blind safety and immunogenicity trial of *Plasmodium falciparum* malaria merozoite surface protein FMP1 vaccine, adjuvanted with AS02A, in adults in western Kenya. Vaccine 25(1):176–184. doi:10.1016/j.vaccine.2005.11.037
17. Sagara I, Dicko A, Ellis RD, Fay MP, Diawara SI, Assadou MH, Sissoko MS, Kone M, Diallo AI, Saye R, Guindo MA, Kante O, Niambele MB, Miura K, Mullen GED, Pierce M, Martin LB, Dolo A, Diallo DA, Doumbo OK, Miller LH, Saul A (2009) A randomized controlled phase 2 trial of the blood stage AMA1-C1/Alhydrogel malaria vaccine in children in Mali. Vaccine 27(23):3090–3098. doi:10.1016/j.vaccine.2009.03.014
18. Barry AE, Schultz L, Buckee CO, Reeder JC (2009) Contrasting population structures of the genes encoding ten leading vaccine-candidate antigens of the human malaria parasite, *Plasmodium falciparum*. PLoS One 4(12), e8497. doi:10.1371/journal.pone.0008497
19. Collins WE, Jeffery GM (1999) A retrospective examination of secondary sporozoite- and trophozoite-induced infections with *Plasmodium falciparum*: development of parasitologic and clinical immunity following secondary infection. Am J Trop Med Hyg 61(1 Suppl):20–35
20. Winkel KD, Good MF (1991) Inability of *Plasmodium vinckei*-immune spleen cells to transfer protection to recipient mice exposed to vaccine 'vectors' or heterologous species of *Plasmodium*. Parasite Immunol 13(5):517–530. doi:10.1111/j.1365-3024.1991.tb00548.x

21. Gupta S, Snow RW, Donnelly CA, Marsh K, Newbold C (1999) Immunity to non-cerebral severe malaria is acquired after one or two infections. Nat Med 5(3):340–343. doi:10.1038/6560
22. Dal-Bianco MP, Köster KB, Kombila UD, Kun JFJ, Grobusch MP, Ngoma GM, Matsiegui PB, Supan C, Ospina Salazar CL, Missinou MA, Issifou S, Lell B, Kremsner P (2007) High prevalence of asymptomatic *Plasmodium falciparum* infection in Gabonese adults. AmJTrop Med Hyg 77(5):939–942
23. Ndungu FM, Urban BC, Marsh K, Langhorne J (2005) Regulation of immune response by *Plasmodium*-infected red blood cells. Parasite Immunol 27(10–11):373–384. doi:10.1111/j.1365-3024.2005.00771.x
24. Stanisic DI, Good MF (2016) Examining cellular immune responses to inform development of a blood-stage malaria vaccine. Parasitology 143(2):208–223. doi:10.1017/S0031182015001092
25. Patiño JAG, Holder AA, McBride JS, Blackman MJ (1997) Antibodies that inhibit malaria merozoite surface protein-1 processing and erythrocyte invasion are blocked by naturally acquired human antibodies. J Exp Med 186(10):1689–1699. doi:10.1084/jem.186.10.1689
26. Kyes S, Horrocks P, Newbold C (2001) Antigenic variation at the infected red cell surface in malaria. Annu Rev Microbiol 55:673–707
27. Smith JD, Craig AG (2005) The surface of the *Plasmodium falciparum*-infected erythrocyte. Curr Issues Mol Biol 7(1):81–93
28. Butler NS, Moebius J, Pewe LL, Traore B, Doumbo OK, Tygrett LT, Waldschmidt TJ, Crompton PD, Harty JT (2011) Therapeutic PD-L1 and LAG-3 blockade rapidly clears established blood-stage *Plasmodium* infection. Nat Immunol 13(2):188–195. doi:10.1038/ni.2180
29. Hirunpetcharat C, Good MF (1998) Deletion of *Plasmodium berghei*-specific $CD4^+$ T cells adoptively transferred into recipient mice after challenge with homologous parasite. Proc Natl Acad Sci U S A 95(4):1715–1720
30. Horne-Debets JM, Faleiro R, Karunarathne DS, Liu XQ, Lineburg KE, Poh CM, Grotenbreg GM, Hill GR, MacDonald KP, Good MF (2013) PD-1 dependent exhaustion of $CD8^+$ T cells drives chronic malaria. Cell Rep 5(5):1204–1213. doi:10.1016/j.celrep.2013.11.002
31. Xu HJ, Wipasa J, Yan HR, Zeng M, Makobongo MO, Finkelman FD, Kelso A, Good MF (2002) The mechanism and significance of deletion of parasite-specific $CD4^+$ T cells in malaria infection. J Exp Med 195(7):881–892. doi:10.1084/jem.20011174
32. Pombo DJ, Lawrence G, Hirunpetcharat C, Rzepczyk C, Bryden M, Cloonan N, Anderson K, Mahakunkijcharoen Y, Martin LB, Wilson D, Elliott S, Eisen DP, Weinberg JB, Saul A, Good MF (2002) Immunity to malaria after administration of ultra-low doses of red cells infected with *Plasmodium falciparum*. Lancet 360(9333):610–617. doi:10.1016/S0140-6736(02)09784-2
33. Elliott SR, Kuns RD, Good MF (2005) Heterologous immunity in the absence of variant-specific antibodies after exposure to subpatent infection with blood-stage malaria. Infect Immun 73(4):2478–2485. doi:10.1128/iai.73.4.2478-2485.2005
34. Belnoue E, Voza T, Costa FT, Grüner AC, Mauduit M, Rosa DS, Depinay N, Kayibanda M, Vigário AM, Mazier D (2008) Vaccination with live *Plasmodium yoelii* blood stage parasites under chloroquine cover induces cross-stage immunity against malaria liver stage. J Immunol 181(12):8552–8558. doi:10.4049/jimmunol.181.12.8552
35. Nahrendorf W, Spence PJ, Tumwine I, Lévy P, Jarra W, Sauerwein RW, Langhorne J (2015) Blood-stage immunity to *Plasmodium chabaudi* malaria following chemoprophylaxis and sporozoite immunization. Elife 4, e05165. doi:10.7554/eLife.05165
36. Edstein MD, Kotecka BM, Anderson KL, Pombo DJ, Kyle DE, Rieckmann KH, Good MF (2005) Lengthy antimalarial activity of atovaquone in human plasma following atovaquone-proguanil administration. Antimicrob Agents Chemother 49(10):4421–4422. doi:10.1128/aac.49.10.4421-4422.2005
37. Stils HF (2005) Adjuvants and antibody production: dispelling the myths associated with Freund's Complete and other adjuvants. ILAR J 46(3):280–293. doi:10.1093/ilar.46.3.280
38. Pinzon-Charry A, McPhun V, Kienzle V, Hirunpetcharat C, Engwerda C, McCarthy J, Good MF (2010) Low doses of killed parasite in CpG elicit vigorous $CD4^+$ T cell responses against blood-stage malaria in mice. J Clin Invest 120(8):2967–2978. doi:10.1172/jci39222

39. Corradetti A, Verolini F, Bucci A (1966) Resistanza a *Plasmodium berghei* da parte di ratti albini precedentement immunizzati con *Plasmodium berghei* irradiato. Parassitologia 8: 133–145
40. Waki S, Tamura J, Imanaka M, Ishikawa S, Suzuki M (1982) *Plasmodium berghei*: isolation and maintenance of an irradiation attenuated strain in the nude mouse. Exp Parasitol 53(3):335–340. doi:10.1016/0014-4894(82)90076-5
41. Miyagami T, Igarshi I, Suzuki M (1987) *Plasmodium berghei*: long lasting immunity induced by a permanent attenuated mutant. Zentralbl Bakteriol Mikrobiol Hyg A 264(3):502–512. doi:10.1016/S0176-6724(87)80074-3
42. Waki S, Yonome I, Suzuki M (1986) *Plasmodium yoelii*: induction of attenuated mutants by irradiation. Exp Parasitol 62(3):316–321
43. Gerald NJ, Majam V, Mahajan B, Kozakai Y, Kumar S (2011) Protection from experimental cerebral malaria with a single dose of radiation-attenuated, blood-stage *Plasmodium berghei* parasites. PLoS One 6(9), e24398. doi:10.1371/journal.pone.0024398
44. Waki S, Yonome I, Suzuki M (1983) *Plasmodium falciparum*: attenuation by irradiation. Exp Parasitol 56(3):339–345. doi:10.1016/0014-4894(83)90079-6
45. Oakley MS, Gerald N, Anantharaman V, Gao Y, Majam V, Mahajan B, Pham PT, Lotspeich-Cole L, Myers TG, McCutchan TF, Morris SL, Aravind L, Kumar S (2013) Radiation-induced cellular and molecular alterations in asexual intraerythrocytic *Plasmodium falciparum*. J Infect Dis 207(1):164–174. doi:10.1093/infdis/jis645
46. Ting LM, Gissot M, Coppi A, Sinnis P, Kim K (2008) Attenuated *Plasmodium yoelii* lacking purine nucleoside phosphorylase confer protective immunity. Nat Med 14(9):954–958. doi:10.1038/nm.1867
47. Madrid DC, Ting L-M, Waller KL, Schramm VL, Kim K (2008) *Plasmodium falciparum* purine nucleoside phosphorylase is critical for viability of malaria parasites. J Biol Chem 283(51):35899–35907. doi:10.1074/jbc.M807218200
48. El Bissati K, Zufferey R, Witola WH, Carter NS, Ullman B, Ben Mamoun C (2006) The plasma membrane permease PfNT1 is essential for purine salvage in the human malaria parasite *Plasmodium falciparum*. Proc Natl Acad Sci U S A 103(24):9286–9291. doi:10.1073/pnas.0602590103
49. Aly ASI, Downie MJ, Mamoun CB, Kappe SHI (2010) Subpatent infection with nucleoside transporter 1-deficient *Plasmodium* blood stage parasites confers sterile protection against lethal malaria in mice. Cell Microbiol 12(7):930–938. doi:10.1111/j.1462-5822.2010.01441.x
50. Spaccapelo R, Janse CJ, Caterbi S, Franke-Fayard B, Bonilla JA, Syphard LM, Di Cristina M, Dottorini T, Savarino A, Cassone A, Bistoni F, Waters AP, Dame JB, Crisanti A (2010) Plasmepsin 4-deficient *Plasmodium berghei* are virulence attenuated and induce protective immunity against experimental malaria. Am J Pathol 176(1):205–217. doi:10.2353/ajpath.2010.090504
51. Spaccapelo R, Aime E, Caterbi S, Arcidiacono P, Capuccini B, Di Cristina M, Dottorini T, Rende M, Bistoni F, Crisanti A (2011) Disruption of plasmepsin-4 and merozoites surface protein-7 genes in *Plasmodium berghei* induces combined virulence-attenuated phenotype. Sci Rep 1:39. doi:10.1038/srep00039
52. Good MF, Reiman JM, Rodriguez IB, Ito K, Yanow SK, El-Deeb IM, Batzloff MR, Stanisic DI, Engwerda C, Spithill T, Hoffman SL, Moses L, McPhun V (2013) Cross-species malaria immunity induced by chemically attenuated parasites. J Clin Invest 123(8):3353. doi:10.1172/JCI66634
53. Sato A, McNulty L, Cox K, Kim S, Scott A, Daniell K, Summerville K, Price C, Hudson S, Kiakos K, Hartley JA, Asao T, Lee M (2005) A novel class of in vivo active anticancer agents: achiral seco-amino- and seco-hydroxycyclopropylbenz[e]indolone (seco-CBI) analogues of the duocarmycins and CC-1065. J Med Chem 48(11):3903–3918. doi:10.1021/jm050179u
54. Su X, Wellems TE (1996) Toward a high-resolution *Plasmodium falciparum* linkage map: polymorphic markers from hundreds of simple sequence repeats. Genomics 33(3):430–444. doi:10.1006/geno.1996.0218

55. Yanow SK, Purcell LA, Pradel G, Sato A, Rodriguez A, Lee M, Spithill TW (2008) Potent antimalarial and transmission-blocking activities of centanamycin, a novel DNA-binding agent. J Infect Dis 197(4):527–534. doi:10.1086/526788
56. Purcell LA, Wong KA, Yanow SK, Lee M, Spithill TW, Rodriguez A (2008) Chemically attenuated *Plasmodium* sporozoites induce specific immune responses, sterile immunity and cross-protection against heterologous challenge. Vaccine 26(38):4880–4884. doi:10.1016/j.vaccine.2008.07.017
57. Purcell LA, Yanow SK, Lee M, Spithill TW, Rodriguez A (2008) Chemical attenuation of *Plasmodium berghei* sporozoites induces sterile immunity in mice. Infect Immun 76(3):1193–1199. doi:10.1128/iai.01399-07
58. Stanisic DI, Liu XQ, De SL, Batzloff MR, Forbes T, Davis CB, Sekuloski S, Chavchich M, Chung W, Trenholme K, McCarthy JS, Li T, Sim BKL, Hoffman SL, Good MF (2015) Development of cultured *Plasmodium falciparum* blood-stage malaria cell banks for early phase in vivo clinical trial assessment of anti-malaria drugs and vaccines. Malar J 14:143. doi:10.1186/s12936-015-0663-x
59. Raja AI, Cai Y, Reiman JM, Groves P, Chakravarty S, McPhun V, Doolan DL, Cockburn I, Hoffman SL, Stanisic DI, Good MF (2016) Chemically attenuated blood-stage *Plasmodium yoelii* parasites induce long-lived and strain-transcending protection. Infect Immun 84(8):2274–88. doi:10.1128/IAI.00157.16

Subunit Blood-Stage Malaria Vaccines

Alexander D. Douglas

Contents

1 Introduction ... 212
2 Mechanisms of BSV-Inducible Protection: Effectors and Assessment ... 214
2.1 Naturally Acquired Immunity, Non-Natural Immunity, Markers and Causes of Protection ... 214
2.2 Fc-Receptor-Independent Merozoite Neutralisation by Antibody ... 215
2.3 Fc-Receptor-Dependent Activity of Anti-Merozoite Antibodies ... 216
2.4 Antibody Against iRBC-Surface Antigens ... 217
2.5 T Cell Responses Against the Blood-Stage ... 218
3 Assessing and Prioritising BSVs In Vivo ... 219
3.1 Mouse Models ... 219
3.2 Non-Human Primate (NHP) Models ... 220
3.3 Controlled Human Malaria Infection (CHMI) ... 220
4 Antigens Which Have Entered Clinical Trials ... 221
4.1 Apical Membrane Antigen 1 (AMA1) ... 221
4.2 Merozoite Surface Protein 1 (MSP1) ... 222
4.3 Merozoite Surface Protein 3 (MSP3) ... 223
4.4 Serine Repeat Antigen 5 (SERA5/SE36) ... 224
4.5 Combination Vaccines ... 224
4.6 Other Antigens Which Have Entered Clinical Trials ... 225
5 Future Prospects: A Personal View ... 226
5.1 Blood-Stage Antigens Which Are More 'Antibody Sensitive' ... 227
5.2 New Vaccine Technologies of Relevance to BSV Development ... 229
5.3 Candidate Prioritisation ... 229
6 Concluding Remarks ... 230
References ... 231

Electronic supplementary material: The online version of this chapter (doi:10.1007/978-3-319-45210-4_11) contains supplementary material, which is available to authorized users.

A.D. Douglas (✉)
Nuffield Department of Medicine, Jenner Institute, University of Oxford, Oxford OX3 7DQ, UK
e-mail: sandy.douglas@ndm.ox.ac.uk

M.M. Mota, A. Rodriguez (eds.), *Malaria*, DOI 10.1007/978-3-319-45210-4_11

1 Introduction

As has been reviewed in Chap. 3 of this book and elsewhere, malaria infection results in immune responses against the parasite's asexual blood-stage which are capable of protecting against clinical disease [1, 2]. In particular, seminal human passive transfer studies demonstrated that naturally acquired IgG antibodies are capable of clearing blood-stage *P. falciparum* parasites, independent of other donor immune effectors or the action of antibody against other parasite life-cycle stages [3, 4]. It has long been considered that the development of an immunogen capable of eliciting a response mimicking this effect is one of the most attractive approaches to an efficacious malaria vaccine. A further attraction of the approach is the potential for 'natural boosting', i.e. the reinforcement of partial or waning vaccine-induced immunity by exposure of the individual to sub-clinical blood-stage infection. This attraction has been brought into particularly sharp focus by recent concerns regarding rapid waning of the immunity of the RTS,S vaccine and age-shifting of clinical disease by interventions such as RTS,S which may reduce the development of blood-stage immunity [5, 6].

Balancing these arguments in favour of the blood-stage vaccine (BSV) approach is a series of challenges. BSV developers share a series of problems with those targeting other parasite life-cycle stages—notably the difficulties associated with producing conformationally accurate recombinant *Plasmodium* spp. antigens and accessing immunogenic adjuvants with which to formulate them [7, 8]. There are, however, additional challenges which are, perhaps, more prominent in the blood-stage field than elsewhere. The principal disadvantage, of course, of attempting to emulate natural immunity to a parasite which establishes chronic and repeated infection is that the parasite has well-evolved immune evasion mechanisms. Antigenic polymorphism among the major parasite molecules on the infected RBC (iRBC) surface is of a different order of magnitude from that among other parasite molecules, notably via the *var* multi-gene family encoding *Plasmodium falciparum* erythrocyte membrane protein-1 (PfEMP1) proteins [9]. Although the extent of diversity among the merozoite antigens which have been the major targets of BSV development is less than that among iRBC-surface antigens, antigenic polymorphism has been a critical obstacle which has hindered the BSV field to a much greater extent than it has affected pre-erythrocytic or transmission-blocking vaccines. This problem may have been inadvertently exacerbated by the focus of the field upon merozoite surface protein 1 (MSP1) and apical membrane antigen-1 (AMA1), both of which were originally identified via their immunogenicity in the context of exposure of rodents to whole *Plasmodium* spp. parasites [10–12]. It is perhaps unsurprising that the parasite has evolved in such a way that the immuno-dominant antigens of its chronically infecting, high biomass stage are challenging targets for vaccine developers.

A second challenge for the blood-stage field (and in particular for approaches dependent upon anti-merozoite antibody) arises from the brief window of extracellular exposure of the merozoite and the resulting kinetic constraints upon antibody binding to the parasite. Although the duration of this period in vivo is not accurately known, in vitro video-microscopy suggests a period of around 60 s [13, 14]. Given that the rate of binding of antibody to antigen (or, in other terms, the half-life of unbound antigen after exposure to antibody) is determined largely by the product of antibody concentration and the antibody–antigen association rate constant, relatively simple biophysical calculations can demonstrate that high antibody concentrations are essential in order to complex the majority of antigen within the available time [15]. Empirical data suggests that (at least using the immunogens studied to date) monoclonal antibody concentrations in excess of 10 μg/mL or polyclonal antibody concentrations in excess of 50 μg/mL are needed to neutralise >50 % of parasites in the widely used in vitro assay of growth inhibitory activity (GIA) [16–19]; concentrations of anti-merozoite antibody required to achieve protection against *P. falciparum* in vivo appear to be well in excess of 100 μg/mL [20, 21]. Although current vaccine technologies can achieve such levels of antigen-specific antibody in the short term (weeks to a few months), they cannot sustain them over a period of years. Success in the blood-stage field therefore appears likely to require either a step-change in immunogenicity via advances in adjuvant/formulation technology, the identification of merozoite targets with substantially different antibody concentration-effect relationships from those previously studied, or a change from anti-merozoite antibody-based approaches to completely different strategies such as those targeting the iRBC surface.

Subunit BSV development began more than 35 years ago [12]. Clinical evaluation of various blood-stage candidates has been ongoing for around 25 years [22]. Trials of at least five candidates have produced 'efficacy signals', typically involving secondary endpoints and typically not reproduced by follow-up studies [23–28]. In contrast, to the author's knowledge, no BSV has demonstrated reproducible or clinically meaningful efficacy as assessed using a pre-specified primary endpoint. BSV development is not currently a funding priority for the PATH Malaria Vaccine Initiative (which is explicitly focussing upon pre-erythrocytic and transmission-blocking approaches). Although other funders continue to support the field, BSV investigators face a tough financial environment at the same time as they attempt to confront thorny scientific challenges. It is striking that the number of publications of BSV clinical trials has dwindled in recent years (Fig. 1).

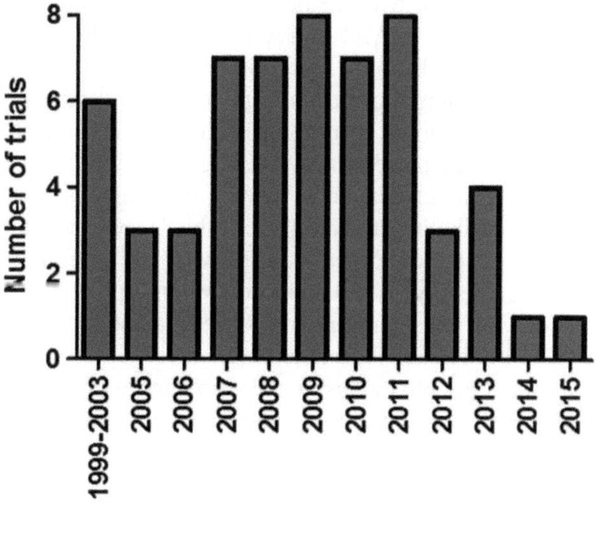

Fig. 1 Number of BSV clinical trials by year of publication. The number of original publications reporting clinical trials of BSV candidates is shown. Data drawn from Supplementary Table 1

At this difficult time for the BSV field, this chapter will attempt to review both past and current BSV development efforts, and briefly look forward at the prospects for overcoming these challenges.

2 Mechanisms of BSV-Inducible Protection: Effectors and Assessment

For an in-depth review of the immunological response to blood-stage infection, readers are referred to the chapter by Cockburn. This section aims to provide a brief overview of the variety of vaccine-inducible immune effector mechanisms which might confer protection against blood-stage infection or disease, and, linked to this, a summary of the experimental systems available for the assessment and prioritisation of vaccine candidates thought to act via each mechanism.

2.1 Naturally Acquired Immunity, Non-Natural Immunity, Markers and Causes of Protection

Given the lack of BSV candidates with unambiguous clinical efficacy, it is clear that there cannot yet be any validated immunological surrogate of BSV protection. Instead, possible links between each immunological effector and in vivo protection of humans are supported by a variety of sources of evidence, all of them imperfect.

It seems likely that more than one immunological mechanism contributes causally to naturally acquired immunity (NAI) [1, 2]. It is certainly clear that multiple immune responses are *associated* with NAI—but, given that these responses tend to correlate with exposure and each other, it is difficult to unpick which responses are *markers* and which are *causes* of protection.

Pregnancy provides a natural 'experiment' in which it is thought that previously acquired anti-PfEMP1 responses become ineffective due to the expression of the pregnancy-specific VAR2CSA antigen [29]. This appears to be sufficient for pregnant women to become susceptible to placental malaria (these women presumably retain something close to their previous level of anti-merozoite immunity, do not become susceptible to non-placental malaria, and clear parasitemia rapidly after delivery of the placenta) [29]. Along with other strands of evidence, this is a fairly strong argument that anti-PfEMP1 immunity is a major contributor—if not *the* major contributor—to NAI [30]. If this is the case, blood-stage vaccine approaches directed to targets other than PfEMP1 are attempting to induce a 'non-natural' immune phenotype, and many of the sero-epidemiological efforts to associate protection with anti-merozoite responses may be focussed upon non-causal markers of NAI or minor contributors to NAI.

Mimicking NAI is just one possible route to a BSV. It seems reasonable to think that there may be multiple valid routes via which subunit vaccines might protect, most of them aiming to induce 'non-natural' responses which differ in quality or quantity from that seen in NAI. If this is the case, it is quite possible that, in time, very different responses measured in different assays could each prove to be valid surrogates of protection. It is also important to acknowledge that responses which are *not* associated with naturally acquired protection could prove protective if induced in greater quantity/quality. Conversely, some responses which do make minor causal contributions to NAI may not be sufficient to protect if induced by subunit vaccination in the absence of the other contributors to NAI.

Many roads may lead to an effective BSV. At present we do not know which of the roads being followed by the community are 'dead ends'—effector mechanisms which might contribute to protection in some settings but cannot be induced by vaccination in sufficient quantity or quality to achieve protection. We are far from knowing which is the 'route of least resistance', i.e. the protective immune response which can most readily be induced and maintained in sufficient quantity by available vaccination platforms.

2.2 Fc-Receptor-Independent Merozoite Neutralisation by Antibody

In vitro assays of the effect of anti-parasite antibodies upon a simple culture comprising parasite-infected and uninfected red cells (and lacking complement or Fc-receptor-bearing immune effector cells) have been used for many years and have recently been reviewed elsewhere [31, 32]. The assay of 'growth inhibitory activity' (GIA) has been widely used and, importantly, methodology for this assay was standardised by Long and colleagues and, for a number of years, made available to the community via the PATH-MVI GIA reference laboratory [18]. Although antibodies against antigens with a variety of subcellular localisations and with a variety of modes of action upon the parasite can exert GIA, the assay has been used principally to evaluate vaccine candidates which induce antibody acting upon antigens on the merozoite surface and involved in the invasion of parasites into RBCs.

It is contentious whether the activity measured by the assay of GIA makes a significant contribution to naturally acquired protection [33]. Strikingly, however, observations that antibodies against the AMA1 and RH5 antigens mediated Fc-independent in vitro parasite neutralisation led to the prioritisation of these molecules as vaccine candidates, and in both cases proved to be predictive of the ability of vaccines based upon them to induce in vivo protection in non-human primates [10, 20, 34, 35]. Moreover, strong relationships between vaccine-induced GIA and protection have been observed in non-human primate studies [20, 36]. Efforts are currently under way to ascertain whether in vitro GIA is also predictive of the protective capacity of passively transferred monoclonal antibodies in the *Aotus* model (the author's unpublished work).

On current evidence, it seems at least plausible that a sufficient level of parasite neutralising activity could be protective in vivo; there is considerably greater doubt about the quantitative relationship between GIA and protection. It seems naïve to expect that 50 % GIA under a given set of in vitro conditions would predict a 50 % reduction in the in vivo parasite multiplication rate. Indeed, recent controlled human malaria infection (CHMI) trials suggest that induction of antibody responses capable of achieving 50 % in vitro GIA at a physiological antibody concentration has no detectable effect upon in vivo PMR [21, 25]. Vaccinologists targeting other pathogens are familiar with the idea that protection is often attained when the in vivo antibody concentration is many-fold higher than that which achieves a prescribed level of activity in an in vitro assay: for example, protection is known to correlate with a serum neutralisation titer of 1/4 to 1/8 for polio, or a hemagglutination inhibition titer of 1/40 for influenza [37]. The situation may well be similar for the relationship between GIA and protection: the ability of antibody to achieve 50 % GIA at 1/5 of the in vivo concentration was found to be predictive of efficacy of an RH5 vaccine in *Aotus* [20]. One might speculate that this could readily arise from differences in the speed of invasion in vitro and in vivo, altering the kinetic constraints upon antibody–antigen binding (see above).

Although a certain level of GIA-inducing antibody is naturally acquired, it seems that protection which is largely dependent upon GIA will require the induction by vaccines of a level of this activity substantially higher than that observed in most naturally exposed- and NAI-protected- individuals. It remains unclear what 'GIA_{50}' titer would predict protection in humans—or whether levels of antibody sufficient to achieve this can be attained with current vaccine/adjuvant technology.

2.3 Fc-Receptor-Dependent Activity of Anti-Merozoite Antibodies

The relative ease of measurement and conceptual simplicity of direct parasite neutralisation by antibody contrasts with the considerably more complex field of investigation around Fc-receptor (FcR) dependent anti-merozoite antibody activity. A variety of in vitro assays have been developed, measuring a variety of effector mechanisms induced by the ligation of FcR by antibody-merozoite complexes (Table 1).

Activity in all of these assays has been associated with natural immunity to malaria [38, 40, 42, 43]. It is less clear whether this association arises because these activities are simply readily measured markers of a broad and strong anti-malaria antibody response, or whether they play a substantial causal role in protection, independent of other immune effectors. It is worth noting that the ADRB and phagocytosis assays do not measure effects upon parasite multiplication, but instead use the parasites almost as 'antigen beads'. The ADCI assay is conceptually attractive but has proven challenging for many laboratories to implement in a robust and reproducible fashion, hindering its widespread adoption [32].

Table 1 Assays of FcR-dependent activity of anti-merozoite antibody

Assay	Conditions	Effector mechanism	Typical readout
Antibody dependent cellular inhibition (ADCI) [38]	Culture of parasites, red cells, antibody and human monocytes	Soluble mediators, e.g. TNFα released by monocytes upon FcR engagement with antibody-bound merozoite [39]	Parasite growth
Antibody dependent respiratory burst (ADRB) [40]	Mixture of frozen parasites, antibody and human neutrophils	Reactive oxygen species (ROS) produced by neutrophils upon FcR engagement with antibody-bound merozoite	Magnitude of ROS production
Merozoite opsonisation/ phagocytosis assays [41, 42]	Mixture of purified merozoites with antibody and human monocytes or PBMCs	Phagocytosis of antibody-bound merozoites	Percentage of phagocytes containing merozoites

A further Fc-dependent (though FcR-independent) effector mechanism which has recently attracted increasing interest is the fixation of complement by merozoite-binding antibody [44]; once again, such activity has been associated with NAI but convincing evidence of complement-dependent in vivo vaccine efficacy has not yet been presented.

It seems possible that the various assays outlined above are measuring multiple downstream effects of similar upstream events (namely the binding of non-neutralising antibody to the merozoite). Clear demonstration that such non-neutralising antibody can achieve protection in vivo—in the absence of GIA-inducing antibody or other effectors—would seem to be of considerable importance for those involved in this area of BSV research.

2.4 *Antibody Against iRBC-Surface Antigens*

iRBC-surface antigens, including the PfEMP1, Rifin, and Stevor families, may well be the principal targets of naturally acquired immunity to malaria [45, 46], as has been particularly clearly shown in the case of pregnancy-associated malaria [47]. Antibodies recognising these antigens may act by a variety of mechanisms including blockade of cyto-adherence and opsonisation resulting in phagocytosis, and different assays capable of measuring these activities in vitro have been reported [48, 49].

Unlike the brief window of exposure of merozoite antigens, iRBC surface antigens are exposed to circulating antibody for several hours during the trophozoite and schizont stages of each intra-erythrocytic parasite multiplication cycle. As a result, antibodies binding these antigens have plentiful time in which to reach equilibrium, and hence relatively low concentrations of antibody will achieve high levels of antigen saturation; 50 % antigen saturation will be achieved by a typical antibody with an equilibrium monovalent binding constant of 10 nM at a concentration of only 1.5 μg/mL (or less, in the event of bivalent binding). Such concentrations are readily attained—and maintained for several years—by modern subunit vaccine/adjuvant approaches.

While the potential for efficacy at relatively low antibody concentrations is an attraction of the iRBC-surface targeting approach, the major challenge it faces is the extreme variability of these antigens. This will be discussed further in the section covering specific PfEMP1-targeting approaches.

2.5 T Cell Responses Against the Blood-Stage

For any antibody-mediated mechanism of protection, it is quite likely that $CD4^+$ T cells will play a role in the causal chain leading to protection (via help for B cell responses). Given that the first generation of asexual merozoites are produced in the liver (and the fact that many 'blood-stage' antigens are in fact also expressed by sporozoites [50]), it is also quite possible that $CD8^+$ T cells reacting to antigens generally considered to be 'blood-stage' could contribute to pre-erythrocytic protection [51].

The possibility that T cell responses themselves may be proximate causes of protection against blood-stage parasite multiplication, independent of antibody, has also attracted the interest of BSV developers. With the exception of the results of a controlled human infection study which was later found to be seriously compromised by persistent anti-malarial drug [52, 53], data to support this possibility has come largely from rodent malaria models of infection. The elegant work of Langhorne and colleagues in the *P. chabaudi* model has demonstrated that infection-induced immunity is contributed to by cytokines including IFNγ, IL-10 and IL-22 which are produced by $CD4^+$ and $CD8^+$ T cells [54–56]. A role for cytotoxic $CD8^+$ T-cell killing of *P. yoelii*-infected MHC-I-expressing erythroblasts via Fas ligation has also been demonstrated, although it is doubtful this mechanism could contribute to control of *P. falciparum* in non-MHC-I-expressing mature RBCs [57].

It remains unclear whether the induction by a subunit vaccine of a T cell response against a blood-stage antigen, in the absence of a protective antibody response, could mediate clinically meaningful protection against *P. falciparum* in humans. The principal subunit vaccine approach which has been explored as a possible means of achieving such an effect has been the use of DNA and viral vector vaccines expressing MSP1 and AMA1 antigens. Depletion and adoptive transfer experiments suggested a statistically significant but relatively modest role for vaccine-induced $CD4^+$ cells in protecting against *P. chabaudi* after vaccination with viral vectors expressing PcAMA1 [58]. Clinical trials with adenovirus and poxvirus vectors have not demonstrated significant efficacy against the blood stage, despite the induction of robust T cell responses as assessed using ELISPOT and flow cytometric assays [59]. Sterile protection of a small number of volunteers after immunisation with a DNA prime-adenovirus boost regime combining CSP and AMA1 has been reported: although this was reported to be associated with cellular responses to the AMA1 component, this observation arose from an exploratory analysis which has not been reproduced, and it is unclear whether the observed protection was mediated at the liver or blood stage [60]. To the author's knowledge, no new subunit vaccines designed to act primarily via direct T cell effects against the blood-stage have entered clinical trials or advanced pre-clinical development in recent years or are projected to do so in the near future.

3 Assessing and Prioritising BSVs In Vivo

3.1 Mouse Models

Candidate BSVs have been extensively evaluated in rodent malaria models. The commonly used model species—*P. yoelii*, *P. chabaudi*, and *P. berghei*—were originally isolated from African thicket rats (i.e. the mouse, *Mus musculus*, is not their natural host). They differ from each other and from *P. falciparum* in important respects relevant to BSV development, notably differing patterns of cytoadherence, erythrocyte invasion receptor-ligand usage and circulation of viable extra-cellular 'latent merozoites' [61, 62]. Some BSV concepts simply cannot be tested in rodent malaria models due to the absence of direct rodent malaria homologues of the target antigens (notably PfRH5 and PfEMP1).

Where homologues do exist, testing of BSV candidates in these models is commonly undertaken, but it is not clear how the results should be interpreted. In short, a large number of MSP1 and AMA1 formulations have been shown to be protective against *P. yoelii* and *P. chabaudi*—yet wherever equivalent *P. falciparum* formulations have been evaluated in Phase IIa/b clinical trials, they have failed to achieve clinically meaningful protection. It has therefore been argued that these models are not particularly stringent tests of the protective potential of a candidate formulation [63]. The *P. berghei* blood-stage model, in contrast, is highly stringent—to the point that there are very limited numbers of reports of formulations achieving protection in this model, none of which have, to the author's knowledge, been replicated outside the original laboratory [63].

'Humanised mouse' models of the *P. falciparum* blood-stage are now available, offering a variety of ways to bring together *P. falciparum* infected human RBCs (provided either by infusion of human RBCs or produced by transferred human haematopoietic stem cells [hHSCs]) and vaccine-induced immune effectors (provided either by passive transfer of antibodies, or in situ active responses derived from hHSCs) [64]. Although rapid development continues, these models do not yet fully recapitulate the interaction of the parasite with a normal host (i.e. with normal immunity, erythropoiesis and human RBC haematocrit). As a result of this (coupled with the relative ease of studying the *P. falciparum* blood-stage in vitro as compared to the liver-stage) humanised mice have yet to find quite as central a role in BSV development as they now occupy in the liver-stage field. One might speculate that they may play a valuable future role in modelling the *P. vivax* blood-stage, which remains challenging to study in vitro.

3.2 Non-Human Primate (NHP) Models

A series of elegant studies—notably by the late Bill Collins—established New World monkeys (*Aotus* and *Saimiri* spp.) as models of the *P. falciparum* and *P. vivax* blood stages [65, 66]. Unlike humanised mice, NHPs offer the opportunity to study the pathogen in the context of a fully immunocompetent host. Largely because 'clinical-grade' (cGMP) vaccine material is not needed, such studies can be performed considerably more rapidly and with lesser resources than clinical trials, although there are only a few centres globally with access to these models. There is clearly a substantial ethical responsibility upon investigators to design NHP studies with care, and a commensurate regulatory burden upon the use of the model. It is also important to note that some aspects of human–pathogen interaction are probably not fully recapitulated in these models.

The potential role of these models in making go/no-go decisions on the path of a BSV candidate towards clinical trial has previously been debated in depth [67, 68]. In the case of GIA-inducing vaccines (principally targeting AMA1 and MSP1), the negative predictive value of the model seems reasonable: vaccine formulations which failed to protect in the *Aotus* model have failed to protect in clinical trials. The positive predictive value is less clear: to the author's knowledge, only one human-compatible BSV formulation has demonstrated statistically significant protection in non-human primates, and has not yet reached clinical efficacy trials [20]. Where GIA *is* thought likely to be the primary mechanism of a candidate's action, it could be argued that outperformance of the current leading candidate in this model (and in vitro studies) is a reasonable pre-requisite for clinical progression.

Fewer NHP studies have been performed for vaccines thought to act via mechanisms other than GIA. It is, perhaps, worth noting that NHPs provide particular opportunities to dissect the contribution of different immune effectors to protection—including the ability to perform antibody passive transfer, depletion of cellular subsets, and cytokine blockade within the context of an otherwise normal immune system—which are difficult to replicate in human or humanised mouse studies. This opportunity for mechanistic studies has yet to be fully exploited by the field and may be of particular value in building the case for vaccines acting via less widely accepted effector mechanisms.

3.3 Controlled Human Malaria Infection (CHMI)

Mosquito-bite CHMI has long enjoyed a pivotal role in the evaluation of pre-erythrocytic vaccine candidates [69, 70]: in contrast to field trials, CHMI studies typically involve <50 participants and are completed within 6 months, allowing the safe, cost-effective and rapid discrimination of promising candidates from those with insufficient efficacy. There has, however, been a degree of doubt about the value of CHMI studies for the evaluation of BSV candidates, leading several candidates to advance to field studies without demonstrating efficacy in CHMI.

One strand of this argument has related to the belief that BSV immunity may be detectable only at high levels of parasitemia which cannot be studied in CHMI studies (in which participants receive anti-malarial treatment as soon as parasitemia is microscopically patent). In particular, it has been proposed that ADCI may provide a parasite 'density-dependent' mechanism of parasite control, which would not be detected in CHMI [71]. Measurement of sub-patent parasite growth in naturally immune adults suggests that NAI, at least, *is* active in the sub-patent period [72]. Moreover, there is no obvious reason to suppose that GIA should be density dependent, and NHP data is suggestive that GIA-inducing BSVs are efficacious in the pre-patent period [20].

A second problem relating to the use of CHMI for BSV evaluation relates to the lesser ability of mosquito-bite CHMI studies to detect partial BSV effects than to detect partial pre-erythrocytic effects. Although blood-stage parasite multiplication rate (PMR) after mosquito-bite challenge can be quantified by combining quantitative polymerase chain reaction (qPCR) data with simple curve-fitting techniques, there are large uncertainties in such estimates, arising from the fact that the liver-to-blood inoculum is not accurately known and the duration of blood-stage replication is typically only two to three blood-stage cycles [73]. Blood-stage CHMI—in which a small and known number of iRBCs from an infected donor are injected IV into vaccinated challengees—largely overcomes this problem, providing accurate estimation of PMRs and greatly enhanced statistical power to detect partial BSV-induced immunity [21, 74, 75]. The power provided by such a study including 15 vaccinees and 15 controls is sufficient to detect PMR reductions of around 30 % [21]; it is doubtful that PMR reductions of less than this magnitude would be clinically meaningful.

A recent blood-stage CHMI study has considerably clarified the discussion around the potential efficacy of a BSV candidate which had produced ambiguous efficacy signals in mosquito-bite CHMI and field trials [21, 24, 25]. The author's view is that field efficacy trials of BSV are now hard to justify without prior demonstration of efficacy against CHMI.

4 Antigens Which Have Entered Clinical Trials

Supplementary Table 1 sets out all clinical trials of subunit vaccines including BSV components of which the author is aware. Antigens which have entered clinical trials are each briefly considered in the following section.

4.1 Apical Membrane Antigen 1 (AMA1)

AMA1 is implicated in erythrocyte invasion, and is among the best studied targets of Fc-independent antibody neutralisation (i.e. GIA-inducing vaccine approaches). A wide variety of AMA1 formulations have been evaluated in rodent, NHP, Phase

I, Phase IIa and Phase IIb clinical studies [34, 76, 77] (see also Supplementary Table 1). Of the AMA1 candidates which have reached clinical trial, the one which has appeared most promising has been FMP2.1, a mono-allelic *E. coli*-produced protein formulated with GlaxoSmithKline's AS01 or AS02 adjuvants [25, 78]. The immunogenicity of the formulation is excellent, attaining AMA1 specific IgG concentrations well in excess of 100 μg/mL in many volunteers [21, 25]. Efficacy against vaccine-homologous parasites was reported in a Phase IIb field study, but this was a secondary analysis and the result was of relatively weak statistical significance ($p=0.03$) [24]. A subsequent blood-stage CHMI study showed no trend towards a PMR reduction in vaccinees as compared to controls, although antibody responses in this study (conducted in UK adults) were lower than previously seen in US adults or Malian children, possibly explaining the discrepancy with the Phase IIb results [21].

Ongoing development of AMA1-based vaccines appears to face twin difficulties: a quantitative challenge, relating to the exceptionally high AMA1 concentration which seems to be necessary to achieve protection even against vaccine-homologous parasites, and a qualitative challenge, relating to overcoming the antigen's high level of polymorphism among parasite strains. The most promising recent effort to tackle the former has involved a structure-based approach in which an AMA1—RON2-peptide complex is used as an immunogen: this appears to reduce the concentration of induced antibody needed to attain a given level of GIA [79]. A variety of approaches to tackle AMA1 antigenic diversity are also being explored, including multi-allelic immunisation, the generation of 'immunodampening' antigens in which polymorphic residues are mutated to glycine, alanine or serine, and the design of 'diversity covering' (DiCo) protein combinations consisting of chimeric proteins which together include the majority of variants at each locus present in circulating parasites [17, 80, 81]. A Phase I trial of the DiCo approach is currently in progress (clinicaltrials.gov identifier NCT02014727).

Prospects for the future success of AMA1 vaccines depend upon bringing together solutions for both of the challenges discussed above. If this can be achieved, the protein's high immunogenicity in the context of natural infection—which led to its initial identification, and probably also to one of its main weaknesses, i.e. problematic polymorphism—may become an asset in that there is clear evidence for infection-induced boosting of vaccine-induced anti-AMA1 responses, potentially aiding in the maintenance of efficacy [20].

4.2 *Merozoite Surface Protein 1 (MSP1)*

Like AMA1, MSP1 has been a leading BSV candidate antigen since the early 1980s, primarily as a result of the fact that anti-MSP1 responses are readily induced by infection in rodent models of infection. Most attention has focussed upon the relatively conserved C-terminal $MSP1_{42}$ and $MSP1_{19}$ fragments, which have been studied mostly as targets of Fc-independent merozoite neutralisation (GIA). Similar to AMA1, MSP1 candidates have proven protective in NHP models, but only when formulated with Freund's adjuvant and only against vaccine-homologous parasites—in other words, MSP1 and AMA1 share a need to reach extreme antibody titers to achieve protection, and a problem of antigenic variability (though the latter is perhaps a lesser issue for the MSP1 C-terminus) [82].

Excluding combination vaccines (see below) two $MSP1_{42}$ formulations have reached Phase II trial, with neither proving efficacious (one of these, a viral-vectored formulation, had yielded results suggesting efficacy in a pilot study which were not replicated in a subsequent larger Phase IIa trial) [28, 59, 83].

Although MSP1 has been investigated mostly as a GIA-inducing candidate, it is a major constituent of the surface coat of the merozoite and hence a tempting target for FcR-dependent antibody activity; this approach, and the use of the full-length MSP1 ectodomain (which is polymorphic, but can now be expressed in heterologous protein production systems) are relatively unexplored [84, 85].

4.3 *Merozoite Surface Protein 3 (MSP3)*

MSP3 has been investigated principally as a target of ADCI. In the absence of MSP3 homologues in rodent malarias, much of the evidence in support of its candidacy comes from sero-epidemiological studies of NAI [86]. As discussed above, many laboratories have found the ADCI assay difficult to implement in reproducible form. The *P. falciparum*—SCID mouse—human erythrocyte infusion model has provided further support for the antigen, but like ADCI, is technically challenging and has not been adopted widely [87].

In NHP challenge studies, full-length MSP3 formulated with Freund's adjuvant has demonstrated a degree of protection against vaccine-homologous parasites [88, 89]. It is, however, worth noting that, unlike similar studies with a number of other leading candidates, no MSP3 vaccinated NHPs were able to self-cure parasitemia (all 'protected' animals required treatment for anaemia).

Two MSP3-based candidates have entered clinical trials. MSP3 'long synthetic peptide' is, as the name suggests, a chemically synthesised 96 amino acid fragment of the antigen, which has been tested in formulation with aluminium hydroxide adjuvant in Phase Ia and Phase Ib studies (Supplementary Table 1). A secondary analysis of a small Phase Ib study, presented in a single-page follow-up article, suggested efficacy of the candidate against clinical malaria [26]. Given the nature of this analysis and the lack of supporting NHP, CHMI or external-laboratory preclinical data for this candidate, it is difficult to interpret this result without replication in a further study with efficacy as the primary endpoint.

A region of MSP3 also forms part of the 'GMZ2' BSV candidate, which is a fusion protein expressed in Lactococcus and also including part of the glutamate rich protein (GLURP). GMZ2 has entered Phase I trials formulated with alum, again with a rationale founded mostly upon sero-epidemiological data and ADCI.

4.4 Serine Repeat Antigen 5 (SERA5/SE36)

SE36 is an immunogen derived from the N-terminal P47 fragment of the SERA5 protein [90]. SERA5 is secreted into the parasitophorous vacuole in late blood-stage development, followed by proteolytic processing around the time of parasite egress, leaving the P47 fragment associated with the merozoite surface [91]. Antigenic polymorphism in the regions included in SE36 appears modest (12 SNPs across 445 isolates in one report) [92]. There are multiple reports that antibodies against it can mediate GIA in vitro and protection against parasite challenge in vivo in NHPs [90]. In prospectively specified follow-up analysis of a Phase Ib trial in Uganda, SE36 formulated with alum appeared to mediate efficacy against clinical malaria [27]. As others have recently commented, this result deserves further study in a Phase II trial, or possibly blood-stage CHMI [32]. Given the relatively modest potency of alum, there is likely to be considerable scope for improvement upon the immunogenicity of SE36 by formulation with other adjuvants.

4.5 Combination Vaccines

A number of clinical trials of multi-antigen malaria vaccines have included one or more blood-stage immunogen (Supplementary Table 1). Of these, the early candidate SPf66 is now generally regarded to have been ineffective [22]. The NMRC-M3V-D/Ad-PfCA candidate displayed possible efficacy in a Phase IIa study which has not subsequently been replicated, and which may have been directed against the pre-erythrocytic stage [60].

The most extensively evaluated combination BSV candidate was 'Combination B', comprising MSP1, MSP2 and RESA antigens formulated in Montanide ISA720 adjuvant. In a Phase IIb study, a reduction in parasite density was observed in one group of the study, along with a reduction in prevalence of parasites expressing the 3D7 (vaccine-homologous) MSP2 allele [23]. The relatively complex design of the study and the multiple analyses conducted make the interpretation of these results challenging, and the study has not been replicated. The effect observed was not of sufficient magnitude to be clinically meaningful, and indeed there was a trend towards higher incidence of clinical malaria in vaccinees as compared to controls [23].

4.6 Other Antigens Which Have Entered Clinical Trials

There has been intense interest in recent years in the erythrocyte binding antigen (EBA) and reticulocyte binding protein homolog (RH) antigen families, stemming largely from investigation of the ligand–receptor interactions implicated in merozoite-erythrocyte invasion [93, 94]. EBA-175 was the first member of these families to attract substantial interest as a vaccine candidate, reaching NHP studies (in which it appeared to achieve modest efficacy) and a Phase Ia clinical trial [95, 96]. Enthusiasm for EBA-175 as a mono-valent vaccine candidate has, however, been dampened by the realisation that it is non-essential in some parasite strains due to invasion ligand redundancy [97].

More recently, RH5 was identified an apparently essential member of the RH family, followed soon after by the demonstrations that it mediates an essential ligand–receptor interaction with the host protein basigin and is susceptible to vaccine-inducible strain-transcending neutralising antibody [35, 98, 99]. Interestingly, the RH proteins are homologs of the *P. yoelii* Py235 protein family, which were among the earliest identified BSV candidates (along with MSP1 and AMA1) [12]. RH5, however, differs from these other candidates in important respects: it does not appear to be particularly immunogenic in the context of natural infection, and it is highly antigenically conserved [19, 35]. Unlike other BSV candidates, RH5 has been shown to protect NHPs against challenge with a vaccine-heterologous parasite, including in a human-compatible vaccine formulation [20]. Clinical trials of viral-vector and protein-adjuvant RH5 vaccine formulations are under way (ClinicalTrials.gov identifiers NCT02181088 and NCT02927145).

Despite the apparent advantages of RH5 over previous candidates, substantial difficulties remain. The concentrations of anti-RH5 antibody required to neutralise parasites in vitro and for protection in NHPs appear somewhat lower than with anti-AMA1 but remain substantial [19, 20]. Achieving these in humans—let alone maintaining them for the duration of one or more malaria transmission seasons—will be a considerable challenge unless there are major advances in adjuvant/formulation technology. Efforts are therefore underway to achieve protection via the induction and maintenance of more manageable antibody concentrations, by focusing the response onto protective epitopes and by seeking synergistic parasite neutralisation assisted by antibodies against other antigens [19].

Trophozoite exported protein 1 (Tex1) was identified on the basis of in silico predictions that it would adopt an alpha-helical coiled coil structure, which it was argued was a desirable characteristic in a vaccine candidate [100]. P27A, a fragment of Tex1, has been noted to induce ADCI [101], and has recently entered Phase I trials (Clinicaltrials.gov identifier NCT01949909). As far as the author is aware, it has not been shown to induce protection in any in vivo challenge model.

Finally, a viral-vector vaccine targeting *Plasmodium vivax* Duffy-binding protein (DBP) has recently entered a Phase I trial (Clinicaltrials.gov identifier NCT01816113). The development of *P. vivax* BSVs is discussed in Box 1.

Box 1: *P. vivax* BSVs

There is increasing interest in the development of vaccines targeting *P. vivax*, which is both more geographically widespread than *P. falciparum* and—due to differing vector ecology and the existence of the dormant hypnozoite stage—more difficult to control using existing techniques [102]. Despite this, *P. vivax* has attracted only a small fraction of the research effort and expenditure devoted to *P. falciparum*.

P. vivax BSV developers face further obstacles in addition to those familiar from the *P. falciparum* field. In vitro culture of the *P. vivax* blood-stage is difficult, largely due to the parasite's preference for immature RBCs. Strenuous efforts have been made to develop in vitro culture systems, typically via approaches which enrich reticulocytes in the culture [8]. Nonetheless, *P. vivax* growth/invasion inhibition assays remain challenging and can only be performed by a few laboratories [103]. NHP studies are slightly more challenging than for *P. falciparum*, as splenectomy is usually necessary in order to achieve consistent parasitemia in *Aotus* or *Saimiri* [104] (it is worth noting, though, that the closely related parasite *P. cynomolgi*, which infects macaques, provides an alternative NHP model [105]). Finally, mosquito-bite CHMI with *P. vivax* is complicated by the need to avoid hypnozoite-driven relapses and the fact that it is not currently possible to obtain mosquitoes carrying *P. vivax* of a known genotype [106, 107]. There is an opportunity to circumvent these problems—and allow more accurate assessment of *P. vivax* BSV efficacy—by the development of an inoculum suitable for *P. vivax* blood-stage CHMI studies.

The most advanced *P. vivax* BSV candidate—and indeed the only candidate to enter clinical trials to date—is the region II (RII) fragment of the Duffy-binding protein (DBP). This antigen, which is structurally related to the *P. falciparum* EBA family, mediates an interaction with the Duffy-antigen Receptor for Chemokines (DARC) host protein. Individuals and populations who are Duffy-antigen-negative (such as the majority of Africans) are resistant to *P. vivax* [108]. Antibodies to DBP inhibit erythrocyte invasion, and DBP-RII formulated in Freund's antigen is protective against *P. vivax* challenge of *Aotus* [109, 110]. The formulation which has entered Phase Ia clinical trial consists of adenovirus and poxvirus vectors expressing DBP-RII (Clinicaltrials.gov identifier NCT01816113) [111].

5 Future Prospects: A Personal View

As outlined above, no BSV candidate has yet achieved unambiguous and reproducible efficacy in a clinical trial. Even in NHP models, extreme antibody titers are needed to attain protection, and only RH5 has demonstrated efficacy against a vaccine-heterologous challenge [20]. Recent experience with the RTS,S vaccine's rapidly waning efficacy and immunogenicity (antibody titers fall by around 90 % in the first year after vaccination [112]) suggests that even candidates which *do* achieve protection against challenges conducted a few weeks after vaccination but are dependent upon extreme antibody titers may face disappointment in field trials.

Difficulties for the field can be divided into those specific to the biology of the *Plasmodium* blood-stage (relating to antigenic polymorphism and the rapid kinetics of merozoite invasion) and those shared with other targets (relating to the expression of antigens in compliance with GMP, and formulation of protein immunogens with appropriate immunostimulating adjuvants). Prospects for tackling each of these obstacles are discussed in the following section.

5.1 Blood-Stage Antigens Which Are More 'Antibody Sensitive'

The antigens for which the relationship between antibody concentration, in vitro effects and in vivo protection have been most closely studied are probably AMA1 and RH5. Both appear to require antigen-specific antibody concentrations substantially in excess of 100 μg/mL to achieve protection (based upon evidence from CHMI and NHP trials, respectively) [20, 21]. There is no known vaccine technology which has been shown to maintain such concentrations in humans over periods of many months. There is therefore a need to identify antigens—or antigen combinations—which can achieve protection with substantially lower total vaccine-induced antibody concentrations, such that those concentrations can realistically be maintained in the medium-to-long-term in human vaccinees.

The sections relating to AMA1 and RH5 above alluded to a number of strategies which are being adopted to try to meet this goal: synergistic antigen combinations, structure-guided focussing of responses upon neutralising epitopes, and structure-guided design of multi-protein complexes which may present more 'native-like' epitopes. In parallel with this, efforts are ongoing to identify other merozoite antigens which may have more favourable antibody concentration—clinical response relationships. Such screens have been greatly facilitated by recent improvements in recombinant protein expression technology [85, 113], but unless it is possible for antigen to 'kill' a merozoite with a very low level of antigen occupancy, kinetic constraints arising from the speed of merozoite invasion seem likely to impose a limit upon the success of this strategy.

An alternative to the identification or improvement of merozoite antigens is to target iRBC-surface antigens. Unlike merozoite antigens, these should be largely free from kinetic constraints and could be protective with very low antibody concentrations (see Sect. 2.4). Understanding of PfEMP1 proteins is steadily advancing—including knowledge about which variants are associated with severe disease, and which features are shared among proteins which were previously seen as intractably variable [30, 114]. A number of PfEMP1-targeting approaches have been explored pre-clinically [49, 115, 116]; this is a complex area but one with potential for transformative developments in coming years. At present, the leading PfEMP1-targeting approach is focussed upon pregnancy-associated malaria (PAM; see Box 2).

Whether targeting merozoite or iRBC surface antigens, a key principle in trying to overcome antigenic variability is to identify an epitope or set of epitopes which are functionally critical (hence vulnerable to blockade by antibody and possibly constrained in their ability to evolve diversity). Typically, such epitopes will not be immuno-dominant in natural infection—otherwise the parasite would be unable to achieve chronic infection. The vaccine developer therefore faces the task of skewing the response in a non-natural way. At the simplest level, of course, this is accomplished by any subunit vaccine. A more challenging task is to skew the response to a particular conserved epitope within a protein with a high overall level of variability. This demands a high degree of knowledge of the structure of antigen-neutralising antibody complexes, as well as antigen engineering approaches (for example, using glycans to mask undesirable epitopes, or displaying the immunogen in a particular orientation on a virus-like particle). Initial attempts to employ such approaches in the BSV field have yielded interesting results [114, 117].

Box 2: Vaccines Against Pregnancy-Associated Malaria (PAM)

As has been reviewed elsewhere, PAM is believed to result from the fact that a woman's first pregnancy makes a new host molecule, chondroitin sulphate A (CSA), available on the placental endothelium [29, 30]. Among its repertoire of PfEMP1 proteins, *P. falciparum* has one ('Var2CSA') which is capable of mediating adhesion to CSA and hence cytoadherence in the placenta. Men and nulligravid women lack anti-Var2CSA responses (probably because the lack of CSA selects strongly against Var2CSA-expressing parasites in non-pregnant hosts), but a protective response is typically acquired by multigravidae [30]. Var2CSA-targeting vaccines aim to protect specifically against PAM by blocking cytoadherence in the placenta, and would therefore be targeted at adolescent girls [118]. They would not be predicted to have any effect against malaria in other contexts.

Challenges for this approach include the lack of an in vivo model of PAM, the large size of the Var2CSA molecule, and antigenic variability within it [118]. As for other PfEMP1-targeting approaches, there is interest in understanding conserved epitopes that may contribute to the design of immunogens capable of inducing strain-transcending responses [119]. The first Var2CSA-targetting vaccines are likely to enter Phase I clinical trials within the coming year (Clinicaltrials.gov identifiers NCT02647489 and NCT02658253).

5.2 New Vaccine Technologies of Relevance to BSV Development

A comprehensive review of vaccine platform technologies which may prove useful in BSV research is clearly beyond the scope of this chapter. It is, however, worth highlighting a few developments which may be of broad interest.

Firstly, protein expression has been a major bottleneck for malaria vaccine developers, particularly when entering GMP antigen production: among other issues *P. falciparum's* AT-rich genome and the presence of (often numerous) disulphide bonds in its proteins have proven problematic for protein expression in E. coli and yeast. Recent work by Gavin Wright and colleagues has demonstrated that transient transfection of mammalian cells is a powerful tool for the production of *P. falciparum* proteins [85]. There is no reason why this approach could not be translated to GMP for proof-of-concept clinical trials.

Secondly, a number of new virus-like particle platforms have been developed recently, some of which have the capacity to display large, folded, conformationally accurate antigens in a chosen orientation—and hence to favour antibody responses to chosen conformational epitopes [120].

Thirdly—and of relevance to the need to induce and maintain extremely high antibody concentrations—it is possible that existing adjuvant platforms may become more widely accessible in future, as GSK's 'adjuvant system' (AS) family begin to come 'off-patent'. Clearly this will depend upon other manufacturers taking the initiative to produce high-quality biosimilar products. In parallel, some interesting novel immunostimulators and antigen-delivery platforms have entered pre-clinical studies: the inter-bilayer cross-linked multi-lamellar vesicle strategy, for example, appears to improve antibody maintenance as compared to other approaches [121].

Finally, vectored immunoprophylaxis (VIP, in which an adeno-associated virus vector is used to drive expression of a chosen monoclonal antibody from within the 'vaccinees' own cells) has the potential to revolutionise vaccine development if it can be proven to be safe, cost-effective and ethically acceptable [122]. VIP has the potential to largely overcome problems of antigenic variability by allowing the expression of a carefully chosen strain-transcending antibody. The approach will, perhaps, be most attractive where the concentration of antibody needed is low, and therefore in the BSV field, it may find a niche in PfEMP1 and PAM approaches.

5.3 Candidate Prioritisation

In a time of scarce resources for BSV development, it is more important than ever to make the correct decisions regarding which candidates should progress to successive stages of development—and which should not.

Section 2 has already discussed the varying levels of evidence that each of the in vitro assays in use for BSV assessment is predictive of vaccine efficacy. At present, it is striking that some candidates have advanced to field efficacy trials on the basis of activity in an in vitro assay without either the immunogen itself demonstrating protection in any in vivo model, or a clear causal relationship between the measured in vitro activity and in vivo protection being demonstrated (as distinct from studies of NAI—including passive transfer of naturally acquired IgG, in which causation of protection by a particular effector cannot be unpicked from unmeasured covariates).

With NHP studies possible to conduct for <USD 150,000, CHMI studies costing c. USD 3 million (including GMP antigen production), and field studies usually considerably more expensive, it is clear that clinical trials of inappropriate candidates come at substantial cost. The author's view is that vaccine developers hoping to advance a candidate into clinical trials should carefully consider:

1. Demonstration in a rigorously quantitative, externally replicable assay that the candidate induces responses superior to those against previously trialled candidates thought to act via the same mechanism.
2. Demonstration that the candidate can achieve protection in an in vivo model—at present, although imperfect, *Aotus* seems most suitable.
3. Prioritising efforts to establish the validity of their chosen in vitro assay as a surrogate of protection *in the context of vaccination*—this requires in vivo efficacy studies of multiple candidates to demonstrate a fixed relationship between the measured activity and protection, and possibly also passive transfer studies.

For candidates that enter clinical trials, the incremental cost of blood-stage CHMI as compared to a Phase I trial is modest. There is a strong financial, practical and ethical case for the broader use of the blood-stage CHMI model to demonstrate—or rule out—efficacy prior to field trials: it would be highly surprising if a vaccine failed to achieve a detectable effect in this model (i.e. a 30 % PMR reduction at the peak of the immune response) and yet went on to demonstrate clinically meaningful efficacy in a field efficacy study. The model could be readily extended to assess efficacy against vaccine-heterologous parasites, the relationship of efficacy with time after vaccination, and the impact of vaccination of subjects with pre-existing NAI. Armed with such in-depth understanding of a candidate's efficacy profile, the field might not have to confront again the difficulty of interpreting ambiguous results of an unrepeatable field trial.

In some ways analogous to the desire to advance studies rapidly to field trials, there is often a strong drive to test antigens in combination. The author's view is that such studies should be driven by careful examination of the effects of such combinations in pre-clinical models, looking for true synergy [19]; merely additive or sub-additive effects are common, and outright antagonism via antigenic competition is a frequent problem.

6 Concluding Remarks

Our understanding of parasite biology and immunology is constantly improving, as are the tools at the disposal of BSV developers to produce and test novel candidates. On the other hand, BSVs are currently facing a tougher scientific and funding environment than for many years. Resolving this impasse—if it is possible—is likely to require careful critical thought regarding the substantial obstacles facing the field. Is it possible to overcome the kinetic constraints upon antibody binding to the merozoite? Is it possible to overcome the antigenic variability of antigens which do not suffer these kinetic constraints? And, finally, how should the community compare and prioritise candidates as objectively as possible?

References

1. Langhorne J, Ndungu FM, Sponaas AM, Marsh K (2008) Immunity to malaria: more questions than answers. Nat Immunol 9:725–732
2. Riley EM, Stewart VA (2013) Immune mechanisms in malaria: new insights in vaccine development. Nat Med 19:168–178
3. Cohen S, McGregor IA, Carrington S (1961) Gamma-globulin and acquired immunity to human malaria. Nature 192:733–737
4. Sabchareon A, Burnouf T, Ouattara D, Attanath P, Bouharountayoun H, Chantavanich P, Foucault C, Chongsuphajaisiddhi T, Druilhe P (1991) Parasitological and clinical human response to immunoglobulin administration in falciparum malaria. Am J Trop Med Hyg 45:297–308
5. Bejon P, White MT, Olotu A, Bojang K, Lusingu JP, Salim N, Otsyula NN, Agnandji ST, Asante KP, Owusu-Agyei S et al (2013) Efficacy of RTS, S malaria vaccines: individual-participant pooled analysis of phase 2 data. Lancet Infect Dis 13:319–327
6. Pemberton-Ross P, Smith TA, Hodel EM, Kay K, Penny MA (2015) Age-shifting in malaria incidence as a result of induced immunological deficit: a simulation study. Malar J 14:287
7. Draper SJ, Angov E, Horii T, Miller LH, Srinivasan P, Theisen M, Biswas S (2015) Recent advances in recombinant protein-based malaria vaccines. Vaccine 33(52):7433–7443
8. Udomsangpetch R, Kaneko O, Chotivanich K, Sattabongkot J (2008) Cultivation of *Plasmodium vivax*. Trends Parasitol 24:85–88
9. Bull PC, Abdi AI (2016) The role of PfEMP1 as targets of naturally acquired immunity to childhood malaria: prospects for a vaccine. Parasitology 143:171–186
10. Deans JA, Alderson T, Thomas AW, Mitchell GH, Lennox ES, Cohen S (1982) Rat monoclonal antibodies which inhibit the in vitro multiplication of *Plasmodium knowlesi*. Clin Exp Immunol 49:297–309
11. Freeman RR, Trejdosiewicz AJ, Cross GA (1980) Protective monoclonal antibodies recognising stage-specific merozoite antigens of a rodent malaria parasite. Nature 284:366–368
12. Holder AA, Freeman RR (1981) Immunization against blood-stage rodent malaria using purified parasite antigens. Nature 294:361–364
13. Dvorak JA, Miller LH, Whitehouse WC, Shiroishi T (1975) Invasion of erythrocytes by malaria merozoites. Science 187:748–750
14. Gilson PR, Crabb BS (2009) Morphology and kinetics of the three distinct phases of red blood cell invasion by *Plasmodium falciparum* merozoites. Int J Parasitol 39:91–96
15. Saul A (1987) Kinetic constraints on the development of a malaria vaccine. Parasite Immunol 9:1–9
16. Douglas AD, Williams AR, Knuepfer E, Illingworth JJ, Furze JM, Crosnier C, Choudhary P, Bustamante LY, Zakutansky SE, Awuah DK et al (2014) Neutralization of *Plasmodium falciparum* merozoites by antibodies against PfRH5. J Immunol 192:245–258
17. Dutta S, Dlugosz LS, Drew DR, Ge X, Ababacar D, Rovira YI, Moch JK, Shi M, Long CA, Foley M et al (2013) Overcoming antigenic diversity by enhancing the immunogenicity of conserved epitopes on the malaria vaccine candidate apical membrane antigen-1. PLoS Pathog 9, e1003840

18. Miura K, Zhou H, Diouf A, Moretz SE, Fay MP, Miller LH, Martin LB, Pierce MA, Ellis RD, Mullen GE et al (2009) Anti-apical-membrane-antigen-1 antibody is more effective than anti-42-kilodalton-merozoite-surface-protein-1 antibody in inhibiting *Plasmodium falciparum* growth, as determined by the in vitro growth inhibition assay. Clin Vaccine Immunol 16:963–968
19. Williams AR, Douglas AD, Miura K, Illingworth JJ, Choudhary P, Murungi LM, Furze JM, Diouf A, Miotto O, Crosnier C et al (2012) Enhancing blockade of *Plasmodium falciparum* erythrocyte invasion: assessing combinations of antibodies against PfRH5 and other merozoite antigens. PLoS Pathog 8, e1002991
20. Douglas AD, Baldeviano GC, Lucas CM, Lugo-Roman LA, Crosnier C, Bartholdson SJ, Diouf A, Miura K, Lambert LE, Ventocilla JA et al (2015) A PfRH5-based vaccine is efficacious against heterologous strain blood-stage *Plasmodium falciparum* infection in Aotus monkeys. Cell Host Microbe 17:130–139
21. Payne RO, Milne KH, Elias SC, Edwards NJ, Douglas AD, Brown RE, Silk SE, Biswas S, Miura K, Roberts R et al (2016) Demonstration of the blood-stage controlled human malaria infection model to assess efficacy of the *Plasmodium falciparum* AMA1 vaccine FMP2.1/AS01. J Infect Dis 213(11):1743–1751
22. Graves P, Gelband H (2006) Vaccines for preventing malaria (SPf66). *Cochrane Database Syst Rev* CD005966
23. Genton B, Betuela I, Felger I, Al-Yaman F, Anders RF, Saul A, Rare L, Baisor M, Lorry K, Brown GV et al (2002) A recombinant blood-stage malaria vaccine reduces *Plasmodium falciparum* density and exerts selective pressure on parasite populations in a phase 1-2b trial in Papua New Guinea. J Infect Dis 185:820–827
24. Thera MA, Doumbo OK, Coulibaly D, Laurens MB, Ouattara A, Kone AK, Guindo AB, Traore K, Traore I, Kouriba B et al (2011) A field trial to assess a blood-stage malaria vaccine. N Engl J Med 365:1004–1013
25. Spring MD, Cummings JF, Ockenhouse CF, Dutta S, Reidler R, Angov E, Bergmann-Leitner E, Stewart VA, Bittner S, Juompan L et al (2009) Phase 1/2a study of the malaria vaccine candidate apical membrane antigen-1 (AMA-1) administered in adjuvant system AS01B or AS02A. PLoS One 4, e5254
26. Sirima SB, Cousens S, Druilhe P (2011) Protection against malaria by MSP3 candidate vaccine. N Engl J Med 365:1062–1064
27. Palacpac NM, Ntege E, Yeka A, Balikagala B, Suzuki N, Shirai H, Yagi M, Ito K, Fukushima W, Hirota Y et al (2013) Phase 1b randomized trial and follow-up study in Uganda of the blood-stage malaria vaccine candidate BK-SE36. PLoS One 8, e64073
28. Sheehy SH, Duncan CJ, Elias SC, Collins KA, Ewer KJ, Spencer AJ, Williams AR, Halstead FD, Moretz SE, Miura K et al (2011) Phase Ia clinical evaluation of the *Plasmodium falciparum* blood-stage antigen MSP1 in ChAd63 and MVA vaccine vectors. Mol Ther 19:2269–2276
29. Rogerson SJ, Hviid L, Duffy PE, Leke RF, Taylor DW (2007) Malaria in pregnancy: pathogenesis and immunity. Lancet Infect Dis 7:105–117
30. Hviid L (2010) The role of *Plasmodium falciparum* variant surface antigens in protective immunity and vaccine development. Hum Vaccin 6:84–89
31. Duncan CJ, Hill AV, Ellis RD (2012) Can growth inhibition assays (GIA) predict blood-stage malaria vaccine efficacy? Hum Vaccin Immunother 8:706–714
32. Miura K (2016) Progress and prospects for blood-stage malaria vaccines. Expert Rev Vaccines 15(6):765–781
33. Crompton PD, Miura K, Traore B, Kayentao K, Ongoiba A, Weiss G, Doumbo S, Doumtabe D, Kone Y, Huang CY et al (2009) In vitro growth inhibitory activity and malaria risk in a cohort study in mali. Infect Immun 78(2):737–745
34. Dutta S, Sullivan JS, Grady KK, Haynes JD, Komisar J, Batchelor AH, Soisson L, Diggs CL, Heppner DG, Lanar DE et al (2009) High antibody titer against apical membrane antigen-1 is required to protect against malaria in the Aotus model. PLoS One 4, e8138

35. Douglas AD, Williams AR, Illingworth JJ, Kamuyu G, Biswas S, Goodman AL, Wyllie DH, Crosnier C, Miura K, Wright GJ et al (2011) The blood-stage malaria antigen PfRH5 is susceptible to vaccine-inducible cross-strain neutralizing antibody. Nat Commun 2:601
36. Singh S, Miura K, Zhou H, Muratova O, Keegan B, Miles A, Martin LB, Saul AJ, Miller LH, Long CA (2006) Immunity to recombinant *Plasmodium falciparum* merozoite surface protein 1 (MSP1): protection in Aotus nancymai monkeys strongly correlates with anti-MSP1 antibody titer and in vitro parasite-inhibitory activity. Infect Immun 74:4573–4580
37. Plotkin SA (2008) Vaccines: correlates of vaccine-induced immunity. Clin Infect Dis 47:401–409
38. Bouharoun-Tayoun H, Attanath P, Sabchareon A, Chongsuphajaisiddhi T, Druilhe P (1990) Antibodies that protect humans against *Plasmodium falciparum* blood stages do not on their own inhibit parasite growth and invasion in vitro, but act in cooperation with monocytes. J Exp Med 172:1633–1641
39. Bouharoun-Tayoun H, Oeuvray C, Lunel F, Druilhe P (1995) Mechanisms underlying the monocyte-mediated antibody-dependent killing of *Plasmodium falciparum* asexual blood stages. J Exp Med 182:409–418
40. Joos C, Marrama L, Polson HE, Corre S, Diatta AM, Diouf B, Trape JF, Tall A, Longacre S, Perraut R (2010) Clinical protection from falciparum malaria correlates with neutrophil respiratory bursts induced by merozoites opsonized with human serum antibodies. PLoS One 5, e9871
41. Hill DL, Eriksson EM, Carmagnac AB, Wilson DW, Cowman AF, Hansen DS, Schofield L (2012) Efficient measurement of opsonising antibodies to *Plasmodium falciparum* merozoites. PLoS One 7, e51692
42. Osier FH, Feng G, Boyle MJ, Langer C, Zhou J, Richards JS, McCallum FJ, Reiling L, Jaworowski A, Anders RF et al (2014) Opsonic phagocytosis of *Plasmodium falciparum* merozoites: mechanism in human immunity and a correlate of protection against malaria. BMC Med 12:108
43. Hill DL, Eriksson EM, Li Wai Suen CS, Chiu CY, Ryg-Cornejo V, Robinson LJ, Siba PM, Mueller I, Hansen DS, Schofield L (2013) Opsonising antibodies to *P. falciparum* merozoites associated with immunity to clinical malaria. PLoS One 8, e74627
44. Boyle MJ, Reiling L, Feng G, Langer C, Osier FH, Aspeling-Jones H, Cheng YS, Stubbs J, Tetteh KK, Conway DJ et al (2015) Human antibodies fix complement to inhibit *Plasmodium falciparum* invasion of erythrocytes and are associated with protection against malaria. Immunity 42:580–590
45. Bull PC, Lowe BS, Kortok M, Molyneux CS, Newbold CI, Marsh K (1998) Parasite antigens on the infected red cell surface are targets for naturally acquired immunity to malaria. Nat Med 4:358–360
46. Marsh K, Howard RJ (1986) Antigens induced on erythrocytes by *Plasmodium falciparum*: expression of diverse and conserved determinants. Science 231:150–153
47. Duffy PE, Fried M (2003) Antibodies that inhibit *Plasmodium falciparum* adhesion to chondroitin sulfate A are associated with increased birth weight and the gestational age of newborns. Infect Immun 71:6620–6623
48. Saveria T, Duffy PE, Fried M (2015) Evaluation of pregnancy malaria vaccine candidates: the binding inhibition assay. Methods Mol Biol 1325:231–239
49. Ghumra A, Khunrae P, Ataide R, Raza A, Rogerson SJ, Higgins MK, Rowe JA (2011) Immunisation with recombinant PfEMP1 domains elicits functional rosette-inhibiting and phagocytosis-inducing antibodies to *Plasmodium falciparum*. PLoS One 6, e16414
50. Silvie O, Franetich JF, Charrin S, Mueller MS, Siau A, Bodescot M, Rubinstein E, Hannoun L, Charoenvit Y, Kocken CH et al (2004) A role for apical membrane antigen 1 during invasion of hepatocytes by *Plasmodium falciparum* sporozoites. J Biol Chem 279:9490–9496
51. Draper SJ, Goodman AL, Biswas S, Forbes EK, Moore AC, Gilbert SC, Hill AV (2009) Recombinant viral vaccines expressing merozoite surface protein-1 induce antibody- and T cell-mediated multistage protection against malaria. Cell Host Microbe 5:95–105

52. Pombo DJ, Lawrence G, Hirunpetcharat C, Rzepczyk C, Bryden M, Cloonan N, Anderson K, Mahakunkijcharoen Y, Martin LB, Wilson D et al (2002) Immunity to malaria after administration of ultra-low doses of red cells infected with *Plasmodium falciparum*. Lancet 360:610–617
53. Edstein MD, Kotecka BM, Anderson KL, Pombo DJ, Kyle DE, Rieckmann KH, Good MF (2005) Lengthy antimalarial activity of atovaquone in human plasma following atovaquone-proguanil administration. Antimicrob Agents Chemother 49:4421–4422
54. Suss G, Eichmann K, Kury E, Linke A, Langhorne J (1988) Roles of CD4- and CD8-bearing T lymphocytes in the immune response to the erythrocytic stages of *Plasmodium chabaudi*. Infect Immun 56:3081–3088
55. Mastelic B, do Rosario AP, Veldhoen M, Renauld JC, Jarra W, Sponaas AM, Roetynck S, Stockinger B, Langhorne J (2012) IL-22 protects against liver pathology and lethality of an experimental blood-stage malaria infection. Front Immunol 3:85
56. Freitas do Rosario AP, Lamb T, Spence P, Stephens R, Lang A, Roers A, Muller W, O'Garra A, Langhorne J (2012) IL-27 promotes IL-10 production by effector Th1 $CD4^+$ T cells: a critical mechanism for protection from severe immunopathology during malaria infection. J Immunol 188:1178–1190
57. Imai T, Ishida H, Suzue K, Taniguchi T, Okada H, Shimokawa C, Hisaeda H (2015) Cytotoxic activities of $CD8^+$ T cells collaborate with macrophages to protect against blood-stage murine malaria. Elife 4, e04232
58. Biswas S, Spencer AJ, Forbes EK, Gilbert SC, Holder AA, Hill AV, Draper SJ (2012) Recombinant viral-vectored vaccines expressing *Plasmodium chabaudi* AS apical membrane antigen 1: mechanisms of vaccine-induced blood-stage protection. J Immunol 188:5041–5053
59. Sheehy SH, Duncan CJ, Elias SC, Choudhary P, Biswas S, Halstead FD, Collins KA, Edwards NJ, Douglas AD, Anagnostou NA et al (2012) ChAd63-MVA-vectored blood-stage malaria vaccines targeting MSP1 and AMA1: assessment of efficacy against mosquito bite challenge in humans. Mol Ther 20:2355–2368
60. Chuang I, Sedegah M, Cicatelli S, Spring M, Polhemus M, Tamminga C, Patterson N, Guerrero M, Bennett JW, McGrath S et al (2013) DNA prime/adenovirus boost malaria vaccine encoding *P. falciparum* CSP and AMA1 induces sterile protection associated with cell-mediated immunity. PLoS One 8, e55571
61. Perkins SL, Sarkar IN, Carter R (2007) The phylogeny of rodent malaria parasites: simultaneous analysis across three genomes. Infect Genet Evol 7:74–83
62. Beaute-Lafitte A, Altemayer-Caillard V, Gonnet-Gonzalez F, Ramiaramanana L, Chabaud AG, Landau I (1994) The chemosensitivity of the rodent malarias—relationships with the biology of merozoites. Int J Parasitol 24:981–986
63. Goodman AL, Forbes EK, Williams AR, Douglas AD, de Cassan SC, Bauza K, Biswas S, Dicks MD, Llewellyn D, Moore AC et al (2013) The utility of *Plasmodium berghei* as a rodent model for anti-merozoite malaria vaccine assessment. Sci Rep 3:1706
64. Siu E, Ploss A (2015) Modeling malaria in humanized mice: opportunities and challenges. Ann N Y Acad Sci 1342:29–36
65. Collins WE, Galland GG, Sullivan JS, Morris CL (1994) Selection of different strains of *Plasmodium falciparum* for testing blood-stage vaccines in Aotus nancymai monkeys. Am J Trop Med Hyg 51:224–232
66. Collins WE (2002) Nonhuman primate models. II. Infection of Saimiri and Aotus monkeys with *Plasmodium vivax*. Methods Mol Med 72:85–92
67. Heppner DG, Cummings JF, Ockenhouse C, Kester KE, Lyon JA, Gordon DM (2001) New World monkey efficacy trials for malaria vaccine development: critical path or detour? Trends Parasitol 17:419–425
68. Stowers AW, Miller LH (2001) Are trials in New World monkeys on the critical path for blood-stage malaria vaccine development? Trends Parasitol 17:415–419
69. Epstein JE, Rao S, Williams F, Freilich D, Luke T, Sedegah M, de la Vega P, Sacci J, Richie TL, Hoffman SL (2007) Safety and clinical outcome of experimental challenge of human

volunteers with *Plasmodium falciparum*-infected mosquitoes: an update. J Infect Dis 196:145–154
70. Roestenberg M, O'Hara GA, Duncan CJ, Epstein JE, Edwards NJ, Scholzen A, van der Ven AJ, Hermsen CC, Hill AV, Sauerwein RW (2012) Comparison of clinical and parasitological data from controlled human malaria infection trials. PLoS One 7, e38434
71. Druilhe P, Perignon JL (1997) A hypothesis about the chronicity of malaria infection. Parasitol Today 13:353–357
72. Douglas AD, Andrews L, Draper SJ, Bojang K, Milligan P, Gilbert SC, Imoukhuede EB, Hill AV (2011) Substantially reduced pre-patent parasite multiplication rates are associated with naturally acquired immunity to *Plasmodium falciparum*. J Infect Dis 203:1337–1340
73. Douglas AD, Edwards NJ, Duncan CJ, Thompson FM, Sheehy SH, O'Hara GA, Anagnostou N, Walther M, Webster DP, Dunachie SJ et al (2013) Comparison of modeling methods to determine liver-to-blood inocula and parasite multiplication rates during controlled human malaria infection. J Infect Dis 208:340–345
74. Cheng Q, Lawrence G, Reed C, Stowers A, Ranford-Cartwright L, Creasey A, Carter R, Saul A (1997) Measurement of *Plasmodium falciparum* growth rates in vivo: a test of malaria vaccines. Am J Trop Med Hyg 57:495–500
75. Sanderson F, Andrews L, Douglas AD, Hunt-Cooke A, Bejon P, Hill AV (2008) Blood-stage challenge for malaria vaccine efficacy trials: a pilot study with discussion of safety and potential value. Am J Trop Med Hyg 78:878–883
76. Remarque EJ, Faber BW, Kocken CH, Thomas AW (2008) Apical membrane antigen 1: a malaria vaccine candidate in review. Trends Parasitol 24:74–84
77. Stowers AW, Kennedy MC, Keegan BP, Saul A, Long CA, Miller LH (2002) Vaccination of monkeys with recombinant *Plasmodium falciparum* apical membrane antigen 1 confers protection against blood-stage malaria. Infect Immun 70:6961–6967
78. Dutta S, Lalitha PV, Ware LA, Barbosa A, Moch JK, Vassell MA, Fileta BB, Kitov S, Kolodny N, Heppner DG et al (2002) Purification, characterization, and immunogenicity of the refolded ectodomain of the *Plasmodium falciparum* apical membrane antigen 1 expressed in *Escherichia coli*. Infect Immun 70:3101–3110
79. Srinivasan P, Ekanem E, Diouf A, Tonkin ML, Miura K, Boulanger MJ, Long CA, Narum DL, Miller LH (2014) Immunization with a functional protein complex required for erythrocyte invasion protects against lethal malaria. Proc Natl Acad Sci U S A 111:10311–10316
80. Harris KS, Adda CG, Khore M, Drew DR, Valentini-Gatt A, Fowkes FJ, Beeson JG, Dutta S, Anders RF, Foley M (2014) Use of immunodampening to overcome diversity in the malarial vaccine candidate apical membrane antigen 1. Infect Immun 82:4707–4717
81. Remarque EJ, Faber BW, Kocken CH, Thomas AW (2008) A diversity-covering approach to immunization with *Plasmodium falciparum* apical membrane antigen 1 induces broader allelic recognition and growth inhibition responses in rabbits. Infect Immun 76:2660–2670
82. Lyon JA, Angov E, Fay MP, Sullivan JS, Girourd AS, Robinson SJ, Bergmann-Leitner ES, Duncan EH, Darko CA, Collins WE et al (2008) Protection induced by *Plasmodium falciparum* MSP1(42) is strain-specific, antigen and adjuvant dependent, and correlates with antibody responses. PLoS One 3, e2830
83. Ogutu BR, Apollo OJ, McKinney D, Okoth W, Siangla J, Dubovsky F, Tucker K, Waitumbi JN, Diggs C, Wittes J et al (2009) Blood stage malaria vaccine eliciting high antigen-specific antibody concentrations confers no protection to young children in Western Kenya. PLoS One 4, e4708
84. Zong S, Kron MW, Epp C, Engler T, Bujard H, Kochanek S, Kreppel F (2011) DeltaE1 and high-capacity adenoviral vectors expressing full-length codon-optimized merozoite surface protein 1 for vaccination against *Plasmodium falciparum*. J Gene Med 13:670–679
85. Crosnier C, Wanaguru M, McDade B, Osier FH, Marsh K, Rayner JC, Wright GJA (2013) A library of functional recombinant cell-surface and secreted *P. falciparum* merozoite proteins. Mol Cell Proteomics 12:3976–3986
86. Oeuvray C, Bouharoun-Tayoun H, Gras-Masse H, Bottius E, Kaidoh T, Aikawa M, Filgueira MC, Tartar A, Druilhe P (1994) Merozoite surface protein-3: a malaria protein inducing

antibodies that promote *Plasmodium falciparum* killing by cooperation with blood monocytes. Blood 84:1594–1602
87. Badell E, Oeuvray C, Moreno A, Soe S, van Rooijen N, Bouzidi A, Druilhe P (2000) Human malaria in immunocompromised mice: an in vivo model to study defense mechanisms against *Plasmodium falciparum*. J Exp Med 192:1653–1660
88. Hisaeda H, Saul A, Reece JJ, Kennedy MC, Long CA, Miller LH, Stowers AW (2002) Merozoite surface protein 3 and protection against malaria in Aotus nancymai monkeys. J Infect Dis 185:657–664
89. Tsai CW, Duggan PF, Jin AJ, Macdonald NJ, Kotova S, Lebowitz J, Hurt DE, Shimp RL Jr, Lambert L, Miller LH et al (2009) Characterization of a protective *Escherichia coli*-expressed *Plasmodium falciparum* merozoite surface protein 3 indicates a non-linear, multi-domain structure. Mol Biochem Parasitol 164:45–56
90. Horii T, Shirai H, Jie L, Ishii KJ, Palacpac NQ, Tougan T, Hato M, Ohta N, Bobogare A, Arakaki N et al (2010) Evidences of protection against blood-stage infection of *Plasmodium falciparum* by the novel protein vaccine SE36. Parasitol Int 59:380–386
91. Stallmach R, Kavishwar M, Withers-Martinez C, Hackett F, Collins CR, Howell SA, Yeoh S, Knuepfer E, Atid AJ, Holder AA et al (2015) *Plasmodium falciparum* SERA5 plays a non-enzymatic role in the malarial asexual blood-stage lifecycle. Mol Microbiol 96:368–387
92. Tanabe K, Arisue N, Palacpac NM, Yagi M, Tougan T, Honma H, Ferreira MU, Farnert A, Bjorkman A, Kaneko A et al (2012) Geographic differentiation of polymorphism in the *Plasmodium falciparum* malaria vaccine candidate gene SERA5. Vaccine 30:1583–1593
93. Tham WH, Healer J, Cowman AF (2012) Erythrocyte and reticulocyte binding-like proteins of *Plasmodium falciparum*. Trends Parasitol 28:23–30
94. Wright GJ, Rayner JC (2014) *Plasmodium falciparum* erythrocyte invasion: combining function with immune evasion. PLoS Pathog 10, e1003943
95. Jones TR, Stroncek DF, Gozalo AS, Obaldia N 3rd, Andersen EM, Lucas C, Narum DL, Magill AJ, Sim BK, Hoffman SL (2002) Anemia in parasite- and recombinant protein-immunized aotus monkeys infected with *Plasmodium falciparum*. Am J Trop Med Hyg 66:672–679
96. El Sahly HM, Patel SM, Atmar RL, Lanford TA, Dube T, Thompson D, Sim BK, Long C, Keitel WA (2010) Safety and immunogenicity of a recombinant nonglycosylated erythrocyte binding antigen 175 Region II malaria vaccine in healthy adults living in an area where malaria is not endemic. Clin Vaccine Immunol 17:1552–1559
97. Stubbs J, Simpson KM, Triglia T, Plouffe D, Tonkin CJ, Duraisingh MT, Maier AG, Winzeler EA, Cowman AF (2005) Molecular mechanism for switching of *P. falciparum* invasion pathways into human erythrocytes. Science 309:1384–1387
98. Baum J, Chen L, Healer J, Lopaticki S, Boyle M, Triglia T, Ehlgen F, Ralph SA, Beeson JG, Cowman AF (2009) Reticulocyte-binding protein homologue 5—an essential adhesin involved in invasion of human erythrocytes by *Plasmodium falciparum*. Int J Parasitol 39:371–380
99. Crosnier C, Bustamante LY, Bartholdson SJ, Bei AK, Theron M, Uchikawa M, Mboup S, Ndir O, Kwiatkowski DP, Duraisingh MT et al (2011) Basigin is a receptor essential for erythrocyte invasion by *Plasmodium falciparum*. Nature 480:534–537
100. Villard V, Agak GW, Frank G, Jafarshad A, Servis C, Nebie I, Sirima SB, Felger I, Arevalo-Herrera M, Herrera S et al (2007) Rapid identification of malaria vaccine candidates based on alpha-helical coiled coil protein motif. PLoS One 2, e645
101. Olugbile S, Kulangara C, Bang G, Bertholet S, Suzarte E, Villard V, Frank G, Audran R, Razaname A, Nebie I et al (2009) Vaccine potentials of an intrinsically unstructured fragment derived from the blood stage-associated *Plasmodium falciparum* protein PFF0165c. Infect Immun 77:5701–5709
102. Mueller I, Shakri AR, Chitnis CE (2015) Development of vaccines for *Plasmodium vivax* malaria. Vaccine 33:7489–7495
103. Russell B, Suwanarusk R, Borlon C, Costa FT, Chu CS, Rijken MJ, Sriprawat K, Warter L, Koh EG, Malleret B et al (2011) A reliable ex vivo invasion assay of human reticulocytes by *Plasmodium vivax*. Blood 118:e74–e81

104. Collins WE, Sullivan JS, Strobert E, Galland GG, Williams A, Nace D, Williams T, Barnwell JW (2009) Studies on the Salvador I strain of *Plasmodium vivax* in non-human primates and anopheline mosquitoes. Am J Trop Med Hyg 80:228–235
105. Dutta S, Kaushal DC, Ware LA, Puri SK, Kaushal NA, Narula A, Upadhyaya DS, Lanar DE (2005) Merozoite surface protein 1 of *Plasmodium vivax* induces a protective response against *Plasmodium cynomolgi* challenge in rhesus monkeys. Infect Immun 73:5936–5944
106. Bennett JW, Pybus BS, Yadava A, Tosh D, Sousa JC, McCarthy WF, Deye G, Melendez V, Ockenhouse CF (2013) Primaquine failure and cytochrome P-450 2D6 in *Plasmodium vivax* malaria. N Engl J Med 369:1381–1382
107. Arevalo-Herrera M, Forero-Pena DA, Rubiano K, Gomez-Hincapie J, Martinez NL, Lopez-Perez M, Castellanos A, Cespedes N, Palacios R, Onate JM et al (2014) *Plasmodium vivax* sporozoite challenge in malaria-naive and semi-immune Colombian volunteers. PLoS One 9, e99754
108. Miller LH, Mason SJ, Clyde DF, McGinniss MH (1976) The resistance factor to *Plasmodium vivax* in blacks. The Duffy-blood-group genotype, FyFy. N Engl J Med 295:302–304
109. Grimberg BT, Udomsangpetch R, Xainli J, McHenry A, Panichakul T, Sattabongkot J, Cui L, Bockarie M, Chitnis C, Adams J et al (2007) *Plasmodium vivax* invasion of human erythrocytes inhibited by antibodies directed against the Duffy binding protein. PLoS Med 4, e337
110. Arevalo-Herrera M, Castellanos A, Yazdani SS, Shakri AR, Chitnis CE, Dominik R, Herrera S (2005) Immunogenicity and protective efficacy of recombinant vaccine based on the receptor-binding domain of the *Plasmodium vivax* Duffy binding protein in Aotus monkeys. Am J Trop Med Hyg 73:25–31
111. de Cassan SC, Shakri AR, Llewellyn D, Elias SC, Cho JS, Goodman AL, Jin J, Douglas AD, Suwanarusk R, Nosten FH et al (2015) Preclinical assessment of viral vectored and protein vaccines targeting the duffy-binding protein region II of *Plasmodium vivax*. Front Immunol 6:348
112. White MT, Bejon P, Olotu A, Griffin JT, Bojang K, Lusingu J, Salim N, Abdulla S, Otsyula N, Agnandji ST et al (2014) A combined analysis of immunogenicity, antibody kinetics and vaccine efficacy from phase 2 trials of the RTS, S malaria vaccine. BMC Med 12:117
113. Tsuboi T, Takeo S, Iriko H, Jin L, Tsuchimochi M, Matsuda S, Han ET, Otsuki H, Kaneko O, Sattabongkot J et al (2008) Wheat germ cell-free system-based production of malaria proteins for discovery of novel vaccine candidates. Infect Immun 76:1702–1708
114. Lau CK, Turner L, Jespersen JS, Lowe ED, Petersen B, Wang CW, Petersen JE, Lusingu J, Theander TG, Lavstsen T et al (2015) Structural conservation despite huge sequence diversity allows EPCR binding by the PfEMP1 family implicated in severe childhood malaria. Cell Host Microbe 17:118–129
115. Ghumra A, Semblat JP, Ataide R, Kifude C, Adams Y, Claessens A, Anong DN, Bull PC, Fennell C, Arman M et al (2012) Induction of strain-transcending antibodies against Group A PfEMP1 surface antigens from virulent malaria parasites. PLoS Pathog 8, e1002665
116. Baruch DI, Gamain B, Barnwell JW, Sullivan JS, Stowers A, Galland GG, Miller LH, Collins WE (2002) Immunization of Aotus monkeys with a functional domain of the *Plasmodium falciparum* variant antigen induces protection against a lethal parasite line. Proc Natl Acad Sci U S A 99:3860–3865
117. Sampath S, Carrico C, Janes J, Gurumoorthy S, Gibson C, Melcher M, Chitnis CE, Wang R, Schief WR, Smith JD (2013) Glycan masking of *Plasmodium vivax* Duffy Binding Protein for probing protein binding function and vaccine development. PLoS Pathog 9, e1003420
118. Fried M, Duffy PE (2015) Designing a VAR2CSA-based vaccine to prevent placental malaria. Vaccine 33:7483–7488
119. Barfod L, Dobrilovic T, Magistrado P, Khunrae P, Viwami F, Bruun J, Dahlback M, Bernasconi NL, Fried M, John D et al (2010) Chondroitin sulfate A-adhering *Plasmodium falciparum*-infected erythrocytes express functionally important antibody epitopes shared by multiple variants. J Immunol 185:7553–7561

120. Brune KD, Leneghan DB, Brian IJ, Ishizuka AS, Bachmann MF, Draper SJ, Biswas S, Howarth M (2016) Plug-and-Display: decoration of Virus-Like Particles via isopeptide bonds for modular immunization. Sci Rep 6:19234
121. Moon JJ, Suh H, Li AV, Ockenhouse CF, Yadava A, Irvine DJ (2012) Enhancing humoral responses to a malaria antigen with nanoparticle vaccines that expand Tfh cells and promote germinal center induction. Proc Natl Acad Sci U S A 109:1080–1085
122. Balazs AB, Chen J, Hong CM, Rao DS, Yang L, Baltimore D (2012) Antibody-based protection against HIV infection by vectored immunoprophylaxis. Nature 481:81–84

Part IV
Immune Response to Malaria Vaccines: Transmission Blocking Vaccines

Antimalarial Transmission-Blocking Vaccines

R.E. Sinden, Sumi Biswas, and A.M. Blagborough

Contents

1 Biology of Transmission to the Human Host ... 242
1.1 The Parasite ... 242
1.2 The Vector ... 245
1.3 The Vertebrate Immune System ... 248
2 Discovery of Targets ... 248
3 Vaccine Development ... 250
3.1 Antigens Currently Under Clinical Consideration ... 250
3.2 Delivery Platforms ... 251
3.3 Clinical Development ... 253
3.4 Future Developments ... 254
4 Evaluation and Potential Impact of TBVs ... 255
4.1 Transmission-Blocking Assays with Immunological Outputs ... 256
4.2 Pre-oocyst Transmission-Blocking Assays Examining Cell Biology ... 256
4.3 Oocyst-Based Transmission-Blocking Assays ... 257
4.4 Sporozoite Assays ... 259
4.5 Population Assays ... 259
References ... 260

The concept that malaria might be attacked by targeting *Plasmodium* as they pass from the human host into the vector was first mooted by Eyles [1], developed by Huff et al. [2] and elegantly endorsed by Gwadz [3] and Carter and Chen [4] whilst working at the NIH Washington. This pioneering work on gametocyte/gamete-based vaccines was then expanded at the London School of Hygiene and Tropical Medicine [5]. Thereafter work at the University of Nijmegen, the NIH and Imperial

R.E. Sinden (✉) • S. Biswas
The Jenner Institute, Old Road Campus Building, Roosevelt Drive, Oxford OX3 7QD, UK
e-mail: robert.sinden@ndm.ox.ac.uk; sumi.biswas@ndm.ox.ac.uk

A.M. Blagborough
The Department of Life Sciences, Imperial College London,
Sir Alexander Fleming Building, Imperial College Road, South Kensington, London SW7 2AZ, UK
e-mail: andrew.blagborough@imperial.ac.uk

M.M. Mota, A. Rodriguez (eds.), *Malaria*, DOI 10.1007/978-3-319-45210-4_12

College London developed the concept yet further to include other parasite stages found in the mosquito gut, notably the ookinete [6–10]. The most recent development has been the identification of targets in the mosquito vector that can be disrupted by vaccination [11–15]. In retrospect it was unfortunate that the early pivotal studies were published at a time when the direction of malaria research was moving away from eradication, to control of disease. A priority target of this new direction was the development of the first protective vaccine targeting the circumsporozoite protein—with the objective of preventing development of disease in the infected/bitten host. Perhaps as a consequence, and despite the undoubted efficacy of sexual-stage antigens demonstrated in the early studies, TBVs were damned by the faint accolade of being 'altruistic' vaccines. This substantially delayed their onward development. A facet of TBVs that has only recently been recognised is that the population targeted is markedly smaller (10^6–10^9-fold lower) than that of asexual blood-stage vaccines, and similar to that of Pre-Erythrocytic Vaccines (PEV) [16], thus either of a TBV or a PEV, would delay the selection of resistant mutations, and their use in combination would be ideal. It is surprising that to date there have been relatively few studies evaluating such a combined vaccine design (e.g. [17]).

In retrospect, it is interesting to note how well the key attributes of TBVs meet the criteria now set out by the WHO for any antiparasitic vaccine, criteria which make clear the central concepts of 'prevention of infection', herd immunity and source-drying (http://www.who.int/bulletin/volumes/86/2/07-040089/en/). In this time of renewed endeavour to eliminate and eradicate these formidable parasites, there are now renewed and exciting efforts to develop effective TBVs. The current understanding of the purpose, regulatory parameters, and PDPs of TBVs has recently been excellently reviewed [18] and will therefore not be revisited here.

1 Biology of Transmission to the Human Host

1.1 The Parasite

Transmission of *Plasmodium* from the human host to the vector is uniquely mediated by the intraerythrocytic gametocytes. These, during their maturation, express stage-specific immunogens on the erythrocyte surface (notably Surfins, Rifins, STEVOR and GEXP5). Whilst lacking the adhesive 'knobs' of the asexual parasites, these surface-expressed proteins include moieties suspected of mediating the sequestration of immature/noninfectious *P. falciparum* gametocytes in the deep tissues of the host [19, 20]. Some have suggested these proteins might represent useful vaccine targets [21, 22]—indeed some naturally occurring antibodies are believed to inhibit the development of immature gametocytes [23]. Recognising that the vast majority of the dimorphic gametocytes are destined to die in the human host, it is inevitable that all their constituent antigens irrespective of their location will be presented to the hosts' immune system. Should the antibodies induced significantly prejudice onward transmission/survival of the parasite, it might be anticipated that the parasites would have evolved effective escape pathways, such as multigene antigenic switching and polymorphism—mechanisms that have hindered the design of useful broad-spectrum asexual blood-stage vaccines. Ample evidence has been gathered demonstrating that natural transmission-blocking antibodies are generated, notably focussing on those against P230 and P48/45 proteins expressed in the parasitophorous vacuole of the gametocyte-infected red blood cell (giRBC) [24–34]. Consistent with the evidence that P230 and P48/45 are transcribed only in the more mature gametocytes [35–37], but in contrast to the analysis of Tongwong et al. [23], evidence suggests that only stage V gametocytes are recognised by these antibodies [21]. It is widely appreciated that natural responses to gametocyte infection might boost vaccine-induced immunity to those TBV antigens synthesised in the human host [38].

Within minutes of entering the blood meal of the female mosquito, the mature gametocytes increase in volume and simultaneously secrete new surface proteins including six members of the pCCP/LAP family [39–42], Pfg377 [43] and proteolytic enzymes [44], e.g. PPLP2 [45] and MDV-1 [46, 47]. The latter weaken the mechanically stressed red cell which then ruptures. Members of the CCP/LAP family demonstrate codependent expression in female gametocytes [42, 48] and are later trafficked through the ookinete crystalloid to become functional in the oocyst [49]. Reports variously suggest these proteins are incorporated into a multimolecular surface complex on both the female and male gametes [50, 51] allegedly anchored via P48/45 (a male-specific protein [52]) to the plasma-membrane [52]. PCCPs1-4 reportedly complexes with Pfs230 where they are susceptible to complement-mediated inhibition of gamete emergence [50, 53, 54]. This disparate data may result from associations formed during promiscuous gamete-gamete binding [35, 36].

The extracellular parasites form motile flagellate male and sessile female gametes. Both the survival and function of the gametes clearly represent aspects of parasite biology vulnerable to attack by immune effectors ingested in the blood meal. Two identified TBV candidates have been shown to be responsible for gamete-gamete recognition (P48/45 and P47) [52, 55]. And one HAP2/CSC1 unquestionably mediates fusion of the gamete membranes at fertilisation [56–58]. Fertilisation occurs within an hour, and the resultant zygote dispenses with the surface complexes essential to fertilisation and adopts a new protein coat [59–61] including the major coat proteins P25 and P28 that will provide defence against digestion by the vector [62]. P25 and P28 show mutual functional redundancy and are encoded by tandemly linked genes, and the *P. falciparum* proteins are reportedly synergistic immunogens [63], although others have failed to demonstrate this synergy in *P. vivax* [62, 64]. The zygote transforms into a motile ookinete that migrates to the periphery of the blood meal. Some 24–36 h later, the ookinete not so much invades, but more 'smashes' the midgut epithelium by the secretion of hydrolase (e.g. chitinase) and protease (e.g. PPLP 3,5) enzymes [65–67]. Recognising that all these stages in the blood meal are extracellular, it is obvious that surface and/or secreted antigens will be fully exposed to potentially deleterious components of the ingested blood meal—including immune effectors of both the host and the vector and the digestive enzymes of the vector. Zygote/ookinete surface and secreted antigens (e.g. P25, P28) are potentially exposed to sustained attack for the 24–36 h sojourn in the blood meal, and this may account for the efficacy of vaccines targeting these proteins.

The contrasting strategies required of the mature gametocyte in the vertebrate and insect hosts may have driven their elegant, yet elaborate, patterns of protein expression. In the human host, the infectious gametocyte ideally circulates 'unrecognised' for extended periods in the peripheral circulation (to optimise the probability of ingestion by the vector), for which 'stealth physiology' would be ideal. Major proteins (e.g. tubulin) required for gamete assembly are pre-synthesised and stored, and then protein synthesis is massively down-regulated, in the male, even the translation machinery itself (ribosomes) is finally dispensed with, whereas in the female the ribosomes are retained (for later rapid zygote development), but here translation is suppressed by sequestration of mRNA in DOZI/CITH/PUF complexes [68–70].

By contrast, in the mosquito, the extracellular gametocytes are highly active and must complete fertilisation and formation of the ookinete rapidly to avoid being digested in the blood meal. We might anticipate that to avoid the induction of transmission-blocking responses, prejudicially immunogenic 'early' zygote/ookinete surface proteins are amongst those under translation control—a search of the relevant transcriptomic and proteomic libraries [48, 71–74] may help select and prioritise new TBV targets. Despite the hypothesis above, male gamete surface moieties, e.g. P230 and P48/45, are synthesised in the gametocyte, and natural antibodies are formed. Are they simply difficult to target, or are they, as evidence suggests, amongst the transient population of proteins rapidly shed from the gamete/zygote surface [60, 61, 75]? This still requires conclusive characterisation.

The search for invariant immunogens has plagued the development of protective blood-stage vaccines. *Plasmodium* has evolved two powerful mechanisms to overcome the host's adaptive immune defences, namely, antigenic variation and antigenic polymorphism. Antigens expressed on the surface of the gametocyte-infected RBC (giRBC), similarly include multigene families [24, 76]. Conversely, many of the zygote/ookinete surface antigens are never expressed in the human host and therefore not exposed to an adaptive immune response; thus, it might be anticipated that they are more conserved, and current data on P25 gene structure supports this conclusion, and it has been demonstrated that vaccine-induced immunity transcends known variants [77–85]. It will be interesting to understand whether proteins synthesised in the gametocyte, but only exposed to the immune response in the blood meal (e.g. P230, P48/45, HAP2) are more diverse than those synthesised following ingestion by the vector [86–96] (see below).

Recognising that many TBV candidates will be secreted/surface parasite proteins, we might anticipate that immunogenicity may highly constrained by post-translational modifications, both conventional, e.g. myristoylation, palmitoylation or protein folding [97, 98], and unconventional, e.g. the absence of N-glycosylation mechanisms [99, 100], and the addition of *Plasmodium*-specific GPI anchors [101]. Addition of GPI anchors, whether from *Plasmodium* or an insect cell, significantly enhanced the immunogenicity of recombinant P28 from *P. berghei* [102–105], as did addition of a mammalian GPI anchor to Pfs230 [106]. Despite significant progress in the refolding of proteins expressed in heterologous systems, which has improved the immunogenicity of Pfs25 [100, 107], it is unlikely that any one heterologous expression system in use today will be universally applicable to all prospective candidates [108–111] (see Sect. 4).

1.2 The Vector

Mosquitoes derive significant energy from plant-derived sugar feeds [112], but the fertilised females at each gonotrophic cycle take and digest a blood meal to support egg production. Following ingestion, the blood meal is rapidly degraded by proteolytic enzymes, e.g. trypsins [113] and carboxy- and amino-peptidases [114–117], and the undigested residue excreted within 96 h. The malarial ookinete is susceptible to these proteases [118, 119]. It has been suggested that one function of the surface proteins P25 and P28, which form tiles on the ookinete surface [120–123], is to provide protection against this proteolytic attack [62]. Within 24 h, many mosquitoes envelope the blood meal in a chitinous peritrophic matrix as a defence against ingested [124–128] or resident microbial pathogens [129–132]. The latter may be responsible for the significant death of blood-fed mosquitoes ~4 days post-feed [133].

The blood-fed mosquito mounts a significant innate immune response to pathogens in the blood meal [134]. Pathways currently identified include the thioester protein (complement-like) protein TEP1 [135], defensins [136], serpins [137], NOS [138] and insulin-like receptors [139]. It has been hypothesised that manipulation of these inhibitory pathways, by ingested antibodies that inactivate regulatory serpins, may offer new routes to block malaria transmission [140]. Intriguingly, recent work has suggested that the malarial gamete surface protein P47 confers resistance to the NOS-mediated response [141, 142] and exhibits global polymorphisms which correlate with local transmission efficiencies [143].

Essential parasite-vector interactions, accessible to ingested antibody, might include recognition and invasion by the ookinete of the midgut peritrophic matrix (e.g. chitinase [144, 145]), of the tubular network [146] or of the midgut epithelium [147, 148] and the recognition and invasion of the salivary gland by the sporozoite [149]. Ookinete-midgut interactions include both carbohydrate [149, 150] and protein moieties [15]. In the view of the authors, parasite-salivary gland interactions are not accessible to *controlled* delivery of antibody and therefore excluded from further consideration as TBV targets (listed in Table 1). Problems in the production of mosquito-derived surface ligands for vaccine formulation despite their significant anticipated glycosylation may not hinder their production simply because diverse insect cell lines with the appropriate synthetic pathways are available for transformation.

Table 1 Parasite molecules considered to be potential candidate transmission-blocking vaccines

	Gametocyte		Gamete		Zygote/Ookinete	
	Antigen	Authors	Antigen	Authors	Antigen	Authors
Tested	Pfg27		**HAP2/GSC1 (m)**	Blagborough et al. (2009), Miura et al. [184, 217]	**P25**	Vermeulen, Kaslow
	PfMR5		**P230 (m)**	Williamson et al. (1995), Tachibana et al. (2011, 2012), Farrance et al. [108, 109]	**P28**	Tirawanchai, Quian et al. (2009), Kim et al. (2011)
	Pfs16		**P48/45 (m)**	Outchkourov et al. (2008)	**WARP**	Abraham et al. [174], Golizadeh et al. (2010)
	Pfs2400/Pf11-1		***PfCCP (assorted proteins)***	Simon and Pradel (unpublished)	**Pf75**	Tsuboi/MVI (2016) (http://www.malariavaccine.org/projects/vaccine-projects/pf75-0)
	Plasmepsin 4	Li et al. (2010) [115]	***PfCCP1/PLAP (f)***	Scholz et al. [50], Carter et al. (2008), Saeed et al. [49]	***CelTOS***	Kariu et al. (2006)
			PfCCP2/PLAP (f)	Scholz et al. [50], Carter et al. (2008), Saeed et al. [49]	***Chitinase***	Shahabuddin (1995), Langer et al. (2002), Li et al. (2005), Takeo et al. (2009)
			PfCCP3/PLAP (f)	Scholz et al. [50], Carter et al. (2008), Saeed et al. [49]	***Enolase***	Ghosh et al. (2011)
			PfCCP4/PLAP (f)	Scholz et al. [50], Carter et al. (2008), Saeed et al. [49]	***PfGAP50***	Beiss et al. (2015), Simon et al. [154]
			PfFPNA/ PLAP (f)	Scholz et al. [50], Carter et al. (2008), Saeed et al. [49]	***PSOP12***	Sala et al. (2015)
			GEST (m)	Talman	***SOAP***	Dessens et al. (2003)
			pfs 47 (f)	van Schaijk et al. [55], Tachibana et al. (2015)	***Plasmepsin 7***	Li et al. [190]
					Plasmepsin 10	Li et al. [190]
					Pgs32	Langer et al. (2002)
					Pgs17	Langer et al. (2002)

	Gametocyte		Gamete		Zygote/Ookinete	
	Antigen	Authors	Antigen	Authors	Antigen	Authors
Honourable mentions	*Pfg377*	Alano et al. (1995)	*PbSR*	Carter et al. (2008)	*CTRP*	Trottein (1995), Ramakrishnan et al. (2011)
	PfPEG3/pfMDV1,	Silvestrini et al. (2005)	*Pf36; Pf38 members of the 6-cys family*	Nikolaeva et al. (2015)	*CWP-WPC-1/ Pf75?*	Kangwanrangsan et al. (2013)
	PfPEG4	Silvestrini et al. (2005)			*MAOP/ PPLP3*	Kadota et al. (2004), Kaiser et al. (2004)
	PHIST family 1-36; pfg14, pfg6	Eksi et al. (2005), Sargeant et al. (2006)			*P40*	Sinden (1993), Rawlings and Kaslow (1992)
	Rifins	Sutherland (2009) [99]			*Pfg 27*	Alano et al. (1991), Lobo et al. (1994, 1999)
	Surfins	Sutherland (2009) [99]			*PfGAP50*	Beiss et al. (2015)
					Pfs16	Moelans et al. (1991), Kongkasuriyachai et al. (2004)
					Pfs41	Rener et al. [180]
					Plasmepsin 4	Li et al. (2010)
					PPLP5	Ecker (2007), Kadota (2004)
					PPLP3	Ecker (2007)
					PSOP2	Ecker et al. (2008)
					PSOP7	Ecker et al. (2008)
					Aspartic protease	Ecker (2007)

Those tested and found to be effective are in bold texts, those showing lower efficacy in bold italics texts and those with no effect in bold underlined texts. Those in roman texts have not yet been tested appropriately. (m) indicates male gamete, (f) female gamete.

1.3 The Vertebrate Immune System

A vaccine targeting the giRBC in either the host or vector can bring to bear all relevant effector arms, but this is not the case for vaccines targeting 'downstream' extracellular parasite stages in the vector. Antibodies and immune cells ingested in the blood meal are digested and inactivated at different rates: Complement survives less than 5 h [151, 152]; interestingly the parasites are initially complement resistant [153], and this has recently been shown to be due to the recruitment of human Factor H onto the parasite surface [154]. Phagocytes ingest as much as 66 % of extracellular gametocytes within 2 h in vitro but only 7–14 % in vivo [155]. Whilst these observations were supported by later studies, it was concluded that phagocytosis played no significant role in the transmission-blocking activity of natural sera [155, 156]. Antibody is active for the entire lifetime of the ookinete, albeit at ever decreasing titre, and can enter the haemocoele possibly due to the destruction of the epithelium), where it can reduce sporozoite infection of the salivary glands [157]. Whilst cytokines are known to inhibit parasite development in the midgut [158–160], there is no published data as to the persistence of this activity. Interestingly it was shown that monocytes and polymorphonuclear leucocytes are positively chemotactic to extracellular gametes, but not to intracellular gametocytes, and killed exflagellating male gametocytes when 5–15 μm distant [155]. Thus whilst recognising that loss of all the immune activities is progressive and continuous, simply stated any vaccine target expressed more than 12 h after blood feeding (e.g. ookinete 'invasins') will primarily be attacked by antibody, which must directly/indirectly inhibit an essential function. By contrast, those antigens expressed immediately (e.g. gamete surface proteins) can be attacked by all effector mechanisms, and the antibody may act simply to identify the parasite for killing by other routes. Observations to date suggest anti-P230 antibodies reduce transmission by the agglutination of the male gametes [161] and by complement-mediated [162, 163], isotype-dependent [164] lysis of the gametes, whereas antibodies to the ookinete protein P28 (Pbs21) almost exclusively reduce transmission in a complement-independent manner (i.e. Fab fragments), cell-mediated mechanisms play only a minor role [165–167].

2 Discovery of Targets

Whilst 'rediscovered' in the 1970s the true value of transmission-blocking immunity as a tool to control malaria has only been appreciated in the last decade. It is therefore unsurprising that the discovery of potential targets for transmission-blocking vaccines has not yet benefitted from concerted 'omics' screens. Nonetheless the serendipitous observations of scientists fascinated by the biology of parasite transmission discovered the majority of the moieties considered priority targets today. The prime route to antigen identification stemmed from work where often crudely fractionated parasites were used to immunise mice for the development of monoclonal antibodies which were in turn evaluated by Western blot and laborious membrane-feeding assays [5, 8, 60, 168–171]. In retrospect, we should not forget these endeavours are likely to have identified the most immunogenic of the natural antigens present in complex whole-cell preparations. More recently, a concerted effort by one laboratory has made use of genomic data to look for individual recombinant immunogens in the gametocytes of *P. falciparum* [111, 172].

Here we have attempted to compile the data known to us on the antigens (irrespective of species) both proven and hypothesised to be targets of transmission-blocking immunity from both the parasite (see Table 1) and the mosquito (see Table 2). Parasite antigens are divided by the principle phase of the life cycle in which they are expressed/functional (pre-, post-fertilisation), such that probable effector arms of immunity might be inferred. In drawing up these tables, we are acutely aware (see below) that there is no value in ranking the candidates based upon fine but meaningless discrimination between the reported transmission-blocking

Table 2 Mosquito molecules considered to be potential candidate transmission-blocking vaccines. Those tested and found to be effective are in green boxes, those showing lower efficacy in yellow boxes, and those with no effect in red boxes. Those in clear boxes have not yet been tested appropriately

	Mosquito
Tested	Antigen
	APN1
	Dodecapeptide (discontinuous glycotype Manalpha1-6 proximal to Galbeta1-4GlcNAcalpha-O-R glycans)
	Serpin-2
	~100kD (Mab25C)
	~7kD (Mab24C)
	Gut
	Aminopeptidase N
	Haemolymph
	Trypsin
	Chondroitin sulphate
	A.culicifaces A 62 Kda
	A.culicifaces B 97,94,58 Kda
	A.culicifaces C 23 Kda
	Carboxypeptidase B1
	~30kD Mab4B)
	AgSGU
Honourable mentions	
	Carbohydrates
	GPI anchored protein
	Sugar epitopes/glycans

efficacies generated by different laboratories using ill-defined protocols (see critique of Churcher et al. [173]). Antigens are simply given the attribute 'strong inhibitor' if supported by more than one study.

In looking for new and improved vaccine candidates, we can exploit the 'omics' data generated by numerous studies. Transcriptomic and proteomic libraries now exist from both the parasite and vector, including the gametocyte [48, 71, 174–176], gamete [73] and ookinete [177, 178] and the mosquito midgut brush border [146, 148, 179]. It is time that these were subject to concerted investigation as to the potential utility of the relevant molecules. However recognising the key property required is the induction of a potent transmission-blocking response and the difficulty in predicting this from genomic data, perhaps we should also consider revisiting/regenerating new comprehensive monoclonal antibody libraries to the gametocyte and ookinete, screening/identifying the ligands by mass spectrometry and determining the comparative transmission-blocking potential of the functional immunogens revealed. For the latter, we still lack a high-throughput screen.

3 Vaccine Development

3.1 Antigens Currently Under Clinical Consideration

Antibodies against the surface antigens of the sexual stages of the malaria parasite have been identified as the mediators of TBV efficacy mainly using the ex vivo Standard Membrane-Feeding assay (SMFA). The ideal TBV would induce sustained high-titre functional antibody response against target antigens [166, 167, 180]. These surface antigens are categorised into either pre-fertilisation targets, which are expressed in the human host, or post-fertilisation targets expressed exclusively when the parasite is in the mosquito vector. Both kinds of antigens have advantages and disadvantages as TBV candidate antigens. Antibodies against the pre-fertilisation targets could in theory be boosted by natural exposure as malaria-exposed individuals do develop antibodies against some of these targets like Pfs48/45 and Pfs230C [28, 31, 34]. The expression of these antigens in the human host also puts them under immune pressure, and there is sequence polymorphism reported in these antigens in field isolates [81, 95]. On the other hand, post-fertilisation targets do not benefit from natural boosting as they are not expressed in the human host and hence not under immune pressure. It is important to note that the level of antibody responses in endemic areas to pre-fertilisation sexual-stage antigens are much lower than blood-stage antigens, such as AMA1 resulting in a lower incidence of antigenic polymorphism [81, 95].

Pfs48/45 and Pfs230 remain the most studied and advanced pre-fertilisation targets, as they were the earliest identified TBV candidate antigens. Antibodies against both these antigens produced in recombinant expression systems have shown significant transmission-blocking activity in SMFA and DMFA [181, 182]. Antibodies against the pre-fertilisation candidate HAP2 expressed in *E. coli* and wheat-germ cell-free system have also exhibited convincing transmission-blocking activity in preclinical studies [183, 184]. HAP2 is a male-specific protein first identified in plants and shown to be essential for membrane fusion of the male and female gametocyte during fertilisation [58]. The most extensively studied post-fertilisation candidates are Pfs25 and Pfs28 which are paralogous proteins expressed on the surface of zygotes and ookinetes [185]. Pfs25 is the most advanced TBV candidate in terms of clinical development. There has also been an interest in exploring mosquito proteins that are essential for the parasite to colonise the midgut as potential TBV candidate antigen (See Table 2). The most advanced of these antigens is *Anopheles gambiae* alanyl aminopeptidase 1 (AgAPN1) which is thought to be an attachment ligand for the ookinete to penetrate the midgut epithelium. Antibodies against AgAPN1 have been shown to inhibit the development of *P. berghei*, *P. falciparum* and *P. vivax* in multiple *Anopheline* species [186].

3.2 *Delivery Platforms*

3.2.1 Recombinant Protein Vaccines

Subunit vaccines comprised of a protein antigen delivered with adjuvant have been most widely used to generate a robust antibody response in humans, with some success in certain diseases. This has proven more challenging for a malaria vaccine due to the requirement of durable high-titre functional antibodies against target antigens. The production of conformational antigens has also been difficult to achieve in recombinant protein expression systems [110]. In order to achieve high antibody titres in humans, vaccine candidates are likely to be administered with strong chemical adjuvants and/or highly immunogenic delivery platforms. The most potent adjuvants can lead to unacceptable levels of reactogenicity, as reported in the Phase Ia clinical trial of a soluble Pfs25-montanide ISA51 formulation [187]. Future trials of vaccine candidates with leading adjuvants in clinical development, such as AS01B (GlaxoSmithKline) and SE-GLA and MF59 (Novartis), will hopefully show acceptable reactogenicity profiles.

Pfs25 has been successfully produced as a soluble protein in a variety of expression systems, such as *E. coli* after codon harmonisation, the wheat-germ cell-free system, mammalian HEK293 cells (Nikolaeva et al. in preparation), plant-based *N. benthamiana* and *Chlamydomonas reinhardtii*, and in yeast (*P. pastoris* and *S. cerevisiae*). To date, the protein produced in yeast is the best characterised and the one tested in human clinical trials. Anti-Pfs25 antibodies correlate with TBA in animal models and humans the absolute concentration of anti-Pfs25 specific IgG required to achieve significant blocking in humans is high (86 μg/mL IC50 in the SMFA).

The cysteine-rich pre-fertilisation targets (Pfs48/45 and Pfs230 region C) have been more difficult to produce in heterologous expression systems. This has been reviewed in detail in a few recent review articles. The production of Pfs230C has been hampered by its size (approximately 310 kDa), but several groups have worked on dissecting the regions that confer TBA and identified region C to contain TB epitopes. Recently, an even smaller fragment of region C, C0 (443–730 residues), has been produced in *P. pastoris* to GMP was shown to elicit high TBA.

Antibodies against properly folded recombinant Pfs48/45 have been shown to elicit TBA, but the production of conformational immunogen has been challenging. After various failed attempts at producing the recombinant protein in *E. coli*, *S. cerevisiae*, *P. pastoris* and recombinant viral vectors, recently a smaller fragment of the antigen has been produced in *E. coli* after co-expression of periplasmic folding catalyst. This protein was shown to be conformational and elicited functional antibodies. Harmonising the Pfs48/45 codons to those used in *E. coli* and treating the cell lysate with ionic detergent to maintain it in a soluble state also resulted in the generation of protein that was of natural conformation and elicited strong TBA. The production of the carboxy-terminal 10C-fragment of Pfs48/45 (containing three known epitopes for transmission-blocking antibodies) as a chimaera with the N-terminal R0 region of PfGLURP in *Lactococcus lactis* is a promising approach. The protein has been shown to be correctly folded and has elicited broadly inhibiting antibodies against both asexual and transmission stages of *P. falciparum*. More recently, some TBV antigens have been expressed in the human embryonic kidney cell platform and the *Drosophila* S2 insect cell line (Nikolaeva et al. unpublished; Dabbs et al. unpublished).

3.2.2 Viral-Vectored TBVs

Viral vectors have been shown to reliably induce functional antibodies against a range of malaria antigens in both preclinical and clinical studies in addition to being the best means to induce cellular immunity. ChAd63 (chimpanzee adenovirus 63) and MVA (modified vaccinia virus Ankara) viral vectors have been used to express Pfs25, and when administered in a heterologous prime-boost regime elicited anti-Pfs25 antibodies capable of blocking transmission in membrane-feeding assays [188]. Subsequently, this vaccination regime was used to directly compare the abilities of four leading sexual-stage antigens (Pfs25, Pfs230C, Pfs48/45 and AgAPN1) to induce transmission-blocking antibodies. In this study, Pfs25 was the most potent immunogen followed by a fragment of Pfs230 (region C). Anti-Pfs25 antibodies completely blocked the development of *P. falciparum* in the mosquito in the ex vivo SMFA [189]. The antibodies also blocked the development of field isolates (from gametocyte donors in Burkina Faso) of *P. falciparum*. The antibody response induced by these vectors can be further improved by fusing Pfs25 to IMX313, a new heptamerisation technology, leading to the expression of a heptamer from viral vectors (ChAd63 and MVA) [190]. Immunisation with human AdHu5 vector expressing Pvs25 elicits antibodies which significantly reduce the average oocyst numbers per mosquito when tested against gametocytes from *P. vivax* infected volunteers

[191]. Baculovirus vectors (baculovirus dual-expression system) expressing both Pvs25 and PvsCSP have also been used to successfully elicit antibodies that result in significant transmission-blocking activity [17, 192].

3.2.3 Conjugates and VLPs

There has been substantial interest in developing improved delivery platforms for TBVs due to the limited availability of safe and potent adjuvants. Most of this work has been done targeting Pfs25 either by conjugating Pfs25 to carrier proteins or displaying Pfs25 on VLPs (virus-like particles). Pfs25 has been conjugated to itself [193], NANP repeats of the PfCSP [194], or to carrier proteins. Pfs25 and Pvs25 have been covalently conjugated to outer membrane protein complex (OMPC) of *Neisseria meningitidis* [195] and the nontoxic cholera toxin subunit B [196] which are used in licensed vaccines and also to *Pseudomonas aeruginosa* detoxified toxin exoprotein A (EPA) which has been tested extensively in humans [197]. Conjugations of Pfs25 to these carrier proteins have led to the production of naturally folded antigens and significant increase in anti-Pfs25 antibody titre and TBA. In the study where Pfs25 was conjugated to OMPC, the persistence of the antibody response in macaques over 18 months was very encouraging [195] as multiseasonal activity is a highly desirable attribute for any TBV. Pfs25-EPA has been manufactured to GMP and subsequently Pfs28, and a region of Pfs230C has also been conjugated to EPA obtaining similar results. The Fraunhofer Institute generated a VLP by fusion of Pfs25 to the *Alfalfa mosaic virus* coat protein, expressed in *N. benthamiana* [198]. Mice receiving one or two administration of this VLP with Alhydrogel generated functional antibodies which were sustained over a 6-month period. Similar to the construct in viral vectors mentioned above, the Pfs25-IMX313 fusion has also been expressed as a protein-nanoparticle in *P. pastoris* with significant improvement in antibody titre, quality and TBA. This is currently being manufactured to GMP at the Jenner Institute in Oxford. Recently in an exciting programme of work, ‘bacterial superglue’ has been used to establish a platform for irreversibly decorating VLPs simply by mixing with protein antigen. The bacteriophage AP205 genetically fused to SpyCatcher was produced in *E. coli* and mixed with its peptide-partner SpyTag fused to Pfs25 [199]. This spontaneously forms a covalent bond, and the VLPs generated displaying Pfs25 are significantly more immunogenic than soluble Pfs25 protein.

3.3 Clinical Development

Until recently, the only TBV candidate listed on the WHO malaria vaccine rainbow table was Pfs25, which is currently the most developed TBV candidate in the product pipeline [200]. In 1996 volunteers were primed with a highly attenuated vaccinia viral vector expressing seven genes from *P. falciparum* (denoted NYVAC-Pf7), including Pfs25, followed by a boost of Pfs25 recombinant protein. Pfs25 formulated in aluminium hydroxide was tested in humans along with its ortholog Pvs25 from *P. vivax*, but the trial was halted due to hypersensitivity reactions [187]. In a later trial when the same Pfs25 vaccine was used to boost responses primed with a viral vector (NYVAC-Pf7), a few volunteers developed functional antibodies. Anti-Pfs25 antibodies induced in humans after vaccination with soluble Pfs25 protein in montanide ISA51 are also functional in the ex vivo membrane-feeding assays and significantly block the development of both laboratory strain and field isolates (from gametocyte donors) of *P. falciparum* [187]. The Pfs25-EPA conjugate formulated with Alhydrogel has been tested in malaria-naïve adult volunteers in the USA, with extension to Phase Ib field trials in Mali underway. Most recently, a clinical study has been completed in the USA to assess a combination of this vaccine with another consisting of EPA conjugated to a region of the gametocyte antigen Pfs230 (Clinicaltrials.gov NCT02334462). The Pfs25 VLP developed by the Fraunhofer Institute formulated in aluminium hydroxide is also currently being tested in humans. The results of these most recent clinical trials of Pfs25-based conjugates are eagerly awaited. A Phase Ia human clinical trial is currently being conducted in Oxford to test viral-vectored vaccines expressing Pfs25-IMX313 as part of an EU funded project (MultiMalVax).

The REDMAL project funded by the European Commission is supporting the GMP production of a chimeric protein called R0-PF10C, comprising of a region of Pfs48/45 (Pfs48/4510C) fused to a portion of glutamate-rich protein (GLURP.R0).

3.4 Future Developments

The future assessment of the merits of the approaches described above in humans will be a key focus of research in the next few years. There are a number of improved protein delivery platforms (carriers and VLPs) that are currently being pursued for the leading antigens (mainly Pfs25), and it will be important to test these in humans to determine their potential. In future, it is likely there will be a range of new platforms designed to improve antibody immunogenicity in humans, and more candidate antigens could be tested in humans using these platforms. Structural studies in humans will also enable us to design improved second-generation immunogens by dissecting the human immune response to these antigens and focussing on blocking epitopes. There is still a need to establish the amount of antibody required against a particular antigen to achieve significant TBA and work towards developing delivery platforms and adjuvants that can achieve these levels in humans. Amongst the candidates currently being investigated, there is a scope of combining antigens expressed at the different stages of sexual development to test if these antibodies are additive or synergistic keeping in mind that some of these antigens might compete with each other and lead to decreased potency of the individual antigens. Potential new vaccine candidates are likely to emerge from '-omic' datasets. To evaluate rationally the efficacy of vaccines developed in different laboratories it is important to standardise the assays that we use to screen these new antigens and establish the suitability of these assays to progress antigens forward.

4 Evaluation and Potential Impact of TBVs

Assessment of the impact of transmission-blocking vaccines is conceptually challenging. The successful use of a TBV should logically result in a reduced number of malaria-infected humans within an endemic population [18]. Quantifying this key output, by assessing variables such as parasite rate (PR), infectiousness, force of infection (FOI), molecular force of infection (mFOI), multiplicity of infection (MOI) and annual parasite index (API), the basic productive number (R*o*) [201] or slide positivity rate (SPR) is mostly impossible within a lab-derived situation and can be technically difficult within a field context.

The relationship between these clinically relevant metrics and changes in malarial transmission are complex and difficult to quantify [202]. Transmission in the wild is exceptionally variable due to changes in a series of underlying factors, comprising, but not limited to, fluctuations in gametocyte density, seasonality, variation in naturally acquired host immunity to malaria infection, genetic variation within mosquito populations, climate-induced changes in the interactions between parasite and host and the geospatial variability of any host/parasite samples examined. Due to this 'standard' variability in transmission, the conclusive assignment of any change in malarial burden due to impact of TBV implementation within an examined region is likely to be difficult and open to varied interpretation. Allied to this, the collection of these relevant metrics currently lack standardised methodology, need specialised training to analyse, require large sample sizes, and have multiple considerations regarding cost, precision and accuracy [16, 67, 202, 203].

As a result of these issues, a wide range of other 'correlate' assays examining earlier convenient (preclinical) points within the parasite lifecycle have been developed and adapted over the years. The use of multiple assays in combination is common to examine the impact of individual TBV candidates throughout the vaccine development pipeline in both the lab and the field. Within the lab, a wide range of assays to examine the impact of TBVs are available. These assays are typically cost-effective and high throughput when compared to their field counterparts, and combination of these assays can often enable identification of the mode of action of an individual TBV. Most importantly, the ability of researchers to perform these studies within a controlled environment gives lab experiments a potential advantage over field studies, where numerous experimental parameters are simultaneously uncontrollable, variable and often undetectable when assessing the effectiveness of a vaccine; however, care must be taken when considering the extrapolation of lab-derived results to a field context.

4.1 Transmission-Blocking Assays with Immunological Outputs

A successful TBV induces antibodies that target surface antigens on the sexual stages of *Plasmodium*, or targets located on the mosquito midgut. These antibodies can inhibit parasite fertilisation through agglutination, steric hindrance or complement-mediated lysis of gametes, e.g. [151], whereas ookinete development can be inhibited or fully prevented by melanisation, antibody-dependent phagocytosis or by blocking recognition of midgut epithelial cells [10, 166]. Probably the simplest, high-throughput and lowest-cost method of assessing the potential impact of a TBV is to perform a relevant immunological assay to measure the ability of (post-immunisation) derived antibody to bind to parasitic/insect immunogens. At the simplest level, performance of a simple Western blot or IFA can be used to confirm ability of induced antibody to recognise an appropriate immunogen; however, this only gives a semi-quantitative (and subjective) readout. To achieve more quantitative data for the triage of antibodies induced by TBVs, enzyme-linked immunosorbant assays (ELISAs) are often utilised. Previous studies have conclusively identified a link between antibody titre identified by ELISA and efficacy in mosquito feeding assays for many (but not all) of the current lead transmission-blocking immunogens (e.g. anti-Pfs25 [184, 204, 205], Pvs25 [205], Pfs230 [184] and Pfs48/45 antibodies). It is still unclear if titre of an antibody response is *always* reflective of its ability to inhibit transmission, with additional qualitative changes (e.g. isotype and affinity maturation) potentially impacting on the ability of an antibody to block transmission to the mosquito with some antigens. The utility of the ELISA technique is largely dependent on the properties of the protein to be used to coat plates—folding of recombinant protein in native conformation gives more accurate prediction of in vivo efficacy. Alternatively, gametocyte, gamete, ookinete or mosquito midgut lysate can be used in some cases to coat plates and examine the ability of antibody to recognise native parasite protein, avoiding the use of recombinant protein [206]. Despite these robust and cheap immunological assays, there is still a real lack of a relevant and convenient immunological correlate that can predict the field efficacy of an induced anti-TBV response. Generation of such a predictive and standardised method, that is, immunogen, strain and parasite species independent, would be an exceptionally attractive advance and would greatly facilitate the process of accelerated legal and ethical approval for TBV usage in the field [18].

4.2 Pre-oocyst Transmission-Blocking Assays Examining Cell Biology

In terms of pre-fertilisation in vitro assays to assess the impact of a transmission-blocking intervention, multiple techniques have been developed to assess the impact of antimalarial drugs (e.g. early- to late-stage gametocyte assays [203], gamete activation assays measuring intracellular calcium [207]); however, only a limited number of these assays have demonstrated suitability to assess the impact of antibodies derived from TBVs. The process of exflagellation (the production of motile-free swimming male gametes) has previously been used in a standardised low-throughput assay to assess the ability of antibody to bind to exflagellation centres [208]; however, concerns persist regarding the low power and reproducibility of this assay. The narrow and variable observation window (minutes) for this process, allied to the fact that the relationship between motile microgametes, ookinetes, oocysts and subsequent infection remains largely unquantified, means that assays of this type have only a limited predictive power to assess impact on transmission [203].

Post-fertilisation, the tractable and robust ookinete conversion assay can be used to examine the ability of TBV-induced antibodies to inhibit transmission. The application of this assay to multiple plasmodial species is constrained by the species-specific differences in the ability to culture ookinetes in vitro. Attempts to culture ookinetes multiple of rodent malaria species and *P. vivax* have been successful, but *P. falciparum* ookinete culture currently remains impractical for routine application [209–211], although fully in vivo derivatives of this assay may provide valuable to examine *P. falciparum* fertilisation events (Marques unpublished). The use of *P. berghei* in this assay is by far the most advanced, where ookinete conversion can be examined quickly and easily (in medium to high throughput) in simple 24 h cultures. Ookinete conversion rates can be calculated, which express the number of ookinetes (successful fertilisation events) relative to the original/total number of macrogametocytes (unfertilised females), thus indicating the efficiency of fertilisation and/or the progression of the zygote to ookinete stage of the lifecycle. By supplementing these cultures with potentially transmission-blocking antibodies, TB efficacy at the pre-ookinete stage can be assayed exceptionally quickly. Blockade is assessed by comparing conversion rates between cultures containing test antibody in comparison with conversion in feeds supplemented with a negative control exhibiting no specific transmission-blocking activity (e.g. purified IgG2a from murine myeloma, clone UPC10 [183]).

4.3 *Oocyst-Based Transmission-Blocking Assays*

By far the most widely used assay to assess antimalarial transmission-blocking interventions (both vaccines and drugs) is the standard membrane-feeding assay (SMFA), considered by many to be the 'gold standard' of transmission-blocking assays. To examine the efficacy of potentially transmission-blocking antibodies, sexually mature cultured gametocytes are typically mixed with antibody or serum and fed through an artificial membrane to uninfected *Anopheles* mosquitoes. Subsequently, parasite load within the mosquito is quantified by examining oocysts to assess levels of transmission from vertebrate to insect host. Both infection intensity (mean number of oocysts per mosquito midgut) and prevalence (percentage of infected mosquitoes) are recorded and blockade assessed by comparison with a replicate feed performed using an appropriate negative control antibody/serum. The concept of enumerating oocysts has been the mainstay of evaluating transmission to the mosquito since the initial studies of Ross in 1897 [212]. Mature oocysts can be easily identified by classical bright-field or phase microscopy or mecurochrome staining of infected midguts. Observation of fixed (robust) and stained mosquito guts can result in a longer counting window [213]. Within the past decade, multiple technological advances have been made to enhance the utility of the SMFA. The use of automated computer-aided imaging/quantitation methods [214] can improve throughput and reduces significant inter-operator variation. Use of fluorescent-tagged parasites (e.g. GFP under the regulation of the EIF1α promoter [215]) has further enhanced the utility and throughput of this assay. More recently, luminescence-based approaches that use *P. falciparum* strains that express firefly luciferase protein within a SMFA platform [216] have been developed. Within these studies, reduction in oocyst intensity and prevalence is closely related to a robust, observable and reproducible reduction in luciferase activity, potentially increasing the throughput and reproducibility of the traditional SMFA.

A wide range of studies describing the utility and limitations of the SMFA have been published previously [173, 184, 217], with extensive discussion based on the relative accuracy of the assay. Briefly, the majority of SMFAs are performed with comparatively high densities of gametocytes, resulting in high oocyst numbers [173, 218]. These high densities are considered unrepresentative of natural-based infections, making it challenging to directly translate SMFA outputs to predicted field impact. The well-described but complex saturating relationship between reduction in oocyst intensity and reduction in oocyst prevalence can also make interpretation of results challenging [173]. Although prevalence and intensity are positively correlated, significant reductions in intensity are often required to obtain measurable reductions in prevalence. This can also have significant impact on the number of dissected mosquitoes that must be examined to achieve precise estimates of significant reductions in oocyst prevalence. However the SMFA is performed, it is a good practice to record the results in terms of both the reduction in oocyst intensity and the prevalence, and the control (no intervention) oocyst intensity and prevalence should be reported. It is additionally highly advantageous to perform the SMFA at a wide range of control gametocyte/oocyst densities to maximise the utility of any resulting data [173, 184].

It should be noted that there are also multiple alternative SMFA-derivative assays available to examine transmission blockade that examine reductions in oocyst intensity and prevalence, with different formats. The direct feeding assay (DFA) requires direct feeding of uninfected mosquitoes on a host, and the direct membrane-feeding assay (DMFA) involves the withdrawal of blood from infected, gametocyte positive individuals, followed by membrane feeding. Previous studies have reported that the DMFA is the most sensitive reporter of reductions in transmission, whereas the SMFA has greater utility [219]. Despite the multiple advantages and disadvantages of each assay, the SMFA, DFA and SMFA all offer valuable high-biological-content options to assess the efficacy of TBVs. All of these assays additionally have extensive utility when testing TBVs within clinical trials. The SMFA or DMFA has previously been used within Phase I trials to assess the efficacy of serum harvested post-vaccination in endemic or non-endemic settings (e.g. both have been used previously to assess the efficacy of anti-Pfs25 vaccines) (e.g. [187, 189]), whereas the DFA, despite exhibiting conditions that more naturally reflect natural feeding, has traditionally been used less due to ethical issues, limiting the number of mosquito exposures and precluding the use of younger trial subjects [184].

4.4 Sporozoite Assays

Rather than examining oocyst load within the mosquito midgut, comparatively rarely, the presence/density of sporozoites in the salivary glands is sometimes examined to assess the impact of a TBV. This option is technically more challenging than the examination of oocyst intensity/prevalence, however, its location within the lifecycle (resulting in the measurement of the directly infectious form of the parasite), can arguably result in a more predictive and clinically relevant output. Simple dissection of mosquito salivary glands, followed by scoring (typically on a log scale), is quick, MTP, cheap and robust; however, it is relatively crude and can result in a low level of sensitivity [220]. An enzyme-linked immunosorbent assay [221, 222] and an immunoradiometric assay [223, 224] have been developed previously to assess sporozoite load, along with more recent studies that utilise GFP-/luciferase-expressing salivary gland sporozoites to allow quantitation of within insect lysates [225]. Although undoubtedly advances on previous low-tech options, the threshold of detection of many of these methods is relatively low (~1000 sporozoites). To increase practical utility, and given the fact that low numbers of sporozoites can successfully establish a blood-stage infection post-bite, increased sensitivity is required [203].

4.5 Population Assays

The ultimate objective of a successful TBV is to reduce the number of blood-stage infections within a human population. The methods described above are incapable of measuring this vital output and instead (sensibly) measure convenient pre-clinical correlates to assess the potential efficacy of a TBV. A resulting issue is that the links between these lab-based surrogates and subsequent malarial infection are largely uncharacterised [203], not linearly correlated, and are likely to be variable depending on differences in transmission intensities in multiple field settings. This hinders the field translatability of resulting data and prevents the assignment of informed go/no-go efficacy requirements for the clinical development of novel TBVs. Historically, studies have suggested that an >80 % reduction in oocyst intensity might be required to take an antigen/adjuvant combination to clinical trials [226]. More recently, an early-stage population transmission model using a rodent malaria parasite (*P. berghei*) has been used to examine the effects of transmission-blocking interventions over multiple transmission cycles in multiple and distinct parasite populations that reflect varied levels of transmission intensity [220, 227]. This model indicates that the required efficacy for a TBV to be considered effective will be heavily dependent on local transmission levels that prevail. Resulting data also suggests that the current efficacy threshold of >80 % reduction in oocyst intensity may be too stringent and that a TBV with lower efficacy could potentially, when utilised over multiple transmission cycles, achieve elimination in areas with a lower transmission intensity [220]. As a result, vaccine candidates with appropriate TBA that are capable of inducing long-lasting circulating antibody titres should be priotitised. It would be advantageous for future related studies to examine the effect of variable vaccine duration on elimination across multiple transmission settings and the minimum requirements for vaccine coverage and how these metrics link to vaccine efficacy.

References

1. Eyles DE (1952) Studies on *Plasmodium gallinaceum*. III Factors associated with the malaria infection in the vertebrate host which influence the degree of infection in the mosquito. Am J Trop Med Hyg 55:386–391
2. Huff CG, Marchbank DF, Shiroishi T (1958) Changes in infectiousness of malarial gametes II. Analysis of possible causative factors. Exp Parasitol 7:399–417
3. Gwadz RW (1976) Malaria: successful immunization against the sexual stages of *Plasmodium gallinaceum*. Science 193:1150–1151
4. Carter R, Chen DH (1976) Malaria transmission blocked by immunisation with gametes of the malaria parasite. Nature 263:57–60
5. Mendis KN, Targett GAT (1979) Immunisation against gametes and asexual erythrocytic stages of a rodent malaria parasite. Nature 277(5695):389–391
6. Carter R, Grotendorst C (1981) Post fertilization targets of transmission blocking immunity to *Plasmodium gallinaceum*. Am J Trop Med Hyg
7. Kaslow DC, Quakyi IA, Syin C, Raum MG, Keister DB, Coligan JE, McCutchan TF, Miller LH (1988) A vaccine candidate from the sexual stage of human malaria that contains EGF-like domains. Nature 333:74–76
8. Tirawanchai N, Winger LA, Nicholas J, Sinden RE (1991) Analysis of immunity induced by affinity-purified 21-kilodalton zygote-ookinete surface antigen of *Plasmodium berghei*. Infect Immun 59:36–44
9. van Amerongen A, Sauerwein RW, Beckers PJA, Meloen RH, Meuwissen JHET (1989) Identification of a peptide sequence of the 25 kD protein of *Plasmodium falciparum* recognized by transmission-blocking monoclonal antibodies: implications for synthetic vaccine development. Parasite Immunol 11:425–428
10. Vermeulen AN, Ponnudurai T, Beckers PJA, Verhave JP, Smits MA, Meuwissen JHET (1985) Sequential expression of antigens on sexual stages of *Plasmodium falciparum* accessible to transmission-blocking antibodies in the mosquito. J Exp Med 162:1460–1476
11. Armistead JS, Morlais I, Mathias DK, Jardim JG, Joy J, Fridman A, Finnefrock AC, Bagchi A, Plebanski M, Scorpio DG et al (2013) Antibodies to a single, conserved epitope in *Anopheles* APN1 inhibit universal transmission of falciparum and vivax malaria. Infect Immun 82:818–829
12. Atkinson SC, Armistead JS, Mathias DK, Sandeu MM, Tao D, Borhani-Dizaji N, Tarimo BB, Morlais I, Dinglasan RR, Borg NA (2015) The *Anopheles*-midgut APN1 structure reveals a new malaria transmission-blocking vaccine epitope. Nat Struct Mol Biol 22:532–539

13. Dinglasan RR, Fields I, Shahabuddin M, Azad AF, Sacci JB Jr (2003) Monoclonal antibody MG96 completely blocks *Plasmodium yoelii* development in *Anopheles stephensi*. Infect Immun 71:6995–7001
14. Lal AA, Patterson PS, Sacci JB, Vaughan J, Paul C, Collins WE, Wirtz RA, Azad AF (2001) Anti-mosquito midgut antibodies block development of *Plasmodium falciparum* and *Plasmodium vivax* in multiple species of *Anopheles* mosquitoes and reduce vector fecundity and survivorship. PNAS 98:5228–5233
15. Mathias DK, Plieskatt JL, Armistead JS, Bethony JM, Abdul-Majid KB, McMillan A, Angov E, Aryee MJ, Zhan B, Gillespie P et al (2012) Expression, immunogenicity, histopathology, and potency of a mosquito-based malaria transmission-blocking recombinant vaccine. Infect Immun 80(4):1606–1614
16. Sinden RE (2010) A biologist's perspective on malaria vaccine development. Hum Vaccin 6:3–11
17. Mizutani M, Iyori M, Blagborough AM, Fukumoto S, Funatsu T, Sinden RE, Yoshida S (2014) Baculovirus-vectored multistage *Plasmodium vivax* vaccine induces both protective and transmission-blocking immunities against transgenic rodent malaria parasites. Infect Immun 82:4348–4357
18. Nunes JK, Woods C, Carter T, Raphael T, Morin MJ, Diallo D, Leboulleux D, Jain S, Loucq C, Kaslow DC et al (2014) Development of a transmission-blocking malaria vaccine: progress, challenges, and the path forward. Vaccine 32:5531–5539
19. Tibúrcio M, Dixon MWA, Looker O, Younis SY, Tilley L, Alano P (2015) Specific expression and export of the *Plasmodium falciparum* gametocyte exported protein-5 marks the gametocyte ring stage. Malar J 14:334
20. Tiburcio M, Sauerwein R, Lavazec C, Alano P (2015) Erythrocyte remodeling by *Plasmodium falciparum* gametocytes in the human host interplay. Trends Parasitol 31:270–278
21. Saeed M, Roeffen W, Alexander N, Drakeley CJ, Targett GAT, Sutherland CJ (2008) *Plasmodium falciparum* antigens on the surface of the gametocyte-infected erythrocyte. PLoS One 3, e2280
22. Sutherland CJ (2009) Surface antigens of *Plasmodium falciparum* gametocytes—a new class of transmission-blocking vaccine targets? Mol Biochem Parasitol 166:93–98
23. Tonwong N, Sattabongkot J, Tsuboi T, Iriko H, Takeo S, Sirichaisinthop J, Udomsangpetch R (2012) Natural infection of *Plasmodium falciparum* induces inhibitory antibodies against gametocyte development in human hosts. Jpn J Infect Dis 65:152–156
24. Bousema T, Roeffen W, Meijerink H, Mwerinde H, Mwakalinga S, van Gemert G-J, van de Vegte-Bolmer M, Mosha F, Targett G, Riley EM et al (2010) The dynamics of naturally acquired immune responses to *Plasmodium falciparum* sexual stage antigens Pfs230 & Pfs48/45 in a low endemic area in Tanzania. PLoS One 5, e14114
25. Carter R, Graves PM, Quakyi IA, Good MF (1989) Restricted or absent immune responses in human populations to *Plasmodium falciparum* gamete antigens that are targets of malaria transmission-blocking antibodies. J Exp Med 169:135–147
26. Graves PM, Burkot TR, Carter R, Cattani JA, Lagog M, Parker J, Brabin BJ, Gibson FD, Bradley DJ, Alpers MP (1988) Measurement of malarial infectivity of human populations to mosquitoes in the Madang area, Papua New Guinea. Parasitology 96:251–263
27. Graves PM, Carter R, Burkot T, Rener J, Kaushal DC, Williams JL (1985) Effects of different transmission-blocking antibodies on different isolates of *Plasmodium falciparum*. Infect Immun 48:611–616
28. Graves PM, Carter R, Burkot TR, Quakyi IA, Kumar N (1988) Antibodies to *Plasmodium falciparum* gamete surface antigens in Papua New Guinea sera. Parasite Immunol 10:209–218
29. Graves PM, Doubrovsky A, Sattabongkot J, Battistutta D (1992) Human antibody responses to epitopes on the *Plasmodium falciparum* gametocyte antigen PFS 48/45 and their relationship to infectivity of gametocyte carriers. Am J Trop Med Hyg 46(6):711–719

30. Graves PM, Wirtz RA, Carter R, Burkot TR, Looker M, Targett GAT (1988) Naturally occurring antibodies to an epitope on *Plasmodium falciparum* gametes detected by monoclonal antibody-based competitive enzyme-linked immunosorbent assay. Infect Immun 56:2818–2821
31. Healer J, McGuinness D, Carter R, Riley E (1999) Transmission-blocking immunity to *Plasmodium falciparum* in malaria-immune individuals is associated with antibodies to the gamete surface protein Pfs230. Parasitology 119(Pt 5):425–433
32. Ouedraogo AL, Roeffen W, Luty AJ, de Vlas SJ, Nebie I, Ilboudo-Sanogo E, Cuzin-Ouattara N, Teleen K, Tiono AB, Sirima SB et al (2011) Naturally acquired immune responses to *Plasmodium falciparum* sexual stage antigens Pfs48/45 and Pfs230 in an area of seasonal transmission. Infect Immun 79:4957–4964
33. Roeffen W, Beckers P, Fassote A, Sieben M, Meuwissen JHET (1989) Serological *Plasmodium falciparum* transmission blocking assay; results from endemic malaria regions and travellers. Proc Brit Soc Parasitol
34. Roeffen W, Lensen T, Mulder B, Teelen K, Sauerwein R, Eling W, Meuwissen JHET, Beckers P (1994) Transmission blocking immunity as observed in a feeder system and serological reactivity to pfs 48/45 and pfs230 in field sera. Mem Inst Oswaldo Cruz 89:13–15
35. Adjalley SH, Johnston GL, Li T, Eastman RT, Ekland EH, Eappen AG, Richman A, Sim BKL, Lee MCS, Hoffman SL et al (2011) Quantitative assessment of *Plasmodium falciparum* sexual development reveals potent transmission-blocking activity by methylene blue. Proc Natl Acad Sci 108:E1214–E1223
36. Lucantoni L, Fidock DA, Avery VM (2016) A luciferase-based, high-throughput assay for screening and profiling transmission-blocking compounds against *Plasmodium falciparum* gametocytes. Antimicrob Agents Chemother 60(4):2097–2107
37. Silvestrini F, Alano P, Williams JL (2000) Commitment to the production of male and female gametocytes in the human malaria parasite *Plasmodium falciparum*. Parasitology 121:465–471
38. Skinner J, Huang C-Y, Waisberg M, Felgner PL, Doumbo OK, Ongoiba A, Kayentao K, Traore B, Crompton PD, Williamson KC (2015) *Plasmodium falciparum* gametocyte-specific antibody profiling reveals boosting through natural infection and identifies potential markers of gametocyte exposure. Infect Immun 83:4229–4236
39. Frank R (2008) Evaluation of PfCCp multidomain adhesion proteins of *Plasmodium falciparum* as candidates for transmission-blocking vaccines and chacterisation of *Plasmodium berghei* putative ookinete surface proteins. Diplomarbeit–Univesitat Wurzburg, Würzburg, pp 1–93
40. Lavazec C, Moreira CK, Mair GR, Waters AP, Janse CJ, Templeton TJ (2009) Analysis of mutant *Plasmodium berghei* parasites lacking expression of multiple PbCCp genes. Mol Biochem Parasitol 163:1–7
41. Pradel G, Wagner C, Mejia C, Templeton TJ (2006) *Plasmodium falciparum*: co-dependent expression and co-localization of the PfCCp multi-adhesion domain proteins. Exp Parasitol 112:263–268
42. Raine JD, Ecker A, Mendoza J, Tewari R, Stanway RR, Sinden RE (2007) Female inheritance of malarial lap genes is essential for mosquito transmission. PLoS Pathog 3, e30
43. de Koning-Ward TF, Olivieri A, Bertuccini L, Hood A, Sivestrini F, Charvalias K, Diaz PB, Camarda G, McElwain TF, Papenfuss T et al (2008) The role of osmiophilic bodies and Pfg377 expression in female gametocyte emergence and mosquito infectivity in the human malaria parasite *Plasmodium falciparum*. Mol Microbiol 67:278–290
44. Sologub L, Kuehn A, Kern S, Przyborski J, Schillig R, Pradel G (2011) Malaria proteases mediate inside-out egress of gametocytes from red blood cells following parasite transmission to the mosquito. Cell Microbiol 13:897–912
45. Wirth CC, Glushakova S, Scheuermayer M, Repnik U, Garg S, Schaack D, Kachman MM, Weißbach T, Zimmerberg J, Dandekar T et al (2014) Perforin-like protein PPLP2 permeabilizes the red blood cell membrane during egress of *Plasmodium falciparum* gametocytes. Cell Microbiol 16:709–733

46. Lal K, Delves MJ, Bromley E, Wastling JM, Tomley FM, Sinden RE (2009) *Plasmodium* male development gene-1 (mdv-1) is important for female sexual development and identifies a polarised plasma membrane during zygote development. Int J Parasitol 39:755–761
47. Ponzi M, Siden-Kiamos I, Bertuccinin L, Curra C, Kroeze H, Camarda G, Pace T, Franke-Fayard B, Laurentino EC, Louis K et al (2009) Egress of *Plasmodium berghei* gametes from their host erythrocyte is mediated by MDV-1/PEG3 protein. Cell Microbiol 11:1272–1288
48. Khan SM, Franke-Fayard B, Mair GR, Lasonder E, Janse CJ, Mann M, Waters AP (2005) Proteome analysis of separated male and female gametocytes reveals novel sex-specific *Plasmodium* biology. Cell 121:675–687
49. Saeed S, Carter V, Tremp AZ, Dessens JT (2010) *Plasmodium berghei* crystalloids contain multiple LCCL proteins. Mol Biochem Parasitol 170:49–53
50. Scholz SM, Simon N, Lavazec C, Dude M-A, Templeton TJ, Pradel G (2008) PfCCp proteins of *Plasmodium falciparum*: gametocyte-specific expression and role in complement-mediated inhibition of exflagellation. Int J Parasitol 38:327–340
51. Simon N, Scholz SM, Moreira CK, Templeton TJ, Kuehn A, Dude M-A, Pradel G (2009) Sexual stage adhesion proteins form multi-protein complexes in the malaria parasite *Plasmodium falciparum*. J Biol Chem 284(21):14537–14546
52. van Dijk MR, Janse CJ, Thompson J, Waters AP, Braks JAM, Dodemont HJ, Stunnenberg HG, van Gemert GJ, Sauerwein RW, Eling W (2001) A central role for P48/45 in malaria parasite male gamete fertility. Cell 104:153–164
53. Kuehn A, Simon N, Pradel G (2010) Family members stick together: multi-protein complexes of malaria parasites. Med Microbiol Immunol 199:209–226
54. Pradel G (2007) Proteins of the malaria parasite sexual stages: expression, function and potential for transmission blocking strategies. Parasitology 134:1911–1929
55. van Schaijk BCL, van Dijk MR, van de Vegte-Bolmer M, van Gemert GJ, van Dooren MW, Eksi S, Roeffen WFG, Janse CJ, Waters AP, Sauerwein RW (2006) Pfs47, paralog of the male fertility factor Pfs48/45, is a female specific surface protein in *Plasmodium falciparum*. Mol Biochem Parasitol 149:216–222
56. Hirai M, Arai M, Mori T, Miyagishima SY, Kawai S, Kita K, Kuroiwa T, Terenius O, Matsuoka H (2008) Male fertility of malaria parasites is determined by GCS1, a plant-type reproduction factor. Curr Biol 18:607–613
57. Hirai M, Mori T (2010) Fertilization is a novel attacking site for the transmission blocking of malaria parasites. Acta Trop 114:157–161
58. Liu Y, Tewari R, Ning J, Blagborough AM, Garbom S, Pei J, Grishin NV, Steele RE, Sinden RE, Snell WJ et al (2008) The conserved plant sterility gene HAP2 functions after attachment of fusogenic membranes in *Chlamydomonas* and *Plasmodium* gametes. Genes Dev 22:1051–1068
59. Carter R, Miller LH, Rener J, Kaushal DC, Kumar N, Graves PM, Grotendorst CA, Gwadz RW, French C, Wirth D (1984) Target antigens in malaria transmission blocking immunity. Philos Trans R Soc 307:201–213
60. Kaushal DC, Carter R (1984) Characterization of antigens on mosquito midgut stages of *Plasmodium gallinaceum*. II. Comparison of surface antigens of male and female gametes and zygotes. Mol Biochem Parasitol 11:145–156
61. Kaushal DC, Carter R, Howard RJ, McAuliffe FM (1983) Characterization of antigens on mosquito midgut stages of *Plasmodium gallinaceum* I. zygote surface antigens. Mol Biochem Parasitol 8:53–69
62. Tomas A, Margos G, Dimopoulos G, van Lin LHM, de Koning-Ward TF, Sinha R, Lupetti P, Beetsma AL, Rodriguez MC, Karras M et al (2001) P25 and P28 proteins of the malaria ookinete surface have multiple and partially redundant functions. EMBO J 20:3975–3983
63. Duffy PE, Kaslow DC (1997) A novel malaria protein, Pfs28, and Pfs25 are genetically linked and synergistic as falciparum malaria transmission-blocking vaccines. Infect Immun 65:1109–1113
64. Hisaeda H, Collins WE, Saul A, Stowers AW (2001) Antibodies to *Plasmodium vivax* transmission-blocking vaccine candidate antigens Pvs25 and Pvs28 do not show synergism. Vaccine 20:763–770

65. Han YS, Thompson J, Kafatos FC, Barillas-Mury C (2000) Molecular interactions between *Anopheles stephensi* midgut cells and *Plasmodium berghei*: the time bomb theory of ookinete invasion of mosquitoes. EMBO J 19:6030–6040
66. Shahabuddin M, Kaslow DC (1994) *Plasmodium*: parasite chitinase and its role in malaria transmission. Exp Parasitol 79:85–88
67. Sinden RE (2015) The cell biology of malaria infection of mosquito: advances and opportunities. Cell Microbiol 17:451–466
68. Mair G, Braks JAM, Garver LS, Wiegant JCAG, Hall N, Dirks RW, Khan SM, Dimopoulos G, Janse CJ, Waters AP (2006) Regulation of sexual development of *Plasmodium* by translational repression. Science 313:667669
69. Mair GR, Lasonder E, Garver LS, Franke-Fayard BM, Carret CK, Wiegant JC, Dirks RW, Dimopoulos G, Janse CJ, Waters AP (2010) Universal features of post-transcriptional gene regulation are critical for *Plasmodium* zygote development. PLoS Pathog 6, e1000767
70. Miao J, Li J, Fan Q, Li X, Li X, Cui L (2010) The Puf-family RNA-binding protein PfPuf2 regulates sexual development and sex differentiation in the malaria parasite *Plasmodium falciparum.* J Cell Sci 123:1039–1049
71. Akinosoglou KA, Bushell ES, Ukegbu CV, Schlegelmilch T, Cho JS, Redmond S, Sala K, Christophides GK, Vlachou D (2014) Characterization of *Plasmodium* developmental transcriptomes in *Anopheles gambiae* midgut reveals novel regulators of malaria transmission. Cell Microbiol 17:254–268
72. Bushell ES, Ecker A, Schlegelmilch T, Goulding D, Dougan G, Sinden RE, Christophides GK, Kafatos FC, Vlachou D (2009) Paternal effect of the nuclear formin-like protein MISFIT on *Plasmodium* development in the mosquito vector. PLoS Pathog 5, e1000539
73. Talman A, Prieto J, Marques S, Ubaida-Mohien C, Lawniczak M, Wass M, Xu T, Frank R, Ecker A, Stanway R et al (2014) Proteomic analysis of the *Plasmodium* male gamete reveals the key role for glycolysis in flagellar motility. Malar J 13:315
74. Tao D, Ubaida-Mohien C, Mathias DK, King JG, Pastrana-Mena R, Tripathi A, Goldowitz I, Graham D, Moss E, Marti M et al (2014) Sex-partitioning of the *Plasmodium falciparum* stage V gametocyte proteome provides insight into falciparum-specific cell biology. Mol Cell Proteomics 13:2705–2724
75. Kumar N, Carter R (1985) Biosynthesis of two stage-specific membrane proteins during transformation of *Plasmodium gallinaceum* zygotes into ookinetes. Mol Biochem Parasitol 14:127–139
76. Sutherland CJ (2001) Stevor transcripts from *Plasmodium falciparum* gametocytes encode truncated polypeptides. Mol Biochem Parasitol 113:331–335
77. Da DF, Dixit S, Sattabonkot J, Mu J, Abate L, Ramineni B, Ouedraogo JB, MacDonald NJ, Fay MP, Su XZ et al (2013) Anti-Pfs25 human plasma reduces transmission of *Plasmodium falciparum* isolates that have diverse genetic backgrounds. Infect Immun 81:1984–1989
78. Feng H, Zheng L, Zhu X, Wang G, Pan Y, Li Y, Yang Y, Lin Y, Cui L, Cao Y (2011) Genetic diversity of transmission-blocking vaccine candidates Pvs25 and Pvs28 in *Plasmodium vivax* isolates from Yunnan Province, China. Parasit Vectors 4:224
79. González-Cerón L, Alvarado-Delgado A, Martínez-Barnetche J, Rodríguez MH, Ovilla-Muñoz M, Pérez F, Hernandez-Avila JE, Sandoval MA, Rodríguez MDC, Villarreal-Treviño C (2010) Sequence variation of ookinete surface proteins Pvs25 and Pvs28 of *Plasmodium vivax* isolates from Southern Mexico and their association to local anophelines infectivity. Infect Genet Evol 10:645–654
80. Kang J-M, Ju H-L, Moon S-U, Cho P-Y, Bahk Y-Y, Sohn W-M, Park Y-K, Cha S, Kim T-S, Na B-K (2013) Limited sequence polymorphisms of four transmission-blocking vaccine candidate antigens in *Plasmodium vivax* Korean isolates. Malar J 12:144
81. Niederwieser I, Felger I, Beck HP (2001) Limited polymorphism in *Plasmodium falciparum* sexual-stage antigens. Am J Trop Med Hyg 64:9–11
82. Sattabongkot J, Tsuboi T, Hisaeda H, Tachibana M, Suwanabun N, Rungruang T, Cao Y-M, Stowers AW, Sirichaisinthop J, Coleman RE et al (2003) Blocking of transmission to mosqui-

toes by antibody to *plasmodium vivax* malaria vaccine candidates pvs25 and pvs28 despite antigenic polymorphism in field isolates. Am J Trop Med Hyg 69:536–541
83. Tsuboi T, Kaslow DC, Gozar MM, Tachibana M, Cao YM, Torii M (1998) Sequence polymorphism in two novel *Plasmodium vivax* ookinete surface proteins, Pvs25 and Pvs28, that are malaria transmission-blocking vaccine candidates. Mol Med 4:772–782
84. Zakeri S, Razavi S, Djadid ND (2009) Genetic diversity of transmission blocking vaccine candidate (Pvs25 and Pvs28) antigen in *Plasmodium vivax* clinical isolates from Iran. Acta Trop 109:176–180
85. Zheng L, Xu WM, Liu YJ, Yang YM, Cao YM (2004) Transmission-blocking vaccine candidate of *Plasmodium vivax* Pvs25 is highly conservative among Chinese isolates. Zhongguo Ji Sheng Chong Xue Yu Ji Sheng Chong Bing Za Zhi 22:16–19
86. Anthony TG, Polley SD, Vogler AP, Conway DJ (2007) Evidence of non-neutral polymorphism in *Plasmodium falciparum* gamete surface protein genes Pfs47 and Pfs48/45. Mol Biochem Parasitol 156:117–123
87. Conway DJ, Machado RLD, Singh B, Dessert P, Mikes ZS, Povoa MM, Oduola AMJ, Roper C (2001) Extreme geographical fixation of variation in the *Plasmodium falciparum* gamete surface protein gene Pfs48/45 compared with microsatellite loci. Mol Biochem Parasitol 115:145–156
88. Doi M, Tanabe K, Tachibana S-I, Hamai M, Tachibana M, Mita T, Yagi M, Zeyrek FY, Ferreira MU, Ohmae H et al (2011) Worldwide sequence conservation of transmission-blocking vaccine candidate Pvs230 in *Plasmodium vivax*. Vaccine 29:4308–4315
89. Drakeley CJ, Duraisingh MT, Povoa M, Conway DJ, Targett GAT, Baker DA (1996) Geographical distribution of a variant epitope of pfs48/45, a *plasmodium falciparum* transmission-blocking vaccine candidate. Mol Biochem Parasitol 81:253–257
90. Juliano JJ, Parobek CM, Brazeau NF, Ngasala B, Randrianarivelojosia M, Lon C, Mwandagalirwa K, Tshefu A, Dhar R, Das BK et al (2015) Pooled amplicon deep sequencing of candidate *Plasmodium falciparum* transmission-blocking vaccine antigens. Am J Trop Med Hyg 94:143–146
91. Lensen A, Vandruten J, Bolmer M, Vangemert G, Eling W, Sauerwein R (1996) Measurement by membrane feeding of reduction in *plasmodium falciparum* transmission induced by endemic sera. Trans R Soc Trop Med Hyg 90:20–22
92. Mehrizi AA, Zakeri S, Djadid ND (2014) Limited genetic diversity and purifying selection in Iranian *Plasmodium falciparum* Generative Cell Specific 1 (PfGCS1), a potential target for transmission-blocking vaccine. Infect Genet Evol 22:150–156
93. Premawansa S, Peiris JS, Perera KL, Ariyaratne G, Carter R, Mendis KN (1990) Target antigens of transmission blocking immunity of *Plasmodium vivax* malaria—characterization and polymorphism in natural parasite isolates. J Immunol 144:4376–4383
94. Targett G (1990) Immunity to sexual stages of human malaria parasites: immune modulation during natural infections, antigenic determinants, and the induction of transmission-blocking immunity. Scand J Infect Dis Suppl 76:79–88
95. Williamson KC, Kaslow DC (1993) Strain polymorphism of *Plasmodium falciparum* transmission-blocking target antigen Pfs230. Mol Biochem Parasitol 62:125–128
96. Woo MK, Kim KA, Kim J, Oh JS, Han ET, An SSA, Lim CS (2013) Sequence polymorphisms in Pvs48/45 and Pvs47 gametocyte and gamete surface proteins in *Plasmodium vivax* isolated in Korea. Mem Inst Oswaldo Cruz 108:359–367
97. Carter R, Coulson A, Bhatti S, Taylor BJ, Elliott JF (1995) Predicted disulfide-bonded structures for three uniquely related proteins of *plasmodium falciparum*, pfs230, pfs48/ 45 and pf12. Mol Biochem Parasitol 71:203–210
98. Gerloff DL, Creasey A, Maslau S, Carter R (2005) Structural models for the protein family characterized by the gamete surface protein Pfs230 of *Plasmodium falciparum*. Proc Natl Acad Sci 102:13598–13603
99. Cova M, Rodrigues JA, Smith TK, Izquierdo L (2015) Sugar activation and glycosylation in *Plasmodium*. Malar J 14:427
100. Datta D, Bansal GP, Kumar R, Ellefsen B, Hannaman D, Kumar N (2015) Evaluation of the impact of codon optimization and N-linked glycosylation on functional immunogenicity of

Pfs25 DNA vaccines delivered by in vivo electroporation in preclinical studies in mice. Clin Vaccine Immunol 22:1013–1019
101. Gowda DC, Gupta P, Davidson EA (1997) Glycosylphosphatidylinositol anchors represent the major carbohydrate modification in proteins of intraerythrocytic stage *Plasmodium falciparum*. J Biol Chem 272:6428–6439
102. Alejo Blanco AR, Paez A, Gerold P, Dearsly AL, Margos G, Schwarz RT, Barker G, Rodriguez MC, Sinden RE (1999) The biosynthesis and post-translational modification of Pbs21 an ookinete-surface protein of *Plasmodium berghei*. Mol Biochem Parasitol 98:163–173
103. Margos G, Kurtenbach K, Posnett E, Barker GC, Matsuoka H, Paton MG, Sinden RE (1995) Expression of the *Plasmodium berghei* ookinete protein Pbs21 in a baculovirus-insect cell system produces an efficient transmission blocking immunogen. Parasite Immunol 17:167–176
104. Martínez AP, Margos G, Barker G, Sinden RE (2000) The roles of the glycosylphosphatidylinositol anchor on the production and immunogenicity of recombinant ookinete surface antigen Pbs21 of *Plasmodium berghei* when prepared in a baculovirus expression system. Parasite Immunol 22:493–500
105. Matsuoka H, Kobayashi J, Barker GC, Miura K, Chinzei Y, Miyajima S, Ishii A, Sinden RE (1996) Induction of anti-malarial transmission blocking immunity with a recombinant ookinete surface antigen of *Plasmodium berghei* produced in silkworm larvae using the baculovirus expression vector system. Vaccine 14:120–126
106. Fanning SL, Czesny B, Sedegah M, Carussi DJ, van Gemert GJEW, Williamson KC (2003) A glycosylphosphatidylinositol anchor signal sequence enhances the immunogenicity of a DNA vaccine encoding *Plasmodium falciparum* sexual-stage antigen, Pfs230. Vaccine 21:3228–3235
107. Kumar R, Angov E, Kumar N (2014) Potent malaria transmission blocking antibody responses elicited by *Plasmodium falciparum* Pfs25 expressed in *E. coli* after successful protein refolding. Infect Immun 82(4):1453–1459
108. Farrance CE, Chichester JA, Musiychuk K, Shamloul M, Rhee A, Manceva SD, Jones RM, Mamedov T, Sharma S, Mett V et al (2011) Antibodies to plant-produced *Plasmodium falciparum* sexual stage protein Pfs25 exhibit transmission blocking activity. Hum Vaccin 7(Suppl):191–198
109. Farrance CE, Rhee A, Jones RM, Musiychuk K, Shamloul M, Sharma S, Mett V, Chichester JA, Streatfield SJ, Roeffen W et al (2011) A plant-produced Pfs230 vaccine candidate blocks transmission of *Plasmodium falciparum*. Clin Vaccine Immunol 18(8):1351–1357
110. Mehlin C, Boni E, Buckner FS, Engel L, Feist T, Gelb MH, Haji L, Kim D, Liu C, Mueller N et al (2006) Heterologous expression of proteins from *Plasmodium falciparum*: results from 1000 genes. Mol Biochem Parasitol 148:144–160
111. Tsuboi T, Takeo S, Arumugam TU, Otsuki H, Torii M (2010) The wheat germ cell-free protein synthesis system: a key tool for novel malaria vaccine candidate discovery: Sweden-Japan joint seminar "Malaria research: diversity and control" in 11 June 2008 at Nobel Forum, Karolinska Institutet, Stockholm. Acta Trop 114:171–176
112. Billingsley PF (1990) The midgut ultrastructure of haematophagous insects. Annu Rev Entomol 35:219–248
113. Muller HM, Crampton JM, Dellatorre A, Sinden R, Crisanti A (1993) Members of a trypsin gene family in *Anopheles gambiae* are induced in the gut by blood meal. EMBO J 12:2891–2900
114. Bokharaei H, Raz A, Zakeri S, Djadid ND (2012) 3′-RACE amplification of aminopeptidase N gene from *Anopheles stephensi* applicable in transmission blocking vaccines. Avicenna J Med Biotechnol 4:131–141
115. Lavazec C, Boudin C, Lacroix R, Bonnet S, Diop A, Thiberge S, Boisson B, Tahar R, Bourgouin C (2007) Carboxypeptidases B of *Anopheles gambiae* as targets for a *Plasmodium falciparum* transmission-blocking vaccine. Infect Immun 75:1635–1642
116. Lavazec C, Bourgouin C (2008) Mosquito-based transmission blocking vaccines for interrupting *Plasmodium* development. Microbes Infect 10:845–849

117. Raz A, Dinparast Djadid N, Zakeri S (2013) Molecular characterization of the carboxypeptidase B1 of *Anopheles stephensi* and its evaluation as a target for transmission-blocking vaccines. Infect Immun 81:2206–2216
118. Gass RF (1977) Influences of blood digestion on the development of *Plasmodium gallinaceum* (Brumpt) in the midgut of *Aedes aegypti* (L.). Acta Trop 34:127–140
119. Gass RF, Yeates RA (1979) In vitro damaged of cultured ookinetes of *Plasmodium gallinaceum* by digestive proteinases from susceptible *Aedes aegypti*. Acta Trop 36:243–252
120. Saxena AK, Saul A, Garboczi DN (2004) Crystallization and preliminary X-ray analysis of the *Plasmodium vivax* sexual stage 25 kDa protein Pvs25, a transmission-blocking vaccine candidate for malaria. Acta Cryst D60:706–708
121. Saxena AK, Singh K, Long CA, Garboczi DN (2004) Preparation, crystallization and preliminary X-ray analysis of a complex between the *Plasmodium vivax* sexual stage 25 kDa protein Pv25 and a malaria transmission-blocking antibody Fab fragment. Acta Cryst D60:2054–2057
122. Saxena AK, Singh K, Su HP, Klein MM, Stowers AW, Saul AJ, Long CA, Garboczi DN (2005) The essential mosquito-stage P25 and P28 proteins from *Plasmodium* form tile-like triangular prisms. Nat Struct Mol Biol 13:90–91
123. Saxena AK, Wu Y, Garboczi DN (2007) *Plasmodium* P25 and P28 surface proteins: potential transmission-blocking vaccines. Eukaryot Cell 6:1260–1265
124. Berner R, Rudin W, Hecker H (1983) Peritrophic membrane and protease activity in the midgut of the malaria mosquito *Anopheles stephensi* (Liston) (Inseide: Distera) under normal and experimental conditions. J Ultrastruc Res 83:195–204
125. Billingsley PF, Rudin W (1992) The role of the mosquito peritrophic membrane in bloodmeal digestion and infectivity of *Plasmodium* species. J Parasitol 78:430–440
126. Briegel H, Lea AO (1975) Relationship between protein and proteolytic activity in the midgut of mosquitoes. J Insect Physiol 21:1597–1604
127. Horler E, Briegel H (1995) Proteolytic enzymes of female *Anopheles*: biphasic synthesis, regulation, and multiple feeding. Arch Insect Biochem Physiol 28:189–205
128. Rudin W, Billingsley PF, Saladin S (1991) The fate of *Plasmodium gallinaceum* in *Anopheles stephensi* Liston and possible barriers to transmission. Ann Soc Belg Med Trop 71:167–177
129. Dimopoulos G, Richman A, Muller HM, Kafatos FC (1997) Molecular immune responses of the mosquito *Anopheles gambiae* to bacteria and malaria parasites. Proc Natl Acad Sci U S A 94:11508–11513
130. Pumpuni CB, Demaio J, Kent M, Davis JR, Beier JC (1996) Bacterial population dynamics in three anopheline species: the impact on *Plasmodium* sporogonic development. Am J Trop Med Hyg 54:214–218
131. Seitz HM, Maier WA, Rottok M, Becker-Feldman H (1987) Concomitant infections of *Anopheles stephensi* with *Plasmodium berghei* and *Serratia marcescens* additive detrimental effects. Zentralbl Bakteriol Mikrobiol Hyg A 266:155–166
132. Yilmaz B, Portugal S, Tran TM, Gozzelino R, Ramos S, Gomes J, Regalado A, Cowan PJ, d'Apice AJ, Chong AS et al (2014) Gut microbiota elicits a protective immune response against malaria transmission. Cell 159:1277–1289
133. Dawes E, Churcher T, Zhuang S, Sinden R, Basanez M-G (2009) *Anopheles* mortality is both age- and *Plasmodium*-density dependent: implications for malaria transmission. Malar J 8:228
134. Osta MA, Christophides GK, Kafatos FC (2004) Effects of mosquito genes on *Plasmodium* development. Science 303:2030–2032
135. Blandin S, Shiao SH, Moita LF, Janse CJ, Waters AP, Kafatos FC, Levashina EA (2004) Complement-like protein TEP1 is a determinant of vectorial capacity in the malaria vector *Anopheles gambiae*. Cell 116:661–670
136. Shahabuddin M, Fields I, Bulet P, Hoffmann JA, Miller LH (1998) *Plasmodium gallinaceum*: differential killing of some mosquito stages of the parasite by insect defensin. Exp Parasitol 89:103–112
137. Michel K, Budd A, Pinto S, Gibson TJ, Kafatos FC (2005) *Anopheles gambiae* SRPN2 facilitates midgut invasion by the malaria parasite *Plasmodium berghei*. EMBO Rep 6:1–7

138. Luckhart S, Vodovotz Y, Cui L, Rosenberg R (1998) The mosquito *Anopheles stephensi* limits malaria parasite development with inducible synthesis of nitric acid. Proc Natl Acad Sci U S A 95:5700–5705
139. Pakpour N, Corby-Harris V, Green GP, Smithers HM, Cheung KW, Riehle MA, Luckhart S (2012) Ingested human insulin inhibits the mosquito NF-KB-dependent immune response to *Plasmodium falciparum*. Infect Immun 80:2141–2149
140. Williams AR, Zakutansky SE, Miura K, Dicks MD, Churcher TS, Jewell KE, Vaughan AM, Turner AV, Kapulu MC, Michel K et al (2013) Immunisation against a serine protease inhibitor reduces intensity of *Plasmodium berghei* infection in mosquitoes. Int J Parasitol 43:869–874
141. Molina-Cruz A, Garver LS, Alabaster A, Bangiolo L, Haile A, Winikor J, Ortega C, van Schaijk BCL, Sauerwein RW, Taylor-Salmon E et al (2013) The human malaria parasite Pfs47 gene mediates evasion of the mosquito immune system. Science 340:984–987
142. Smith RC, Jacobs-Lorena M (2015) Malaria parasite Pfs47 disrupts JNK signaling to escape mosquito immunity. Proc Natl Acad Sci 112:1250–1251
143. Molina-Cruz A, Canepa GE, Kamath N, Pavlovic NV, Mu J, Ramphul UN, Ramirez JL, Barillas-Mury C (2015) *Plasmodium* evasion of mosquito immunity and global malaria transmission: the lock-and-key theory. Proc Natl Acad Sci U S A 112:15178–15183
144. Shahabuddin M, Toyoshima T, Aikawa M, Kaslow DC (2000) Transmission-blocking activity of a chitinase inhibitor and activation of malarial parasite chitinase by mosquito protease. Proc Natl Acad Sci 90:4266–4270
145. Tsai YL, Hayward RE, Lange RC, Fidock DA, Vinetz JM (2001) Disruption of the *Plasmodium falciparum* chitinase prevents parasite invasion of the mosquito midgut. Infect Immun 69:4048–4054
146. Zieler H, Garon CF, Fischer ER, Shahabuddin M (2000) A tubular network associated with the brush-border surface of *Aedes aegypti* midgut: implications for pathogen transmission by mosquitoes. J Exp Biol 203:1599–1611
147. Mathias DK, Jardim JG, Parish LA, Armistead JS, Trinh HV, Khumpitak C, Sattabongkot J, Dinglasan RR (2014) Differential roles of an Anopheline midgut GPI-anchored protein in mediating *Plasmodium falciparum* and *Plasmodium vivax* ookinete invasion. Infect Genet Evol 28:635–647
148. Parish LA, Colquhoun DR, Mohien CU, Lyashkov AE, Graham DR, Dinglasan RR (2011) Ookinete-interacting proteins on the microvillar surface are partitioned into detergent resistant membranes of *Anopheles gambiae* midguts. J Proteome Res 10:5150–5162
149. Ghosh AK, Jacobs-Lorena M (2009) *Plasmodium* sporozoite invasion of the mosquito salivary gland. Curr Opin Microbiol 12:394–400
150. Zieler H, Nawrocki JP, Shahabuddin M (1999) *Plasmodium gallinaceum* ookinetes adhere specifically to the midgut epithelium of *Aedes aegypti* by interaction with a carbohydrate ligand. J Exp Biol 202:485–495
151. Grotendorst CA, Carter R, Rosenberg R, Koontz L (1986) Complement effects on the infectivity of *Plasmodium gallinaceum* to *Aedes aegypti* mosquitoes I. resistance of zygotes to the alternative pathway of complement. J Immunol 136:4270–4274
152. Margos G, Navarette S, Butcher G, Davies A, Willers C, Sinden RE, Lachmann PJ (2001) Interaction between host complement and mosquito-midgut-stage *Plasmodium berghei*. Infect Immun 69:5064–5071
153. Grotendorst CA, Carter R (1987) Complement effects on the infectivity of *Plasmodium gallinaceum* to *Aedes aegypti* mosquitoes II. Changes in sensitivity to complement-like factors during zygote development. J Parasitol 73:980–984
154. Simon N, Lasonder E, Scheuermayer M, Kuehn A, Tews S, Fischer R, Zipfel PF, Skerka C, Pradel G (2013) Malaria parasites co-opt human factor H to prevent complement-mediated lysis in the mosquito midgut. Cell Host Microbe 13:29–41
155. Sinden RE, Smalley ME (1976) Gametocytes of *Plasmodium falciparum*: phagocytosis by leucocytes in vivo and in vitro. Trans R Soc Trop Med Hyg 70:344–345

156. Healer J, Graszynski A, Riley E (1999) Phagocytosis does not play a major role in naturally acquired transmission-blocking immunity to *Plasmodium falciparum* malaria. Infect Immun 67:2334–2339
157. Do Rosario VE, Appiah A, Vaughan JA, Hollingdale MR (1989) *Plasmodium falciparum*: administration of anti-sporozoite antibodies during sporogony results in production of sporozoites which are not neutralized by human anti-circumsporozoite protein vaccine sera. Trans R Soc Trop Med Hyg 83:305–307
158. Motard A, Baccam D, Landau I (1990) Temporary loss of *Plasmodium* gametocytes infectivity during schizogony. Ann Parasitol Hum Comp 65:218–220
159. Naotunne TD, Karunaweera ND, Delgiudice G, Kularatne MU, Grau GE, Carter R, Mendis KN (1991) Cytokines kill malaria parasites during infection crisis—extracellular complementary factors are essential. J Exp Med 173:523–529
160. Naotunne TD, Karunaweera ND, Mendis KN, Carter R (1993) Cytokine-mediated inactivation of malarial gametocytes is dependent on the presence of white blood cells and involves reactive nitrogen intermediates. Immunology 78:555–562
161. Aikawa M, Rener J, Carter R, Miller LH (1981) An electron microscopical study of the interaction of monoclonal antibodies with gametes of the malarial parasite *Plasmodium gallinaceum*. J Protozool 28:383–388
162. Healer J, McGuinness D, Hopcroft P, Haley S, Carter R, Riley E (1997) Complement-mediated lysis of *Plasmodium falciparum* gametes by malaria-immune human sera is associated with antibodies to the gamete surface antigen Pfs230. Infect Immun 65:3017–3023
163. Read D, Lensen AHW, Begarnie S, Haley S, Raza A, Carter R (1994) Transmission-blocking antibodies against multiple, non-variant target epitopes of the *Plasmodium falciparum* gamete surface antigen pfs230 are all complement-fixing. Parasite Immunol 16:511–519
164. Roeffen W, Geeraedts F, Eling W, Beckers P, Wizel B, Kumar N, Lensen T, Sauerwein R (1995) Transmission blockade of *Plasmodium falciparum* malaria by anti-Pfs230-specific antibodies is isotype dependent. Infect Immun 63:467–471
165. Ranawaka G, Alejoblanco R, Sinden RE (1993) The effect of Transmission-Blocking antibody ingested in primary and secondary bloodfeeds, upon the development of *Plasmodium berghei* in the mosquito vector. Parasitology 107:225–231
166. Ranawaka G, Fleck SL, Alejo-Blanco A, Sinden RE (1994) Characterisation of the modes of action of anti Pbs21 malaria transmission-blocking immunity upon ookinete to oocyst differentiation in vivo. Parasitology 109:403–411
167. Ranawaka GRR, Alejoblanco AR, Sinden RE (1994) Characterization of the effector mechanisms of a transmission-blocking antibody upon differentiation of *Plasmodium berghei* gametocytes into ookinetes in vitro. Parasitology 109:11–17
168. Grotendorst CA, Kumar N, Carter R, Kaushal DC (1984) A surface protein expressed during transformation of zygotes of *Plasmodium gallinaceum* is a target of transmission-blocking antibodies. Infect Immun 45:775–777
169. Kaushal DC, Carter R (1981) Identification of antigens on the surface of zygotes of *Plasmodium gallinaceum* by radioiodination and immunoprecipitation. In: Federation proceedings 72nd annual meeting of the American Society of Biological Chemists, St. Louis, MO, 40, p 1817
170. Vermeulen AN, Deursen JV, Brakenhof RH, Lensen THW, Ponnudurai T, Meuwissen JHET (1986) Characterization of *Plasmodium falciparum* sexual stage antigens and their biosynthesis in synchronized gametocyte cultures. Mol Biochem Parasitol 20:155–163
171. Winger LA, Tirawanchai N, Nicholas J, Carter HE, Smith JE, Sinden RE (1988) Ookinete antigens of *Plasmodium berghei*. Appearance on the zygote surface of an Mr 21 kD determinant identified by transmission-blocking monoclonal antibodies. Parasite Immunol 10:193–207
172. Tsuboi T, Takeo S, Iriko H, Jin L, Tsuchimochi M, Matsuda S, Han E-T, Otsuki H, Kaneko O, Sattabongkot J et al (2008) Wheat germ cell-free system-based production of malaria proteins for discovery of novel vaccine candidates. Infect Immun 76:1702–1708

173. Churcher TS, Blagborough AM, Delves M, Ramakrishnan C, Kapulu MC, Williams AR, Biswas S, Da DF, Cohuet A, Sinden RE (2012) Measuring the blockade of malaria transmission—an analysis of the Standard Membrane Feeding Assay. Int J Parasitol 42:1037–1044
174. Abraham EG, Islam S, Srinivasan P, Ghosh AK, Valenzuela JG, Ribeiro JMC, Kafatos FC, Dimopoulos G, Jacobs-Lorena M (2004) Analysis of the *Plasmodium* and *Anopheles* transcriptional repertoire during ookinete development and midgut invasion. J Biol Chem 279:5573–5580
175. Hall N, Karras M, Raine JD, Carlton JM, Kooij TW, Berriman M, Florens L, Janssen CS, Pain A, Christophides GK et al (2005) A comprehensive survey of the *Plasmodium* life cycle by genomic, transcriptomic, and proteomic analyses. Science 307:82–86
176. Hayward RE, DeRisi JL, Alfadhli S, Kaslow DC, Brown PO, Rathod PK (2000) Shotgun DNA microarrays and stage-specific gene expression in *Plasmodium falciparum* malaria. Mol Microbiol 35:6–14
177. Lal K, Prieto JH, Bromley E, Sanderson SJ, Yates JR, Wastling JM, Tomley FM, Sinden RE (2009) Characterisation of *Plasmodium* invasive organelles; an ookinete microneme proteome. Proteomics 9:1142–1151
178. Wass MN, Stanway R, Blagborough AM, Lal K, Prieto JH, Raine D, Sternberg MJE, Talman AM, Tomley F, Yates J et al (2012) Proteomic analysis of *Plasmodium* in the mosquito: progress and pitfalls. Parasitology 139:1131–1145
179. Mohien CU, Colquhoun DR, Mathias DK, Gibbons JG, Armistead JS, Rodriguez MC, Rodriguez MH, Edwards NJ, Hartler Jr, Thallinger GG et al (2013) A bioinformatics approach for integrated transcriptomic and proteomic comparative analyses of model and non-sequenced anopheline vectors of human malaria parasites. Mol Cell Proteomics 12:120–131
180. Rener J, Graves PM, Carter R, Williams JL, Burkot TR (1983) Target antigens of transmission-blocking immunity on gametes of *Plasmodium falciparum*. J Exp Med 158(3): 976–981
181. Nikolaeva D, Draper SJ, Biswas S (2015) Toward the development of effective transmission-blocking vaccines for malaria. Expert Rev Vaccines 14(5):653–680
182. Wu Y, Sinden RE, Churcher TS, Tsuboi T, Yusibov V (2015) Development of malaria transmission-blocking vaccines: from concept to product. Adv Parasitol 89:109–152
183. Blagborough AM, Sinden RE (2009) *Plasmodium berghei* HAP2 induces strong malaria transmission-blocking immunity in vivo and in vitro. Vaccine 27(38):5187–5194
184. Miura K, Takashima E, Deng B, Tullo G, Diouf A, Moretz SE, Nikolaeva D, Diakite M, Fairhurst RM, Fay MP, Long CA, Tsuboi T (2013) Functional comparison of *Plasmodium falciparum* transmission-blocking vaccine candidates by the standard membrane-feeding assay. Infect Immun 81(12):4377–4382
185. Hisaeda H, Stowers AW, Tsuboi T, Collins WE, Sattabongkot JS, Suwanabun N, Torii M, Kaslow DC (2000) Antibodies to malaria vaccine candidates Pvs25 and Pvs28 completely block the ability of *Plasmodium vivax* to infect mosquitoes. Infect Immun 68(12): 6618–6623
186. Dinglasan RR, Kalume DE, Kanzok SM, Ghosh AK, Muratova O, Pandey A, Jacobs-Lorena M (2007) Disruption of *Plasmodium falciparum* development by antibodies against a conserved mosquito midgut antigen. Proc Natl Acad Sci U S A 104(33):13461–13466
187. Wu Y, Ellis RD, Shaffer D, Fontes E, Malkin EM, Mahanty S, Fay MP, Narum D, Rausch K, Miles AP, Aebig J, Orcutt A, Muratova O, Song G, Lambert L, Zhu D, Miura K, Long C, Saul A, Miller LH, Durbin AP (2008) Phase 1 trial of malaria transmission blocking vaccine candidates Pfs25 and Pvs25 formulated with montanide ISA 51. PLoS One 3(7), e2636
188. Goodman AL, Blagborough AM, Biswas S, Wu Y, Hill AV, Sinden RE, Draper SJ (2011) A viral vectored prime-boost immunization regime targeting the malaria Pfs25 antigen induces transmission-blocking activity. PLoS One 6(12), e29428
189. Kapulu MC, Da DF, Miura K, Li Y, Blagborough AM, Churcher TS, Nikolaeva D, Williams AR, Goodman AL, Sangare I, Turner AV, Cottingham MG, Nicosia A, Straschil U, Tsuboi T, Gilbert SC, Long CA, Sinden RE, Draper SJ, Hill AV, Cohuet A, Biswas S (2015) Comparative assessment of transmission-blocking vaccine candidates against *Plasmodium falciparum*. Sci Rep 5, 11193

190. Li Y, Leneghan DB, Miura K, Nikolaeva D, Brian IJ, Dicks MD, Fyfe AJ, Zakutansky SE, de Cassan S, Long CA, Draper SJ, Hill AV, Hill F, Biswas S (2016) Enhancing immunogenicity and transmission-blocking activity of malaria vaccines by fusing Pfs25 to IMX313 multimerization technology. Sci Rep 6, 18848
191. Miyata T, Harakuni T, Sugawa H, Sattabongkot J, Kato A, Tachibana M, Torii M, Tsuboi T, Arakawa T (2011) Adenovirus-vectored *Plasmodium vivax* ookinete surface protein, Pvs25, as a potential transmission-blocking vaccine. Vaccine 29(15):2720–2726
192. Blagborough AM, Yoshida S, Sattabongkot J, Tsuboi T, Sinden RE (2010) Intranasal and intramuscular immunization with Baculovirus Dual Expression System-based Pvs25 vaccine substantially blocks *Plasmodium vivax* transmission. Vaccine 28(37):6014–6020
193. Kubler-Kielb J, Majadly F, Wu Y, Narum DL, Guo C, Miller LH et al (2007) Long-lasting and transmission-blocking activity of antibodies to *Plasmodium falciparum* elicited in mice by protein conjugates of Pfs25. Proc Natl Acad Sci U S A 104:293–298
194. Kubler-Kielb J, Majadly F, Biesova Z, Mocca CP, Guo C, Nussenzweig R et al (2010) A bicomponent *Plasmodium falciparum* investigational vaccine composed of protein-peptide conjugates. Proc Natl Acad Sci U S A 107:1172–1177
195. Wu Y, Przysiecki C, Flanagan E, Bello-Irizarry SN, Ionescu R, Muratova O et al (2006) Sustained high-titer antibody responses induced by conjugating a malarial vaccine candidate to outer-membrane protein complex. Proc Natl Acad Sci U S A 103(48):18243–18248
196. Gregory JA, Topol AB, Doerner DZ, Mayfield S (2013) Alga-produced cholera toxin-Pfs25 fusion proteins as oral vaccines. Appl Environ Microbiol 79:3917–3925
197. Shimp RL Jr, Rowe C, Reiter K, Chen B, Nguyen V, Aebig J et al (2013) Development of a Pfs25-EPA malaria transmission blocking vaccine as a chemically conjugated nanoparticle. Vaccine 31:2954–2962
198. Jones RM, Chichester JA, Mett V, Jaje J, Tottey S, Manceva S, Casta LJ, Gibbs SK, Musiychuk K, Shamloul M, Norikane J, Mett V, Streatfield SJ, van de Vegte-Bolmer M, Roeffen W, Sauerwein RW, Yusibov V (2013) A plant-produced Pfs25 VLP malaria vaccine candidate induces persistent transmission blocking antibodies against *Plasmodium falciparum* in immunized mice. PLoS One 8(11), e79538
199. Brune KD, Leneghan DB, Brian IJ, Ishizuka AS, Bachmann MF, Draper SJ, Biswas S, Howarth M (2016) Plug-and-Display: decoration of Virus-Like Particles via isopeptide bonds for modular immunization. Sci Rep 6, 19234
200. Schwartz L, Brown GV, Genton B, Moorthy VS (2012) A review of malaria vaccine clinical projects based on the WHO rainbow table. Malar J 11:11
201. Macdonald G (1956) Theory of the eradication of malaria. Bull World Health Organ 15:369–387
202. Tusting LS, Bousema T, Smith DL, Drakeley C (2014) Measuring changes in *Plasmodium falciparum* transmission: precision, accuracy and costs of metrics. Adv Parasitol 84:151–208
203. Sinden RE, Blagborough AM, Churcher T, Ramakrishnan C, Biswas S, Delves MJ (2012) The design and interpretation of laboratory assays measuring mosquito transmission of *Plasmodium*. Trends Parasitol 28(11):457–465
204. Cheru L, Wu Y, Diouf A, Moretz SE, Muratova OV, Song G et al (2010) The IC_{50} of anti-Pfs25 antibody in membrane-feeding assay varies among species. Vaccine 28:4423–4429
205. Miura K, Keister DB, Muratova OV, Sattabongkot J, Long CA, Saul A (2007) Transmission-blocking activity induced by malaria vaccine candidates Pfs25/Pvs25 is a direct and predictable function of antibody titer. Malar J 6:107
206. Theisen M, Roeffen W, Singh SK, Andersen G, Amoah L, van de Vegte-Bolmer M et al (2014) A multi-stage malaria vaccine candidate targeting both transmission and asexual parasite life-cycle stages. Vaccine 32:2623–2630
207. Billker O, Dechamps S, Tewari R, Wenig G, Franke-Fayard B, Brinkmann V (2004) Calcium and a calcium-dependent protein kinase regulate gamete formation and mosquito transmission in a malaria parasite. Cell 117(4):503–514

208. Delves M, Plouffe D, Scheurer C, Meister S, Wittlin S, Winzeler EA, Sinden RE, Leroy D (2012) The activities of current antimalarial drugs on the life cycle stages of *Plasmodium*: a comparative study with human and rodent parasites. PLoS Med 9(2), e1001169
209. Bounkeua V et al (2011) In vitro generation of *Plasmodium falciparum* ookinetes. Am J Trop Med Hyg 85:207–213
210. Ghosh A et al (2010) An improved method for the in vitro differentiation of *Plasmodium falciparum* gametocytes into ookinetes. Malar J 9:194
211. Carter EH et al (1987) The in vitro cultivation of *P. falciparum* ookinetes and their enrichment on Nycodenz density gradients. Parasitology 95:25–30
212. Ross R (1897) Observations on a condition necessary to the transformation of the malaria crescent. BMJ 1:251–255
213. Usui M et al (2011) Improvement of the observational method for *Plasmodium berghei* oocysts in the midgut of mosquitoes. Parasit Vectors 4:118
214. Delves MJ, Sinden RE (2010) A semi-automated method for counting fluorescent malaria oocysts increases the throughput of transmission blocking studies. Malar J 9:35
215. Franke-Fayard B et al (2004) A *Plasmodium berghei* reference line that constitutively expresses GFP at a high level throughout the complete life cycle. Mol Biochem Parasitol 137:23–33
216. Stone WJ, Churcher TS, Graumans W, van Gemert GJ, Vos MW, Lanke KH et al (2014) A scalable assessment of *Plasmodium falciparum* transmission in the standard membrane-feeding assay, using transgenic parasites expressing green fluorescent protein-luciferase. J Infect Dis 210:1456–1463
217. Miura K, Deng B, Tullo G, Diouf A, Moretz SE, Locke E, Morin M, Fay MP, Long CA (2013) Qualification of standard membrane-feeding assay with *Plasmodium falciparum* malaria and potential improvements for future assays. PLoS One 8(3), e57909
218. van der Kolk M, De Vlas SJ, Saul A, van de Vegte-Bolmer M, Eling WM, Sauerwein RW (2005) Evaluation of the standard membrane feeding assay (SMFA) for the determination of malaria transmission-reducing activity using empirical data. Parasitology 130:13–22
219. Bousema T et al (2012) Mosquito feeding assays to determine the infectiousness of naturally infected *Plasmodium falciparum* gametocyte carriers. PLoS One 7, e42821
220. Blagborough AM, Churcher TS, Upton LM, Ghani AC, Gething PW, Sinden RE (2013) Transmission-blocking interventions eliminate malaria from laboratory populations. Nat Commun 4:1812
221. Burkot TR et al (1984) Identification of malaria-infected mosquitoes by a two-site enzyme-linked immunosorbent assay. Am J Trop Med Hyg 33:227–231
222. Baker EZ et al (1987) Detection and quantification of *Plasmodium falciparum* and *P. vivax* infections on Thai-Kampuchean *Anopheles* (Diptera: Culicidae) by enzyme linked immunosobent assay. J Med Entomol 24:536–541
223. Davis JR et al (1989) Estimate of *Plasmodium falciparum* sporozoite content of *Anopheles stephensi* used to challenge human volunteers. Am J Trop Med Hyg 40:128–130
224. Zavala F et al (1982) Monoclonal antibodies to circumsporozoite proteins identify the species of malarial parasite in infected mosquitoes. Nature 299:737–738
225. Ramakrishnan C et al (2012) Salivary gland-specific *P. berghei* reporter lines enable rapid evaluation of tissue-specific sporozoite loads in mosquitoes. PLoS One 7, e36376
226. malERA Consultation Group on Vaccines (2011) A research agenda for malaria eradication: vaccines. PLoS Med 8, e1000398
227. Upton LM, Brock PM, Churcher TS, Ghani AC, Gething PW, Delves MJ, Sala KA, Leroy D, Sinden RE, Blagborough AM (2015) Lead clinical and preclinical antimalarial drugs can significantly reduce sporozoite transmission to vertebrate populations. Antimicrob Agents Chemother 59(1):490–497

Index

A
Abdulla, S., 143
Abraham, E.G., 246
Adaptive immunity
  CD4 T cells, 36
  CD8 T cells, 32–36
  CXCR6, 35
  liver-stage infection, 28–32
  malaria infections, 28
  preerythrocytic antigens, 29
  WSV, 35
Adenoviruses, 160–161
Adjuvant/formulation technology, 213
Agnandji, S.T., 143
Ajua, A., 143
Alano, P., 247
Alfalfa mosaic virus, 253
Alloueche, A., 142
Alphaviruses, 161
Amante, F.H., 71
Annual parasite index (API), 255
Anopheles, 257
Anopheline, 251
Anopheline midgut alanyl aminopeptidase 1 (AgAPN1), 251
Ansong, D., 143
Antibody and B cell-mediated protection
  candidate approaches, 51
  erythrocyte-binding antigens, 51
  GIAs, 51
  growth inhibition assay (GIA), 49
  mouse models, 49
  P. falciparum, 49, 51
  parasitemia, 49
  PfEMP1, 50
  RIFIN proteins, 50
Antibody-dependent respiratory burst (ADRB), 216, 217
Antibody-dependent cellular inhibition (ADCI), 216, 217, 221, 223–225
Antigen-presenting cells (APCs), 72–73, 75
Antigens, clinical trials
  AMA1, 221–222
  combination vaccines, 224
  DBP, 225
  EBA-175, 225
  MSP1, 222–223
  MSP3, 223–224
  RH5, 225
  SERA5/SE36, 224
  Tex1, 225
Anti-merozoite antibodies, 216–217
Antinuclear antigens (ANAs), 85
Anti-PfEMP1 immunity, 214
Anti-phosphatidylserine (anti-PS), 85
Anti-sporozoite antibodies, 30
Aotus model, 215
APCs. *See* Antigen-presenting cells (APCs)
Apical membrane antigen 1 (AMA1), 51, 164, 215, 218, 219, 221–222
Aponte, J.J., 143
Artemisinin combination treatments (ACTs), 77
Asante, K.P., 143
Asexual blood-stage, 212
Autoimmunity
  autoantibody-mediated pathology, 84–85
  cellular and molecular components, 81
  Fc receptors, 89, 90
  genetic and environmental factors, 82
  host molecules/epitopes, 82
  hygiene hypothesis, 89
  immunological genes, 91

M.M. Mota, A. Rodriguez (eds.), *Malaria*, DOI 10.1007/978-3-319-45210-4

Autoimmunity (*cont.*)
implications, 91–92
inflammation and innate immunity-induced pathology, 83–84
inhibitory receptors, 90, 91
lymphocytes, 87, 88
malaria, 82, 86
mechanisms, 82
Plasmodium, 86–87
Plasmodium falciparum, 91
polyclonal activation, 82
polymorphisms, 91
T-cell-mediated pathology, 86

B

B cell memory, 54–56
Barbosa, A., 143
Barr, M., 72
B-cell receptor (BCR), 89
Bejon, P., 143
Biswas, S., 241–245, 248–260
Blagborough, A.M., 241–246, 248–260
Blood-brain barrier (BBB), 69
Blood-stage malaria parasites, 198–200
Blood-stage vaccines (BSVs), 215–229
antigens, clinical trials
AMA1, 221–222
antibody sensitive, 227–229
combination vaccines, 224
EBA-175, 225
MSP1, 222–223
MSP3, 223–224
P. vivax BSVs, 225, 226
SERA5/SE36, 224
Tex1, 225
BSV-inducible protection, 214
Fc-receptor-dependent activity, 216–217
Fc-receptor-independent merozoite neutralisation, 215–216
iRBC-surface antigens, 217, 218
NAI (*see* Naturally acquired immunity (NAI))
T cell responses, 218, 219
candidate prioritisation, 229–230
clinical trials, 213
in vivo
CHMI, 220–221
mouse models, 219
NHP models, 220
PAM, 228
T cell responses, 218–219
technologies, development, 229
Branched Synthetic Peptides, 175–176
BSVs. *See* Blood-stage vaccines (BSVs)

C

Campo, J.J., 143
Carboxy- and amino-peptidases, 245
Carter, R., 241, 246, 247
Cartilage oligomeric matric protein (COMP), 184
CD4 T cell, 36, 147
CD8 T cell epitopes, 34
Cerebral malaria (CM)
antigen processing, co-stimulation and cross presentation, 73–74
APCs, 72–73
$CD4^+$ and $CD8^+$ T lymphocytes, 68
cells and soluble mediators, 67
endothelial cells, APC, 74–76
experimental cerebral malaria (ECM), 68
innate immune responses, 68–70
MPs, 76
numerous factors, 68
parasite-induced pathology, 67
T cells, 70–72
Chemical attenuation of sporozoites (CAS), 121
Chemoprophylaxis (CPS), 116–120
Chen, D.H., 241
Chimpanzee adenovirus 63 (ChAd63), 252
Chlamydomonas reinhardtii, 251
CHMI. *See* Controlled human malaria infection (CHMI)
Chora, A.F., 4–13
Churcher, T.S., 250
Circumsporozoite protein (CSP), 103, 105, 106, 109, 110, 113, 115, 119, 121, 122, 140
CM-resistant (CM-R) mice, 70
Cockburn, I.A., 48–57
Collins, B., 220
Combination B, BSV candidate, 224
Controlled human malaria infection (CHMI), 52, 53, 141, 216, 220–221
CS Repeat Peptide-Protein Conjugates, 173–175
C-type lectin receptors (CLRs), 73
Cytotoxic CD4 T Cells, 37–38
Cytotoxic T lymphocytes (CTL), 74, 75

D
Damage-associated molecular patterns (DAMPs), 68, 69
DBP. *See* Duffy-binding protein (DBP)
DC immuno-receptor (DCIR), 73
Defensins, 245
Dendritic cells (DCs), 10, 68, 69, 72, 73
Dessens, J.T., 246
Direct feeding assay (DFA), 258
Direct membrane-feeding assay (DMFA), 258
Doll, K.L., 28, 30–38
Duffy-antigen Receptor for Chemokines (DARC), 226
Duffy-binding protein (DBP), 225

E
Ecker, A., 247
Enosse, S., 143
Enzyme-linked immunosorbant assays (ELISAs), 256
Epitopic vaccines, 172, 173, 183–185
Erythrocyte binding antigen (EBA), 225, 226
European Medicines Agency (EMA), 140, 178
Exoerythrocytic parasite, 4
Exoprotein A (EPA), 253
Exported protein 1 (EXP-1), 107
Eyles, D.E., 241

F
Farrance, C.E., 246
Fc receptors, 89, 90
Fernández-Arias, C., 157–166
Flaviviruses, 161–162
Force of infection (FOI), 255
Fowlpox virus, 159

G
Gamete, 244, 248, 256
Gametocyte-infected RBC (giRBC), 243, 244
Gene knockout (GKO), 70
Genetically attenuated parasites (GAPs), 111–116
Geometric mean titers (GMT), 182
Ghosh, A.K., 246
Glutamine-rich protein (GLURP), 51
Glycophosphatidylinositol (GPI), 68
Good, M.F., 197, 198, 200, 202–206
Gordon, D.M., 142
Götz, A., 4–13
Granulocytes, 9–10
Granzyme B (GzmB), 70
Grau, G.E.R., 67–74, 76
Growth inhibitory activity (GIA), 213, 215, 216, 220–224
Gwadz, R.W., 241

H
Haemozoin, 5, 68
Hepatocytes, 9, 30
Heterologous prime-boost regimen, 162
Horowitz, A., 143
Huff, C.G., 241
Human immunodeficiency virus (HIV), 158
Humoral immunity, 119, 144–146

I
Immune responses. *See* Malaria vaccine
Immunobiology, 141–144
Immunoreceptor tyrosine-based inhibitory motif (ITIM), 89, 90
Immunosuppression, 72
Innate immunity
- cytokine response, 6, 12–13
- dendritic cells, 7
- malaria infection, 4
- parasite and host components, 8
- parasite- and host-derived inflammatory molecules, 4–9
- plasmodium RNA, 6
- ROS, 8
- TLR-4 homodimers, 5
- uric acid, 7

Insulin-like receptors, 245
Interferon gamma (IFN-γ), 52, 71
Interferon-stimulated genes (ISGs), 9
Interleukin-10 (IL-10), 53
Intravital microscopy (IVM), 30
iRBC-surface antigens, 217, 218

K
Kaslow, D.C., 246
Kester, K.E., 142
Khan, S.M., 99–123

L
Lalvani, A., 142
Lell, B., 143
Leroux-Roels, G., 142
Li, Y., 246

Liposomes, 182
Liver-stage antigen 1 (LSA-1), 107, 109, 110, 115
Long-lived plasma cell (LLPC), 55
Lumsden, J.M., 142
Lymphocytes, 87, 88

M

Macrophages, 10
Major histocompatibility complex (MHC), 71
Malaria, 48, 49, 51, 52, 212
- BSVs (*see* Blood-stage vaccine (BSVs))

Malaria vaccine, 164
- antibody- or cell-mediated immune protection, 198
- blood-stage malaria parasites, 198–200
- chemical attenuation, 204
- CpG-ODN, 202
- IFN-γ and IL-12, 202
- immuno-epidemiological studies, 198
- morbidity and mortality, 197
- radiation, 202, 203
- red blood cell, 198
- whole blood-stage parasite vaccines, 205–206
- whole-organism vaccines, 198

Male, D.K., 74
Mannose receptor (MR), 74
Mast cells, 10
Mc, G.I., 72
Mendes, A.M., 99–123
Merozoite surface protein (MSP), 51
Merozoite surface protein 1 (MSP1), 222, 223
Merozoite surface protein 3 (MSP3), 223–224
Microparticle epitopic vaccines, 181–183
Microparticles (MPs), 70, 76
Microvesicles, 7
Mitochondrial antiviral-signaling protein (MAVS), 6
Miura, K., 246
Molecular force of infection (mFOI), 255
Monophosphoryl lipid A (MPLA), 181
Montanide ISA720 adjuvant, 224
Mosquito, 249
Mota, M., 4–13
Mueller, A. K., 99–123
Multiple antigen peptide (MAP), 175
Multiplicity of infection (MOI), 255
Myristoylation, 244

N

Nanofibrils, 183
Nardin, E.H., 171, 173–182, 184–186
Natural killer (NK) cells, 11
N. benthamiana, 251, 253
Ndungu, F.M., 143
Neafsey, D.E., 143
Nikolaeva, D., 247
Non-human primate (NHP) models, 220
Non-natural immunity, 214–215
Nucleotide-binding oligomerisation domain (NOD), 68

O

Ockenhouse, C.F., 142
Olotu, A., 143
OMPC, 174
Ookinete, 243–245, 256
Open reading frames (ORFs), 107
Outer membrane protein complex (OMPC), 253
Owusu-Agyei, S., 143
Oxidative stress, 8

P

Palmitoylation, 244
Parasite life cycle, 118
Parasite nucleoside transporter 1 (NT1), 203
Parasite rate (PR), 255
PATH Malaria Vaccine Initiative, 213
Pathogen-associated molecular patterns (PAMPs), 68, 185
Pattern recognition receptors (PRRs), 69
Perforin, 70
Peripheral blood mononuclear cells (PBMCs), 8, 106, 107, 109
PEV. *See* Pre-erythrocytic vaccines (PEV)
Pfs25-EPA, 254
PfSPZ vaccine, 108–110
Pinder, M., 142
Plasmodium, 28, 32–36, 82, 86–87, 241
- B cell memory, 54–56
- field and controlled infection studies, 48–49
- infection, 32
- parasite species, 102
- sporozoites, 100, 103
- T cell memory and exhaustion, 56–57
- T cell-mediated protection, 52–54

Plasmodium berghei, 202, 204, 245, 251
Plasmodium chabaudi, 50, 51, 53, 56, 200, 204
Plasmodium falciparum, 33, 49, 51, 76, 88, 140, 171, 173, 249, 252
Plasmodium interspersed repeats (PIR), 50
Plasmodium knowlesi, 50
Plasmodium pastoris, 251–253

Plasmodium vivax, 252
Plasmodium yoelii, 203
Polhemus, M.E., 142
Polymorphisms, 90
Poxviruses, 159
Poxviruses and adenoviruses, 158
Preerythrocytic antigens, 31
Preerythrocytic infection, 30
Pre-erythrocytic vaccines (PEV), 242
Pregnancy-associated malaria (PAM), 228
Prime-boost heterologous immunization, 165
Programmed cell death-1 (PD-1), 56, 57
Protective immunity, 37–38
Prudêncio, M., 99–123
Pseudomonas aeruginosa, 253
Purine nucleoside phosphorylase (PNP), 203

Q
Quillaja saponaria, 141

R
Radiation-attenuated sporozoite (RAS) immunization, 103–110
Radiation-attenuated sporozoites (RAS), 28, 103–110
Raja, A.I., 197, 198, 200, 202–206
Ramakrishnan, C., 247
Reactive oxygen species (ROS), 8
Red blood cell (RBC), 49, 198
REDMAL project, 254
Rener, J., 247
Rhesus macaques, 174
Rheumatoid arthritis (RA), 82
Rheumatoid factor (RF), 88
Rivera-Correa, J., 81–92
Rodriguez, A., 4–13, 81–92
Ross, R., 258
RTS,S/AS01
  chimeric virus, 141
  CHMI, 141
  CS, 140
  European Medicines Agency, 140
  HBsAg, 141
  humoral immunity, 144–146
  immune memory, 147–149
  immunobiology, 141–144
  parasite genetic diversity, 150
  parasite life cycle, 149–150
  Quillaja saponaria, 141
  Salmonella minnesota, 141
  T-cell epitopes, 141
  T-cell immunity, 147
  translational science, 150–151
  vaccine-induced immunity, 150

S
S. cerevisiae, 251, 252
Saeed, S., 246
Sala, K., 246
Salmonella minnesota, 141
SAPN, 184
Sauerwein, R.W., 99–123
Scholzen, A., 99–123
Scholz, S.M., 246
Schwenk, R., 142
Serine repeat antigen 5 (SERA5), 224
Shahabuddin, M., 246
Silvestrini, F., 247
Simon, N., 246
Sinden, R.E., 241–245, 247–260
Single-stranded DNA (ssDNA), 88
Slide positivity rate (SPR), 255
SMFA. *See* Standard membrane-feeding assay (SMFA)
Sollid, L.M., 73
Sporozoite antigens, 31–32
Sporozoite infection, 248
Sporozoite-neutralizing antibodies, 182
Sporozoites, 30
Standard membrane-feeding assay (SMFA), 250, 257, 258
Stanisic, D.I., 197, 198, 200, 202–206
Stephens, R., 48–57
Sterilizing immunity, 28
Stoute, J.A., 142
Subunit vaccine, 214, 218, 221, 228
Sun, P., 142
Sutherland, C.J., 247
Systemic lupus erythematosus (SLE), 82

T
T- and B-cell epitopes, 171, 175, 180, 184, 185
T cell memory, 56–57
T follicular helper cells (Tfh), 55
Tachibana, M., 246
Takeo, S., 246
Talman, A., 246
T-cell immunity, 147
T-cell responses, 163
Tetrabranched peptide, 176
Thrombospondin-related adhesive protein (TRAP), 159
Tirawanchai, N., 246

TLR-5 agonist flagellin, 178, 186
TLR7 agonist adjuvant, 177–178
Transmission
- blocking epitopes, 254
- circumsporozoite protein, 242
- gametocyte/gamete-based vaccines, 241
- mosquito, 249
- oocyst-based transmission-blocking assays, 257–259
- parasite, 242–245
- parasite molecules, 246–247, 249
- PEV, 242
- *P. falciparum*, 249
- *Plasmodium*, 241
- population assays, 259–260
- pre-oocyst transmission-blocking assays, 256–257
- sporozoite assays, 259
- TBVs, 242
- transcriptomic and proteomic libraries, 250
- transmission-blocking assays, 256
- vector, 245–248
- vertebrate immune system, 248
- western blot and laborious membrane-feeding assays, 249

Trophozoite exported protein 1 (Tex1), 225
Trypanosoma cruzi, 87
Trypsins, 245
Tsuboi, T., 246
Tumor necrosis factor (TNF), 52, 68
Tumor necrosis factor alpha (TNF-α), 83
Ty, M., 4–13
Type I interferons, 83

U

Urban, B.C., 72
Urban, S.L., 28, 30–38

V

Vaccine
- antigens, 250–251
- clinical development, 253–254
- conjugates and VLPs, 253
- efficacy, 140
- recombinant protein vaccines, 251–252
- viral-vectored TBVs, 252–253

Vahey, M.T., 142
van Schaijk, B.C.L., 246
Variant surface antigens (VSAs), 49
Vectored immunoprophylaxis (VIP), 229
Vekemans, J., 140, 141, 144–151
Vermeulen, A.N., 246
Villadangos, J.A., 73
Viral vector vaccines
- Ad35, 160
- Ad capsid, 161
- adenoviruses, 160–161
- DNA vaccines, 157
- fowlpox virus, 159
- FP9, 165
- parasites, 157
- poxviruses and adenoviruses, 158
- VACV, 158
- viral vectors, 158

Virosome, 181, 182
Viruslike particle (VLP), 178–180

W

Waitumbi, J.N., 142
Warimwe, G.M., 143
Wassmer, S C., 67–74, 76
Whole sporozoite vaccination (WSV), 28
Whole-sporozoite malaria vaccines
- antibody and T-cell responses, 103–106
- CD8+ T cells, 104
- GAPs, 111–116
- health-care systems, 100
- immunity, 113–116
- immunization, 116–117
- preerythrocytic immune responses, 100
- RAS, 103–110
- sporozoite administration, 100
- sporozoites and intrahepatic parasite, 105

Williamson, K.C., 246
Woodchuck hepatitis core antigen (WHcAg), 180
World Health Organization, 140
Wright, G., 229
Wykes, M.N., 48–57

Y

Yellow fever (YF) virus, 158

Z

Zuzarte-Luís, V., 4–13

MIX
Papier aus verantwortungsvollen Quellen
Paper from responsible sources
FSC® C105338

If you have any concerns about our products,
you can contact us on
ProductSafety@springernature.com

In case Publisher is established outside the EU,
the EU authorized representative is:
Springer Nature Customer Service Center GmbH
Europaplatz 3, 69115 Heidelberg, Germany

Printed by Libri Plureos GmbH
in Hamburg, Germany